多原发肿瘤与不明原发肿瘤

名誉主编　樊代明
主　　编　廖子君　罗志国

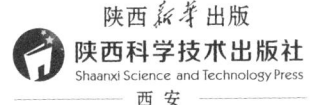

图书在版编目(CIP)数据

多原发肿瘤与不明原发肿瘤 / 廖子君,罗志国主编. 西安：陕西科学技术出版社,2025.4. -- ISBN 978-7-5369-9160-6

Ⅰ. R730.269

中国国家版本馆 CIP 数据核字第 20255E3G60 号

多原发肿瘤与不明原发肿瘤
DUOYUANFA ZHONGLIU YU BUMING YUANFA ZHONGLIU

樊代明　名誉主编
廖子君　罗志国　主编

策　　划	付　琨
责任编辑	潘晓洁
封面设计	曾　珂

出 版 者	陕西科学技术出版社
	西安市曲江新区登高路1388号陕西新华出版传媒产业大厦B座
	电话(029)81205187　传真(029)81205155　邮编710061
	http://www.snstp.com
发 行 者	陕西科学技术出版社
	电话(029)81205180　81205178
印　　刷	陕西金和印务有限公司
规　　格	710mm×1000mm　16开本
印　　张	17.75
字　　数	290千字
版　　次	2025年4月第1版
	2025年4月第1次印刷
书　　号	ISBN 978-7-5369-9160-6
定　　价	98.00元

版权所有　翻印必究

《多原发肿瘤与不明原发肿瘤》
编委会

名誉主编 樊代明
主　　编 廖子君　罗志国
副 主 编 张彦兵　张红梅　李　晟
编　　委（按姓氏拼音排序）
　　　　　　陈　娟（河北省邢台市中医院）
　　　　　　陈仕林（江苏省肿瘤医院）
　　　　　　陈轶洁（福建省肿瘤医院）
　　　　　　顾春东（大连医科大学附属第一医院）
　　　　　　郭克锋（河南科技大学附属黄河医院）
　　　　　　纪广玉（上海交通大学医学院附属第九人民医院）
　　　　　　姜　金（浙江省嘉兴市第一医院）
　　　　　　姜　军（青海大学附属医院）
　　　　　　金立亭（湖北省肿瘤医院）
　　　　　　李　晟（江苏省肿瘤医院）
　　　　　　李　捷（福建省联勤保障部队900医院）
　　　　　　李鹤飞（河北大学附属医院）
　　　　　　李金鹏（武汉大学中南医院）
　　　　　　李索妮（西安交通大学医学院附属陕西省肿瘤医院）
　　　　　　李晓琴（青海大学附属医院）
　　　　　　廖子君（西安交通大学医学院附属陕西省肿瘤医院）
　　　　　　林心琛（福建省人民医院）

刘德林（江苏省肿瘤医院）
刘宇飞（江苏省肿瘤医院）
吕　铮（吉林大学第一医院）
罗志国（复旦大学附属肿瘤医院）
马春华（天津市人民医院）
马婕群（西安交通大学医学院附属陕西省肿瘤医院）
马兆明（江苏省连云港第二人民医院）
潘　军（东部战区总医院）
钱　旭（浙江省肿瘤医院）
邱昌洪（广东省肇庆市人民医院）
邵　军（湖北省肿瘤医院）
史　健（河北医科大学第四医院）
王　青（南通大学附属肿瘤医院）
吴剑秋（江苏省肿瘤医院）
徐　林（中国医学科学院肿瘤医院深圳医院）
徐　琳（四川省肿瘤医院）
袁　渊（江苏省肿瘤医院）
张红梅（空军军医大学西京医院）
张彦兵（西安交通大学医学院附属陕西省肿瘤医院）
赵亚宁（陕西省宝鸡市中心医院）
周　菁（西安交通大学医学院附属陕西省肿瘤医院）
周俊伟（湖北省黄石市中心医院）

前 言

多原发肿瘤（multiple primary neoplasms，MPNs）是指机体同时性或异时性发生2个或2个以上彼此无关的原发恶性肿瘤，可分别来源于同一器官、成对器官、不同系统的器官、同一系统的不同器官；多原发肿瘤的存在不取决于时间，每一个原发肿瘤起源于一个组织或部位，而不是侵袭、复发或转移。确定多原发肿瘤有3个要点，第一，必须是2个及以上的恶性肿瘤；第二，每个恶性肿瘤之间彼此是独立的、原发的；第三，与发生时间没有关系。

同时性多原发肿瘤（synchronous multiple primary neoplasms，S-MPNs）是指2个或2个以上的原发肿瘤明确诊断的间隔时间≤6个月，异时性多原发肿瘤（metachronous multiple primary neoplasms，M-MPNs）是指2个或2个以上的原发肿瘤明确诊断的间隔时间>6个月。

多原发肿瘤相对于其他常见肿瘤而言，发病率较低，临床少见。美国第二原发肿瘤占所有肿瘤的比例为9.3%，欧洲国家为6.3%，中国为0.6%~2.67%。近年来，随着医疗技术的进步，长期生存的肿瘤患者明显增加，而多原发肿瘤的发生率有升高趋势。一般而言，多原发肿瘤以双原发肿瘤为主，三原发肿瘤较少，四原发及以上原发肿瘤临床罕见。

在所有多原发肿瘤中，同时性多原发肿瘤仅占20%左右，而异时性多原发肿瘤近80%。在异时性多原发肿瘤中，第一原发肿瘤与第二原发肿瘤的发生间隔时间多为5~10年，第一原发肿瘤发病后的1~3年内为第二原发肿瘤发生的高峰期。

超过80%的多原发肿瘤发生在不同的器官系统，第二、第三等原发肿瘤与第一原发肿瘤在同一组织或器官的仅占13.2%，最常见的部位是乳腺、结肠、肺、皮肤（如黑色素瘤），另外，有3.8%的第二原发肿瘤起源于第一原发肿瘤的邻近组织或器官；实体肿瘤发生第二原发血液肿瘤主要包括多发性骨髓瘤、骨髓增生异常综合征、非霍奇金淋巴瘤、慢性粒细胞白血病。

多原发肿瘤的发病率通常与年龄相关,年龄越大,发生率越高,50～60岁为高发年龄段,60岁以上人群比例达1/3,中位年龄为59岁(29～80岁);首次被诊断60～69岁的肿瘤患者,10年内患第二原发肿瘤的累积风险可达13%。男性发病率高于女性。

目前,多原发肿瘤的发病因素尚不十分清楚,从现有文献报道来看,多原发肿瘤的发病因素主要包括环境因素、生活方式(如吸烟、酗酒、肥胖等)、内分泌因素、家族遗传因素、免疫因素、治疗因素(如放射治疗、化学治疗等)、年龄因素等。

多原发肿瘤的发病机制目前亦不十分明确,一般认为,多原发肿瘤并非由单个细胞DNA突变引起,而是涉及受同一致癌物质刺激的一个广泛区域范围的细胞,包括同一暴露器官及不同暴露器官,在接受同一致癌物质刺激的同时或异时发生DNA结构及功能的改变,从而产生不同的癌变过程。

多原发肿瘤检查与第一原发肿瘤初始基线检查基本相同,主要包括全身影像学检查、内镜检查(如鼻咽镜、支气管镜、胃镜、肠镜、膀胱镜、宫腔镜等)及新发病灶组织(内镜活检、穿刺活检、腔镜活检等)病理学检查(包括常规病理、免疫组化、分子基因检测等)、遗传学检查及肿瘤标志物检测等。

多原发肿瘤的诊断主要依赖于影像学和组织病理学(包括免疫组化、分子病理等),总体诊断标准为每个肿瘤必须独立存在于不同器官或同一器官的不同部位、每个肿瘤具有各自不同的病理学特征,同一、单一器官及对称性同侧器官肿瘤间须间隔一定距离的正常组织(>2cm),通过影像学及组织病理学检查(包括免疫组化、基因检测)排除了第一原发肿瘤转移。

目前,尚无统一的、公认的多原发肿瘤标准治疗方案,但大多数学者认为,一旦确诊为多原发肿瘤,须组织多学科团队(multidisciplinary team,MDT)讨论,通常应遵照个体化治疗原则,通过对各原发肿瘤的病理类型、临床分期、患者身体耐受情况等进行全面评估，制订各原发肿瘤最佳治疗方案，在治疗方法上达成一致意见或共识。

目前，对于多原发肿瘤患者生存时间的计算方法没有统一标准，且存在一定分歧，尤其是异时性多原发肿瘤患者的生存计算。由于计算方法的不同，文献报道的多原发肿瘤生存率存在较大差异。有学者报道，多原发肿瘤患者的10年生存率为69.3%，还有报道，多原发肿瘤患者3年、5年生存率仅为48.3%、37.5%。多数学者认为，多原发肿瘤患者的预后与各原发肿瘤临床或病理分期、肿瘤分化程度、肿瘤部位分布、两种肿瘤发生的间隔时间、治疗方式以及患者年龄等多种因素相关。

不明原发肿瘤（carcinomas of unknown primary，CUP）是指经组织学确认的转移性上皮来源的癌或神经内分泌肿瘤，且经详细的病史询问、体格检查、肿瘤标志物检测、免疫组化检测，以及多种影像学（如X线、B超、CT、MRI、PET/CT等）检查，并由专家进一步判定，最终仍未确定组织起源的恶性肿瘤。

不同的国家、地区及不同的作者、不同的报道时间，不明原发肿瘤发病率略有差异，一般为（6~16）/10万，占所有恶性肿瘤的2.3%~7.8%，为第八大常见肿瘤，死亡率位列第四。

不明原发肿瘤的转移部位十分广泛，在CUP发现的转移部位中，常见的转移部位有淋巴结、肝脏、肺、骨骼和脑实质，少见的有卵巢、骨髓、脑膜、胸膜、腹膜等。

目前，CUP确切的发病因素、发生机制均不十分清楚，有多种理论或观点。可能是原发灶过小且生长缓慢或微小原发灶生长受宿主免疫抑制，并发生消退；或可能因其原发肿瘤太小或位置隐蔽，现有的检查方法难以发现。

在对可疑CUP患者进行多学科诊断评估时，影像学检查发挥着不可替代的作用。对于可疑CUP常规影像学检查而言，X线、B超、CT、MRI、骨扫描等是寻找原发肿瘤的首选检查方法。目前对于可疑CUP患者初始检查选择PET/CT尚存在争议，在现有指南中尚未被推荐作为CUP初始检查的首选手段。

一般而言，通常根据患者的临床症状、影像学检查结果来选择相应内镜检查，发现可疑病灶，则需活检。

虽然血液中各种肿瘤标志物（如 CEA、AFP、CA125、CA19-9、CA72-4、CA15-3、PSA 等）的升高与其原发肿瘤类型有一定关系，但特异性、敏感性均不强，在确定原发肿瘤部位方面的价值有限，通常不能作为诊断依据。

组织病理学检查结果是 CUP 诊断的金标准，病理学检查首先应明确肿瘤细胞的基本类型，尽可能确定肿瘤的原发部位。

基于大多数原发肿瘤与转移性肿瘤的蛋白表达谱存在一致性，免疫组化检测可提供肿瘤谱系、细胞类型等信息，辅助确定 CUP 的病理类型、肿瘤原发部位等。

转移部位肿瘤细胞的基因表达谱与其原发部位肿瘤的基因表达谱存在一定的相似性，通过对比转移性肿瘤组织样本与已知来源的肿瘤分子特征，一般可推测出转移性肿瘤最可能的组织起源。但因大样本的前瞻性研究较少，且价格昂贵，临床上难以广泛开展，故目前多数指南不建议常规使用基因测序来推测 CUP 原发肿瘤部位。

在临床实践中，对 CUP 的诊断目前仍是一个巨大挑战。一般而言，在完成病理和临床诊断检查后，CUP 的诊断取决于多学科团队对临床表现、病理学、免疫组化和影像学检查结果的仔细解读，通常是根据肿瘤相关信息最终判定是原发肿瘤还是与 CUP 相符的转移瘤。在没有可明确识别原发肿瘤特异性基因组改变的情况下，必须判断其中一个可见病灶是否可能代表原发肿瘤。

迄今为止，CUP 治疗尚缺乏充分的循证医学依据，且无标准治疗方案推荐，故多数学者认为，最好由多学科专家讨论，达成一致意见。

目前，对于 CUP 多主张采取以手术、放射治疗、化学治疗等综合治疗模式。多数 CUP 患者在诊断时常为多发转移，已失去手术机会，但对孤立性转移的 CUP 患者，手术治疗或局部放射治疗仍是首选方法。

对于最终确诊为 CUP 的患者而言，无论是何种类型的组织病理学，内科系统治疗对提高患者生存质量、延长患者生存均具有重要意义，主要包括化学治疗、靶向治疗及免疫治疗等。

目前，没有任何特定的化学治疗方案被推荐为标准治疗方案，主要根据转移性肿瘤组织病理类型选择化学治疗方案，CUP 主要组织病理类型为腺癌、鳞癌与神经内分泌癌。一般而言，对于有症状的、广泛转移的、PS 评分为 0~2 分的 CUP 患者，或无症状的侵袭性强的 CUP 患者，可考虑系统化学治疗。

CUP 肿瘤组织中基因异常改变的发现为部分 CUP 患者提供了靶向治疗的可能性，对靶向治疗潜在获益的 CUP 人群筛查具有重要意义。目前，仅有少数靶向药物适用于 CUP 一线单药治疗，在许多 CUP 治疗中，联合化学疗仍然发挥着重要作用，CUP 单一靶向治疗的有效性仍需进一步临床验证。

随着对免疫检查点抑制剂（immune checkpoint inhibitors，ICIs）预测生物标记物的识别，免疫检查点抑制剂治疗已成为 CUP 患者的另一种选择。

对免疫治疗反应的预测指标目前仍无定论，在已知的肿瘤类型中，肿瘤突变负荷（tumor mutation burden，TMB）、微卫星不稳定性（microsatellite instability，MSI）、错配修复基因（mismatch repairgene，MMR）表达和程序性死亡受体配体 1（programmed death ligand 1，PD－L1）表达等。高度微卫星不稳定性（microsatellite instability－high，MSI－H）、PD－L1 高表达和高肿瘤突变负荷（tumor mutation burden－high，TMB－H）已被确定为免疫治疗有效的泛癌生物标志物。目前，FDA 已批准 pembrolizumab 用于 MSI－H 或错配修复基因缺失（deficient mismatch repair，dMMR）肿瘤患者的二线治疗，其中亦包括 CUP 患者。对于 PD－L1 高表达且无其他治疗选择的复发或难治性 CUP 患者，可考虑选择 ICIs 治疗。

一般而言，CUP 患者的根治性治疗机会较少，多数患者预后不良，约 50% 的患者死亡发生在确诊后的 3 个月内。CUP 患者平均生存期为 2~10 个月，OS 为 8~11 个月，仅 20% 左右预后良好的亚型患者生存期超过 1 年，中位 OS 可达 12~36 个月。

总之，多原发肿瘤与不明原发肿瘤发病率低，临床少见，其诊断、治疗、预后等前瞻性研究较少，在预防、诊断、治疗、康复等方面目前仍处于探索阶段。

查阅大量相关资料，目前全球尚无比较全面、系统介绍多原发肿瘤与不明原发肿瘤方面的专著。鉴于此，中国抗癌协会多原发肿瘤和不明原发肿瘤整合康复专业委员会、陕西省抗癌协会罕见肿瘤专委会组织全国专家编写了《多原发肿瘤与不明原发肿瘤》一书。该书通过对现有文献资料的查阅，系统介绍了多原发肿瘤与不明原发肿瘤基本概念、流行病学、检查与诊断、治疗与预后等，是目前全球唯一系统介绍多原发肿瘤与不明原发肿瘤的专著，可为临床偶遇多原发肿瘤与不明原发肿瘤的一、二线肿瘤医生在其诊断、治疗时提供一定的帮助。然而，因编者水平有限，定有诸多不足与瑕疵，诚望读者不吝赐教，待再版时加以斧正。

樊代明　廖子君　罗志国
乙巳年春于古都长安

目 录

上 篇 多原发肿瘤

第一章 总 论 …………………………………………（ 3 ）

　第一节 基本概念 ……………………………………（ 3 ）

　第二节 流行病学 ……………………………………（ 5 ）

　　一、发病率 …………………………………………（ 5 ）

　　二、发生间隔时间 …………………………………（ 6 ）

　　三、发生部位 ………………………………………（ 8 ）

　　四、性别与年龄 ……………………………………（ 16 ）

　第三节 发病因素 ……………………………………（ 18 ）

　　一、环境因素 ………………………………………（ 19 ）

　　二、家族遗传因素 …………………………………（ 20 ）

　　三、内分泌因素 ……………………………………（ 21 ）

　　四、治疗因素 ………………………………………（ 22 ）

　　五、不良生活方式 …………………………………（ 27 ）

　　六、年龄因素 ………………………………………（ 30 ）

　第四节 发病机制 ……………………………………（ 31 ）

　　一、相关理论学说 …………………………………（ 31 ）

　　二、遗传性癌症综合征 ……………………………（ 34 ）

　　三、主要基因异常 …………………………………（ 36 ）

第二章 预防与筛查 …………………………………（ 86 ）

　第一节 预 防 ………………………………………（ 86 ）

第二节　筛　查 ……………………………………… (89)
　　　一、多原发肿瘤发生风险评估要求 ……………… (89)
　　　二、多原发肿瘤筛查对象与筛查方法 …………… (90)

第三章　检查、诊断与治疗 ……………………………… (97)
　　第一节　检　查 ……………………………………… (97)
　　　一、影像学检查 …………………………………… (97)
　　　二、组织病理学检查 ……………………………… (98)
　　　三、免疫组化检查 ………………………………… (99)
　　　四、分子基因检测 ………………………………… (99)
　　　五、肿瘤标志物检测 ……………………………… (100)
　　第二节　诊　断 ……………………………………… (101)
　　　一、漏诊分析 ……………………………………… (101)
　　　二、总体诊断标准 ………………………………… (102)
　　　三、双侧原发乳腺癌诊断 ………………………… (102)
　　　四、肺内多原发癌诊断 …………………………… (102)
　　　五、多原发肿瘤临床或病理分期 ………………… (104)
　　第三节　治　疗 ……………………………………… (107)
　　　一、治疗原则 ……………………………………… (107)
　　　二、肺内多原发癌的治疗 ………………………… (110)
　　　三、上消化道内多原发肿瘤治疗 ………………… (111)
　　　四、同时性结直肠内多原发癌治疗 ……………… (111)

第四章　预后、随访与康复 ……………………………… (122)
　　第一节　预后情况 …………………………………… (122)
　　　一、生存率的计算 ………………………………… (122)
　　　二、总体预后 ……………………………………… (122)
　　　三、预后相关因素 ………………………………… (123)
　　第二节　医生随访与患者康复 ……………………… (129)

下 篇 不明原发肿瘤

第五章 总 论 (141)
第一节 基本概念 (141)
第二节 流行病学 (142)
一、发病情况 (142)
二、转移部位 (142)
第三节 发生机制 (148)
第四节 临床分型与分期 (149)

第六章 可疑 CUP 检查与诊断 (158)
第一节 可疑 CUP 一般检查 (158)
一、病史询问 (158)
二、临床表现 (158)
三、体格检查 (159)
第二节 可疑 CUP 影像学检查 (160)
一、常规影像学检查 (160)
二、PET/CT 检查 (161)
第三节 可疑 CUP 内镜检查 (167)
第四节 可疑 CUP 肿瘤标志物检测 (168)
第五节 病理学检查 (169)
一、组织或细胞标本 (169)
二、骨髓涂片和（或）骨髓活检 (169)
三、脱落细胞学检查与细胞蜡块技术 (170)
四、液体活检 (171)
五、转移部位肿瘤的主要病理类型 (171)
第六节 免疫组化检测 (172)
一、细胞角蛋白 (175)

二、GATA3 ……………………………………………………（175）
　　三、TTF-1 ……………………………………………………（176）
　　四、GCDFP 15 …………………………………………………（176）
　　五、URO Ⅲ ……………………………………………………（176）
　第七节　可疑CUP分子基因检测 …………………………………（180）
　　一、推测CUP组织起源 ……………………………………（181）
　　二、指导CUP系统治疗方案制订 …………………………（185）
　第八节　诊　断 ……………………………………………………（186）
　　一、尽力明确原发肿瘤 ………………………………………（187）
　　二、CUP诊断标准 ……………………………………………（190）
　　三、几种常见原发肿瘤与可疑CUP鉴别诊断的逻辑推理 ……（191）
　　四、几种特殊转移灶的诊断 …………………………………（195）

第七章　CUP治疗与预后 ……………………………………………（215）
　第一节　治　疗 ……………………………………………………（215）
　　一、治疗原则 …………………………………………………（215）
　　二、外科治疗 …………………………………………………（222）
　　三、放射治疗 …………………………………………………（228）
　　四、内科治疗 …………………………………………………（229）
　第二节　预　后 ……………………………………………………（244）
　　一、总体预后 …………………………………………………（244）
　　二、预后相关因素 ……………………………………………（245）
　　三、随访 ………………………………………………………（248）

附　录 …………………………………………………………………（266）
　附录1　主要名词术语英文缩写、全称、中文名 ………………（266）
　附录2　体能状态（ECOG-PS）评分 ……………………………（270）

上 篇
多原发肿瘤

第一章

总　论

第一节　基本概念

多原发肿瘤(multiple primary neoplasms，MPNs)有"多原发癌"(multiple primary cancer，MPC)、"多重癌"(multiplicity carcinoma，MC)、"重复癌"、"多中心癌"等称谓[1-5]，由 Billroth 于 1871 年首次报道；1961 年，Moertel 等[6]将多原发肿瘤分为同时性多原发肿瘤(synchronous multiple primary neoplasms，S-MPNs)与异时性多原发肿瘤(metachronous multiple primary neoplasms，M-MPNs)，目前这一分类方法已被众多学者所接受，并广泛用于多原发肿瘤诊断与治疗中[7-9]。

第三版《国际疾病分类肿瘤分册》指出[10]，多原发肿瘤的存在不取决于时间，每一个原发肿瘤起源于一个组织或部位，而不是侵袭、复发或转移，可能涉及许多不同的器官系统。

陈舒兰[11]认为，确定多原发肿瘤有 3 个要点，第一，必须是 2 个及以上的恶性肿瘤；第二，恶性肿瘤彼此是独立的、原发的；第三，与发生时间没有关系。

双侧原发性乳腺癌亦分为同时性双侧原发性乳腺癌(synchronous bilateral primary breast cancer，S-BPBC)与异时性双侧原发性乳腺癌(metachronous bilateral primary breast cancer，M-BPBC)，二者间隔时间与 S-MPNs、M-MPNs 相同[12-13]。

同样，多原发肺内癌(multiple primary lung cancers，MPLCs)也分为同时性多原发肺内癌(synchronous MPLCs，S-MPLCs)与异时性多原发肺内癌(metachronous MPLCs，M-MPLCs)，包括同侧肺内、对侧肺内多原发肿瘤[14-18]。

表 1-1 本书常用多原发肿瘤定义

名称	定义	备注
多原发肿瘤	指机体同时性或异时性发生 2 个或 2 个以上、彼此无关系的原发恶性肿瘤，可分别来源于同一器官、成对器官、不同系统的器官、同一系统的不同器官	本书所言多原发肿瘤是指多原发恶性肿瘤，不包括良性肿瘤
同时性多原发肿瘤	指 2 个或 2 个以上原发肿瘤明确诊断的间隔时间≤6 个月	该诊断仅指组织病理学诊断，不包括脱落细胞学诊断
异时性多原发肿瘤	指 2 个或 2 个以上原发肿瘤明确诊断的间隔时间＞6 个月	该诊断仅指组织病理学诊断，不包括脱落细胞学诊断
同侧同时性甲状腺内多原发癌	指具有多种癌成分，且病灶均局限于甲状腺内的癌，可分为 2 种类型。 类型Ⅰ：不同组织学类型的癌分别独立存在于一侧或双侧甲状腺，间隔以正常甲状腺组织。 类型Ⅱ：同一个瘤体中存在 2 种不同组织学类型的癌	同一个器官内、同侧内同时性发生的组织学类型不同的恶性肿瘤
双侧原发性乳腺癌	指两侧乳腺同时性或异时性发生独立的原发性乳腺癌	不包括对侧乳腺癌转移
肺内多原发癌	指单侧或双侧肺同时或异时性确诊 2 个及 2 个以上彼此独立的原发性肺癌	病理类型可以是腺癌、鳞癌、大细胞癌、大细胞神经内分泌癌、小细胞癌，或组织学分类不明的癌，不包括软组织恶性肿瘤、淋巴瘤（如黏膜相关性淋巴瘤）、黑色素瘤等
消化道内多原发肿瘤	指食管、胃、小肠、结直肠同时性或异时性发生 2 个或 2 个以上经组织病理学证实的、独立的恶性肿瘤	属于同一系统不同器官的多原发肿瘤，不包括同时性或异时性发生的消化道外的癌
结直肠内多原发癌	指结直肠内同时性或异时性发生 2 个或 2 个以上的原发癌	不包括同时性或异时性发生的结直肠外的癌
胃内多原发癌	指胃内不同部位存在 2 个或 2 个以上独立的原发癌	不包括同时性或异时性发生的胃外的癌

上篇 多原发肿瘤
第一章 总 论

第二节 流行病学

一、发病率

由于不同国家、不同地区对多原发肿瘤的认识、诊断水平、统计学方法等不一致,以及受地域因素的影响,其多原发肿瘤的发病率报道存在较大差异[19-23]。

2003年,在一项1104269例美国肿瘤患者的研究中,报道多原发肿瘤占所有肿瘤的比例为0.73%~11.7%[24]。1975—2001年,在美国大样本统计的900多万肿瘤患者中,多原发肿瘤的占比为7.9%[25]。SEER(Surveillance,Epidemiology,and End Results)癌症登记报道,美国第二原发肿瘤占比为9.3%(60271/647672)[26]。

在69个欧洲癌症登记处的2919023例恶性肿瘤中发现183683例多原发肿瘤,总体占比为6.3%,范围从0.4%(意大利)到12.9%(冰岛)[27]。

Utada等[28]报道,日本MPNs的占比为8.1%;韩国报道为11.7%(962/8204)[29];多数中国学者报道[30-46],中国多原发肿瘤占比为0.6%~2.67%。

但近年来,随着基础医学与临床医学的快速发展,恶性肿瘤长生存者在不断增加。有报道称,从1971年至2007年美国肿瘤长生存者由原来的300万增加到了1170万[47-48]。据美国癌症协会(American Cancer Society,ACS)报道,截至2019年1月,美国恶性肿瘤长生存者超过1690万,预计到2030年1月,恶性肿瘤长生存者将超过2210万[49]。

相对于普通人群而言,恶性肿瘤长生存者再次罹患恶性肿瘤的风险更高;加之环境污染、医疗辐射暴露增加、现代不良生活习惯(如熬夜、久坐)等影响,以及临床医生对多原发肿瘤的认识逐步加深,从而降低了临床漏诊率与误诊率[5]。因此,近年来多原发肿瘤患者数量亦在明显上升[50-69]。21世纪之前,文献报道的发病率均较低[70]。美国,2005—2009年恶性肿瘤存活患者再发恶性肿瘤风险较1975—1979年上升了10%[71];芬兰,1980年恶性肿瘤存活患者再发恶性肿瘤风险较1950年增加了50%[72]。近5年国内外报道MPNs占所有肿瘤的比例为1.02%~37.25%[73-85]。2023年,陈小良等[86]报道,2000年1月—2021年3月中国深圳市共登记多原发恶性肿瘤4137例，占同期所有恶性肿瘤的1.64%。梁智恒等[87]报道了1970—2019年中国中山市5369例多原发肿瘤，粗发病率、中标率和世标率分别为8.60/10万、6.62/10万和8.62/10万。

一般而言，多原发肿瘤以双原发肿瘤为主，三原发肿瘤较少，四原发及以上原发肿瘤罕见[88-90]。Kilciksiz等[91]报道了土耳其297例多原发肿瘤，53.2%为同时性双原发肿瘤，43.1%为异时性双原发肿瘤；1.7%为同时性三原发肿瘤，1.3%既有同时性肿瘤又有异时性肿瘤，0.7%为异时性三原发肿瘤。Pacheco-Figueiredo等[92]报道了葡萄牙北部1684例多原发肿瘤，95%为双原发肿瘤，4%为三原发肿瘤，1%为四原发及以上原发肿瘤，异时性肿瘤占77.9%。梁智恒等[87]报道了1970—2019年中国中山市5369例多原发肿瘤，双原发肿瘤和三原发肿瘤分别占多原发肿瘤发病总数的94.06%和5.31%，异时性多原发肿瘤占75.79%。在陈小良等[86]报道的深圳市共登记多原发肿瘤4137例者中，双原发、三原发、四原发病例各4021例（97.20%）、110例（2.66%）和6例（0.14%）。Noh等[93]报道了一例女性罹患4种异时性多原发癌，其发生部位为乳腺、直肠、卵巢、子宫内膜。

另外，20世纪80年代有五原发肿瘤的个案报道[94-95]；2015年，中国学者Zhao等[96]报道了一例八原发肿瘤患者。2018年，Arakawa等[97]报道了一名男性患者在67~73岁之间发生了9个原发性恶性肿瘤，3个原发于食管、2个原发于胃、2个原发于结直肠、1个原发于前列腺、1个原发于外耳道，如此多原发肿瘤病例，临床实为罕见。

二、发生间隔时间

有研究报道[98-100]，在所有多原发肿瘤中，同时性多原发肿瘤仅占20%左右，而异时性多原发肿瘤近80%。Jiao等[34]对上海交通大学附属第一人民医院2009年9月至2013年2月6545名肿瘤患者中72例多原发肿瘤进行分析发现，22.2%为同时性MPNs，76.4%为异时性MPNs。

在异时性多原发肿瘤中，第一原发肿瘤与第二原发肿瘤的发生间隔时间多为5~10年[101]，第一原发肿瘤发病后的1~3年为第二原发肿瘤的高峰期[102]，在第一年发生的频率更高[103]。肖彩宏等[104]报道，多原发肿瘤之间发生的间隔时间不超过6年的发生率为65%~80%。日本学者Utada等[28]通过分析长崎区癌症登记中心1985—2007年间的癌症患者数据发现，

上篇 多原发肿瘤

第一章 总　论

对于所有部位的第一原发肿瘤,第二原发肿瘤在第一年发生频率更高,第二年下降,然后在约10年后又出现一个上升趋势。

一项为期9年的回顾性临床研究统计了855例多原发肿瘤[105],结果显示,第一原发肿瘤与第二原发肿瘤的发生间隔时间平均为45个月,异时性多原发肿瘤患者占比超过50%,且在这部分患者中,50%患者第二原发肿瘤发生在第一原发肿瘤诊断后31个月内。中国一项关于152例多原发恶性肿瘤患者的临床研究发现[106],第一原发肿瘤与第二原发肿瘤平均发生间隔的时间为43.1个月。Kilciksiz等[91]报道,在异时性多原发肿瘤患者中,2个肿瘤发生的平均间隔时间是44.4个月。陈小良等[86]报道,中国深圳市4137例多原发肿瘤中,第二原发肿瘤确诊距第一原发肿瘤确诊时间为0~1个月(同时确诊)、1~3个月、3~6个月、0.5~1年、1~3年、3~5年、5~10年、10年及以上的比例分别为19.73%、10.85%、7.90%、9.81%、22.51%、12.01%、14.41%和2.78%,其中,1~3年发生率最高(22.51%)。

相关研究报道[107-110],乳腺癌确诊后的1~5年是MPNs发生的高风险期,而Rosso等[111]对意大利都灵1985—1988年的9233例乳腺癌患者研究发现,乳腺癌患者在第8年至第9年可出现一个再患肿瘤风险的高峰;王成峰等[112]报道,乳腺作为第一原发肿瘤的发病年龄为51.4岁,与第二原发肿瘤间隔时间平均为8.6年,同时性仅占8%。

乳腺癌作为第一原发肿瘤,其与第二原发肿瘤发生的间隔时间似乎与年龄相关。师弘等[36]报道了82例多原发乳腺癌,在发病年龄方面,<50岁的乳腺癌患者其第一原发肿瘤与第二原发肿瘤的中位间隔时间为2.4年;而≥50岁的多原发肿瘤患者,其发病中位间隔时间为8.5年。

奥婷等[113]报道了55例原发性肺癌合并其他原发肿瘤,55例患者中,以肺癌作为第一原发肿瘤,与第二原发肿瘤发生的平均间隔时间31.94个月;以其他肿瘤作为第一原发肿瘤,与发生肺癌的平均间隔时间85.13个月;提示其他第一原发肿瘤发生第二原发肿瘤肺癌的间隔时间较长。Duchateau等[114]的观察结果亦显示,肺癌作为第一原发肿瘤,与第二原发肿瘤发生的间隔时间明显短于其他第一原发肿瘤发生第二原发肿瘤肺癌的间隔时间;而Kim等[68]的研究表明,肺癌先发组和其他肿瘤先发组两次肿瘤发生的时间间隔差异无统计学意义,原发肺癌合并多原发肿瘤的中位发生间隔时间为47.2个月。

三、发生部位

有研究报道[115],超过80%的多原发肿瘤发生在不同的器官系统,第二、第三等原发肿瘤与第一原发肿瘤在同一组织或器官的仅占13.2%,最常见的部位是乳腺、结肠、肺、皮肤(黑色素瘤),另外有3.8%的第二原发肿瘤起源于第一原发肿瘤的邻近组织或器官。

MPNs可发生于人体任何器官,但总体发病部位以胸、腹和头颈部等较多;系统以消化、呼吸和生殖等系统较多;器官则以肺、结直肠和乳腺等较多,最常见的配对器官是结直肠-结直肠和结直肠-肺等[116-123]。

然而,不同地区的作者报道MPNs的好发部位存在一定差异,主要与不同国家或地区的肿瘤发病情况及患者生活环境有关。

欧美国家皮肤、膀胱、前列腺和甲状腺多原发肿瘤发病较高,膀胱癌常伴发肺癌,乳腺癌常伴发甲状腺、妇科和消化道肿瘤[124-126]。Wittekind等[127]报道,在MPNs中,位于头颈部、食管胃肠道、肺部的比例分别为23%~42%、15%~43%、5%~26%。Giardiello等[128]的研究发现,第一原发肿瘤好发器官依次为子宫、乳腺、食管、肺;第二原发肿瘤好发器官依次为肺、食管、乳腺、子宫、直肠。

土耳其MPNs最常见于胃肠道、皮肤、头颈部、女性生殖道和呼吸道[57]。Gursel等[129]的研究结果显示,土耳其第一原发肿瘤好发部位依次为喉、膀胱和乳腺;第二原发肿瘤好发部位依次为肺、乳腺和结肠。

中国、日本、韩国、马来西亚、印度等亚洲国家MPNs的好发部位基本相同,以消化系统、乳腺、生殖系统等多见[130-135]。中国学者陈小良等[86]报道了中国深圳市4137例多原发肿瘤,第一原发肿瘤排名前5位的部位分别为乳腺(11.51%)、支气管和肺(8.12%)、宫颈(7.95%)、结肠(7.76%)和甲状腺(6.70%);第二原发肿瘤排名前10位的部位分别为支气管和肺(14.48%)、结肠(7.78%)、甲状腺(7.69%)、乳腺(6.94%)、胃(4.79%)、宫颈(4.25%)、直肠乙状结肠连接处(4.11%)、肝和肝内胆管(3.07%)、卵巢(2.63%)和膀胱(2.56%),占58.30%;第三原发肿瘤(116例)排前10位的部位分别为支气管和肺(7.76%)、甲状腺(7.76%)、直肠乙状结肠交界处(6.90%)、宫颈(6.03%)、结肠(5.17%)、膀胱(5.17%)、非四肢的其他骨和关节软骨(3.45%)、脑(3.45%)、食管(2.59%)、胃(2.59%);第四原发肿瘤(6例)的好发部位分别是鼻咽、胃、小肠、结肠、子宫和白血病。

Utada 等[28]随访了 174477 例日本肿瘤患者,发生第二原发肿瘤 14167 例,第一原发肿瘤主要为食管癌、喉癌,其次为卵巢癌、下咽癌、口咽癌等;第二原发肿瘤好发部位为甲状腺、食管,其次为乳腺、结肠。如果第一原发肿瘤是口咽/下咽癌,第二原发肿瘤多为食管癌,反之,如果第一原发肿瘤是食管癌,第二原发肿瘤是口咽/下咽癌的概率亦最大。Naik 等[136]的研究发现,马来西亚人群中第一原发肿瘤主要分布在头颈、乳腺;第二原发肿瘤主要分布在头颈、消化道、乳腺。

有研究报道[137-138],同时有非小细胞肺癌的多原发肿瘤患者中,胃肠道肿瘤的发生率居首位。Zhang 等[139]分析了合并有肺癌的 5570 例患者,结果发现,结直肠癌、乳腺癌和甲状腺癌居前三位,无论是第一原发肿瘤,还是第二、第三原发肿瘤,消化道肿瘤均为高发。

实体肿瘤发生第二原发血液肿瘤主要包括多发性骨髓瘤、骨髓增生异常综合征、非霍奇金淋巴瘤、慢性粒细胞白血病[140],王艳峰等[141]进行的恶性实体肿瘤发生第二原发恶性血液病类型分析结果显示,常见第二原发恶性血液病主要为淋巴瘤和髓系白血病。

(一)甲状腺癌为第一原发肿瘤

甲状腺内多原发癌临床极其罕见,国内外报道不足 50 例[142-147];而甲状腺癌作为第一原发肿瘤,继发第二原发肿瘤最常见的是乳腺癌,其继发乳腺癌的风险是普通人群的 1.18 倍,继发病理类型多为浸润性导管癌,分子分型为激素受体阳性型[148-149]。Vanfossen 等[150]的研究发现,女性甲状腺癌患者继发乳腺癌风险较普通人群增加 0.67 倍,男性患者此风险增加 29 倍。

甲状腺癌发病年龄大、甲状腺癌体积小、滤泡状甲状腺癌是甲状腺癌发生第二原发乳腺癌的危险因素,甲状腺癌细胞类似乳腺癌细胞,亦存在 ER、PR 的表达,且其表达水平较正常甲状腺细胞高,雌激素亦可通过性激素受体促进甲状腺癌的形成与发展。Rajoria 等[151]研究发现,在雌激素作用下,甲状腺乳头状癌细胞的黏附能力、迁移能力、侵袭力较对照组分别增加 140%、27%、100%。

(二)头颈部鳞癌为第一原发肿瘤

第一原发肿瘤为头颈部鳞癌(head and neck squamous cell carcinoma,

HN-SCC)发生第二原发肿瘤的概率较高[152],每年占第二原发肿瘤的2%~6%,20年累计发生率可达36%[153],其中原发性下咽癌、口腔癌患者患第二原发肿瘤的风险最高[154-156],第二原发肿瘤中肺癌最常见[157-158]。田慎之等[159]报道,喉鳞状细胞癌多原发癌中有25.9%为肺癌。但也有研究报道[160],第一原发肿瘤为头颈部癌,其最易继发的第二原发肿瘤为食管癌。

(三)肺内多原发癌

肺内多原发癌是指同侧或对侧肺内同时性或异时性发生组织病理学不同或相同的、非转移的、独立的2个或2个以上的肺癌,1924年,Beyreuther[161]首次报道了同时性多原发肺内癌(multiple primary lung cancers,MPLC)。

近年来,随着影像学技术(如PET/CT)的发展,同时性肺内多原发癌检出率不断上升[162-166]。国外报道肺内多原发癌发病率为5%~6%,同时性肺内癌发病率为1.1%~3.1%[167];中国同时性肺内多原发癌发病率为0.2%~2.0%[168-174]。

(四)肺癌与肺外器官多原发肿瘤

以肺癌为第一原发肿瘤,其发生的第二、第三等原发肿瘤主要为上呼吸道癌、乳腺癌、食管癌、结直肠、胃癌、宫颈癌、淋巴瘤等[175],但总体临床少见。第一原发肺癌的病理学类型以肺腺癌为多,肺鳞癌、肺小细胞癌亦有报道[176];多为异时性,同时性少见。李辉等[177]分析了其所在单位的1019例肺癌患者,21例合并其他器官肿瘤,5例为同时性,16例为异时性。

(五)乳腺癌为第一原发肿瘤

较多的研究报道显示[178-179],近年来,随着乳腺癌患者总生存期的明显延长与放射治疗、化学治疗、靶向治疗、内分泌治疗等的广泛使用,第二、第三等原发肿瘤发生的风险亦在增加。一篇关于乳腺癌多原发肿瘤的meta文章中指出[8],女性患者在患乳腺癌后,其患第二原发肿瘤的概率较正常人群高17%,且这一比例在绝经前女性中还有上升趋势[107]。

据相关文献报道[180-184],乳腺癌总体发生率为4.1%~16.4%;国外报道[185-187],乳腺癌相关多原发癌发生率为0.73%~11.70%。Howe等[188]对1994—1998年北美癌症登记中心协会(NAACCR)数据集上登记的乳腺癌数据进行统计分析,结果显示,乳腺多原发肿瘤的患病率约为2.72%。中国报道的发生率为2.6%~8.79%[189]。

乳腺癌发生第二原发肿瘤常见部位有对侧乳腺、甲状腺、肺、子宫内膜、卵巢、肾、骨等,亦有继发黑色素瘤、淋巴瘤、白血病等第二原发肿瘤的报道[190]。一项基于SEER数据库的回顾性研究(2001—2014年)显示[187],乳腺癌再发第二原发肿瘤的发生部位依次为对侧乳腺、消化系统、肺和支气管、生殖系统、淋巴造血系统、泌尿系统和甲状腺。

师弘等[36]报道了82例多原发乳腺癌,以继发肺癌、卵巢癌、甲状腺癌、结直肠癌最常见。杨韵等[191]报道了19例多原发乳腺癌,其中继发妇科系统肿瘤6例,胃癌1例,结肠及直肠癌3例,肺癌3例,原发性肝癌1例,泌尿系统恶性肿瘤2例,血液系统恶性肿瘤1例,甲状腺1例,其他癌1例。郑希希等[35]的研究发现,在第二原发恶性肿瘤中,甲状腺癌最常见,其次为妇科系统恶性肿瘤(包括子宫、宫颈、卵巢、外阴)。

1. 发生对侧第二原发性乳腺癌

对侧乳腺癌是乳腺癌最常见的第二原发恶性肿瘤,与普通人群相比,5年内乳腺癌患者继发对侧乳腺癌风险增加4倍[192],单侧乳腺癌患者发生对侧乳腺癌的概率达2%~12%[195],是健康人群发生乳腺癌的2~6倍[183]。

有研究报道[194-195],乳腺癌再发第二原发肿瘤的最常见部位是对侧乳腺,仅2.02%的乳腺癌患者第二原发肿瘤发生于非乳腺部位,如卵巢、子宫内膜[196]。第一原发乳腺癌与对侧第二原发乳腺癌均以浸润性乳腺癌为最多见,即双侧浸润性乳腺癌[197-199]。

对于一侧乳腺癌组织病理学类型及ER、PR、HER-2表达状态与对侧乳腺癌发生风险的相关性存在一定争议。

有学者认为[200-201],乳腺浸润性小叶癌是发生双侧原发性乳腺癌的危险因素。Reinr等[202]报道,首发病理类型为浸润性小叶癌或ER阴性者,对侧乳腺癌风险各增加30%和40%。陈学燕等[203]报道,双侧乳腺癌ER、PR表达及分子分型一致性较差。荷兰学者发现[204],首发HER-2阴性乳腺癌患者对侧乳腺癌的5年累积风险(1.9%, $95\% CI = 1.8\% \sim 2.0\%$)高于首发HER-2阳性乳腺癌患者($1.5\%$, $95\% CI = 1.3\% \sim 1.7\%$)。

Kurian等[205]的研究显示,4%的女性乳腺癌长期生存者对侧乳腺有发生原发性乳腺癌的风险,若该患者第一原发乳腺癌为激素受体(HR)阴性,则其对侧乳腺发生原发性乳腺癌的风险明显高于 HR 阳性者,且其对侧乳腺发生激素受体阴性乳腺癌的可能性更大。

但有学者认为[206-207],罹患双侧乳腺癌的风险与组织学类型无明显相关性。田青青等[208]报道,第一原发肿瘤与第二原发肿瘤患者的 ER、PR、HER-2 的表达较为一致。一项纳入 419818 名女性乳腺癌患者的美国研究显示,HER-2 状态对于对侧乳腺癌风险无显著影响[209]。

2. 发生第二原发性乳腺外肿瘤

Lee 等[196]报道,乳腺癌合并乳腺外恶性肿瘤的发生率占同期乳腺癌患者的 2.02%。乳腺癌组织类似甲状腺组织,存在促甲状腺激素(thyroid stimulating hormone,TSH)受体的表达,其肿瘤细胞中 FT_4 水平较正常人群和乳腺良性疾病人群显著升高,提示 TSH 可促进乳腺癌的发生和发展,这一假设已在体外实验被证实,TSH 的促癌作用通过激活雌激素依赖信号通路实现[210-211]。

Joseph 等[212]报道,乳腺癌患者发生第二原发性甲状腺癌风险增加 1.59 倍($95\% CI = 1.28\% \sim 1.99\%$),较其他第二原发恶性肿瘤增加 17%。郑希希等[35]报道了 226 例乳腺癌 MPCs 患者,在第二原发恶性肿瘤中,甲状腺癌最常见,占 39.82%(90/226)。

乳腺癌发生第二原发性甲状腺癌在乳腺癌确诊 3 年内风险最高;Nielsen 等[148]的 Meta 分析结果显示,乳腺癌患者罹患第二原发性甲状腺癌的风险较非乳腺癌患者高 1.55 倍。Vanfossen 等[150]的研究发现,女性乳腺癌患者发生第二原发性甲状腺癌风险较普通人群增加 2 倍,男性患者此风险增加 19 倍。Li 等[213]认为,非洲裔女性、乳腺癌原发病灶位于外上象限、病理为高级别、ER 或 PR 阳性为乳腺癌发生第二原发性甲状腺癌的高危因素。

乳腺癌相关多原发肿瘤中,亦易发生第二女性生殖系统肿瘤。王成锋等[214]报道,乳腺癌合并女性生殖系统肿瘤(如子宫内膜癌、宫颈癌、卵巢癌)占乳腺癌相关多原发癌总数的 34.78%~49.49%。刘晨等[215]报道,乳腺癌合并妇科恶性肿瘤患者,占同期收治乳腺癌患者的 1.80%。

Evans 等[190]的研究表明,乳腺癌患者发生第二原发性肺癌的相对危险度为 1.4~1.7。有研究报道[216-217],乳腺癌治疗后发生第二原发性肺癌的风险会随着时间的推移而增加。

瑞典学者在其国家癌症登记处开展了一项基于 1961—2010 年女性乳

腺癌人群的前瞻性队列研究[218]，结果显示，乳腺癌长期生存者中原发性结直肠癌的标准化发病率为1.59%，发生风险较普通人群增加1倍[219]。

（六）消化系肿瘤为第一原发肿瘤

日本与中国均为消化系恶性肿瘤高发的国家，其多原发肿瘤以消化道肿瘤居首[220-224]，其中以食管、胃、结肠多原发肿瘤常见。Uemo等[220]报道，胃肠道是第二种原发肿瘤最为好发的部位，发生率为5.2%，1.9%为同一器官、3.3%为不同器官，多数患者在第一原发肿瘤确诊后3年内发生。张立书等[225]报道，胃肠道多原发肿瘤的发病率为4.3%。张培趁等[226]对5759例经术后病理证实的胃肠道恶性肿瘤患者进行了统计分析，结果显示，确诊为多原发恶性肿瘤48例，发生率为0.83%，其中双原发肿瘤44例、三原发肿瘤4例；第二原发肿瘤按部位分，多原发大肠癌32例，占0.56%；胃多原发癌10例，占0.17%。第一原发癌与第二原发癌间隔时间为7个月~21年。

张献文等[90]文献报道，下咽癌合并食管癌的多原发肿瘤最常见（12.8%），其次为结直肠癌合并胃癌（6.4%）、结直肠癌合并乳腺癌（5.6%）、食管癌合并喉癌（4.8%）。

上消化道多原发肿瘤中，以食管、胃多原发肿瘤最为多见。食管内多原发肿瘤常发于中段与下段[227-228]，胃内多原发肿瘤以食管胃结合部及上1/3胃体最为常见[229]，十二指肠多原发癌高发于球部，与高发于乳头部的单发十二指肠癌存在显著差异[230]。

另外，有研究报道[231-232]，有4.5%~33.0%的胃肠道间质瘤（GIST）可发生同时性多原发肿瘤。

1. 食管多原发肿瘤

食管多原发肿瘤通常包括食管内与食管外同时性或异时性多原发肿瘤，总体食管多原发肿瘤的发生率为9.5%~21.9%[233-241]。章国芬等[242]的研究显示，食管癌发生多原发肿瘤的可能性可高达30%；同时性食管癌多原发肿瘤的发生率为1%~30%[243]。

食管外多原发肿瘤好发部位为头颈部、胃部[244-246]。贺舜等[131]在3104例食管癌中发现合并食管外多原发肿瘤369例，占11.9%，以头颈部肿瘤最常见，占6.8%，其次为胃癌和肺癌，分别占4.2%和0.5%，其中同时性多原发肿瘤占72.4%。Otowa等[239]对273例手术切除的食管癌患者进行分析,结果表明,最常见合并食管外多原发肿瘤的部位是咽部(29.7%),其次是胃(19.8%)。孙洁等[247]报道,食管癌合并食管外多原发肿瘤以胃癌最常见,占食管外多原发肿瘤的55.2%。

食管在解剖上,淋巴组织广泛密集,具有上下双向扩散及跳跃性转移特点,易形成壁内转移灶或多发性病灶。洪明等[248]报道,食管癌向上下段黏膜浸润长度均<3.3cm,跳跃性病灶最长间隔距离为7.4cm。有研究发现[249],多原发食管内癌好发于食管中下段。

有研究报道[250-251],36%的异时性多原发食管内鳞癌第二原发肿瘤出现在第一原发肿瘤的同一节段,食管病灶集中出现于中段。食管内多原发肿瘤的病理类型以鳞癌多见,而腺癌及其他类型肿瘤相对少见[252-253]。Slaughter等[254]认为,这些肿瘤可能来源于不同的癌发中心。

2. 胃多原发肿瘤

随着现代临床诊治技术的不断改进,胃癌患者的预后有所改善,生存时间得以延长,但同时残胃本身或其他器官再次发生肿瘤的风险亦有所增加[255-256]。项武等[257]报道,多原发胃癌发生率为0.35%~2.40%,以双原发肿瘤多见,三原发肿瘤、四原发肿瘤较少见。李小毅等[258]的研究结果显示,同时性或异时性多原发胃癌发生于胃外的恶性肿瘤以结直肠癌最多,为27.43%;其次为肺癌,占15.04%。

3. **原发性肝癌为第一原发肿瘤**

第一原发肿瘤诊断为原发性肝癌的患者发生第二原发肿瘤的概率仅1%[259]。赵岩等[260]报道了56例肝细胞癌合并肝外多原发肿瘤,24例为同时性多原发肿瘤,32例为异时性多原发肿瘤,多原发肿瘤部位最常见的是胃(12例)、结直肠(11例),其次是鼻咽(6例)、肺(5例),其他部位有喉、食管、膀胱、甲状腺、乳腺、口腔、子宫、前列腺和睾丸等,但例数极少。

4. **结直肠内多原发肿瘤**

多数文献报道,结直肠内多原发肿瘤占结直肠癌的2%~10%,同时性多原发结直肠癌占52%,异时性多原发结直肠癌占48%[261-262]。Tomio等[263]报道,大于65岁的大肠癌患者发生肠内多原发肿瘤中,外科手术为8.6%,尸检为9.4%。

多原发结直肠内肿瘤可发生于结直肠任何部位,以直肠、乙状结肠、升结肠最多见[264]。何建军[46]对2025例多原发结直肠内肿瘤进行的Meta

分析表明，30.9%位于直肠，19.9%位于乙状结肠，11.8%位于升结肠，9.1%位于横结肠，9.0%位于降结肠，8.1%位于盲肠，6.1%位于结肠肝曲，5.2%位于结肠脾曲。潘源等[38]对116例消化系统多原发肿瘤的临床分析发现，多原发结直肠内肿瘤高发于结肠，尤其是右半结肠。Ikeda等[265]的研究结果显示，大多数同时性多原发结直肠内肿瘤分布在同一肠段或相邻肠段，其发生倾向于从近端到远端结直肠；相反，异时性多原发结直肠内肿瘤的发生则倾向于从远端到近端结直肠。

另外，结直肠癌发生结直肠外的多原发肿瘤临床较少见，Lee等[266]回顾性分析了758例结直肠癌患者，仅33例(4.6%)发生了结直肠外的多原发肿瘤，其中21例为异时发生、12例为同时发生，多为第二原发肿瘤，出现超过3个肿瘤的患者仅有2例，发生率为0.3%；按照第二原发肿瘤部位出现的概率依次为胃(36.4%)、甲状腺(15.1%)、前列腺(15.1%)、食管(6.0%)。

（七）淋巴瘤为第一原发肿瘤

Brennan等[267]分析了109451例包括非霍奇金淋巴瘤(non Hodgkin's lymphoma，NHL)在内的多原发肿瘤，NHL作为第一原发肿瘤时，其他肿瘤的发生风险率，以及NHL作为第二原发肿瘤时第一原发肿瘤的发病情况。结果显示，在NHL作为第一原发肿瘤发生后，第二原发肿瘤总风险提高了47%，患病风险增加的肿瘤包括唇癌、舌癌、口咽癌、胃癌、小肠癌、结肠癌、肝癌、鼻腔癌、肺癌、软组织肿瘤、皮肤黑色素瘤、非黑色素瘤的皮肤癌、膀胱癌、肾癌、甲状腺癌、霍奇金淋巴瘤(Hodgkin's lymphoma，HL)、淋巴细胞白血病和髓系白血病等。秦燕等[268]统计2668例多原发肿瘤病例，有32例NHL、HL，30例为双原发肿瘤，2例为三原发或四原发肿瘤；32例患者中，以淋巴瘤作为第一原发肿瘤的有7例，同时双原发癌有5例(结直肠腺癌3例、胃癌和甲状腺乳头状癌各1例)。

乳腺癌是霍奇金淋巴瘤患者最常见的第二原发肿瘤，Schaapveld等[269]研究者通过对3905名初始治疗结束5年后的HL患者进行中位19.1年的随访，发现第二原发肿瘤乳腺癌占所有HL患者发生第二原发肿瘤的20.4%(24.9例/1万人年)，占女性HL患者第二原发肿瘤的40.5%(54.3例/1万人年)。有研究发现[269]，初诊HL年龄与第二原发肿瘤乳腺癌发生风险呈负相关，15岁以前发病者发生乳腺癌的风险最高($RR = 68.7$)；发生乳腺癌风险在初诊 HL 后 5～10 年开始升高，在 15～19 年达到高峰，在 20～24 年后开始呈下降趋势，但直到初诊 HL 后 40 年，发生乳腺癌的风险仍处于较高水平，约为一般人群的 2.53 倍。

乳腺癌家族史对于 HL 患者发生第二原发肿瘤乳腺癌的影响目前尚不明确。Hill 等[270]的研究发现，一级或二级亲属罹患乳腺癌家族史未增加 HL 患者乳腺癌发生的风险，甚至有降低风险的可能。但 Sud 等[271]通过对 1965—2012 年诊断为 HL 的 9522 名患者进行回顾性分析，发现有乳腺癌家族史的患者发生乳腺癌的风险为无乳腺癌家族史的 1.85 倍。Moskowitz 等[272]对儿童癌症幸存者的研究发现，HL 幸存者 50 岁乳腺癌累积发生风险为 35%，而该风险在 BRAC1 和 BRCA2 基因突变携带者中分别为 31% 和 10%，提示携带 BRCA 基因突变未增加乳腺癌发生风险。

刘丽等[176]在对 655 例 HL 或 NHL 患者随访中发现，有 6 例发生了第二原发肿瘤肺癌。

B 细胞淋巴瘤同时性发生胃肠道癌，尤其是黏膜相关淋巴瘤与弥漫大 B 细胞淋巴瘤（DLBCL）多有报道。在 Nakamura 等[273]报道与非霍奇金淋巴瘤有关的 10 例同时性双原发肿瘤中，最常见的同时性多原发肿瘤的发生部位为胃（6 例）和结肠（2 例）。

第一原发肿瘤淋巴瘤发生第二原发肿瘤结直肠腺癌临床罕见，发生率 <0.0002%[274-278]。

（八）其他第一原发肿瘤

第一原发肿瘤为前列腺癌的患者，其第二原发肿瘤多为膀胱癌、甲状腺癌[279-280]。第一原发肿瘤为膀胱癌的患者，其第二原发肿瘤多为肺癌、前列腺癌。第一原发肿瘤为宫颈癌的患者，其第二原发肿瘤多为乳腺癌、肺癌[63]。

第一原发肿瘤为子宫内膜癌（endometrial cancer，EC）的患者，其第二原发肿瘤多为结直肠癌（colorectal cancer，CRC），其中部分肿瘤患者表现为 Lynch 综合征（Lynch syndrome，LS）。叶天仪等[281]报道的 34 例子宫内膜癌合并结直肠癌双原发癌，64.7%（22/34）有肿瘤家族史。

四、性别与年龄

就多原发肿瘤在性别上的差异而言，主要体现在男性患者中常见的部位是泌尿生殖系统、呼吸系统、消化系统,而在女性患者中常见的部位是泌尿生殖系统、消化系统和乳腺。

MPNs患者性别的差异可能与地域环境、医院收治相关病种有关[129],美国MPNs发病的男女比例为1.18∶1;在韩国女性乳腺癌患者中,患非乳腺第二原发性肿瘤最常见的是甲状腺肿瘤,其次是妇科肿瘤[11]。在中国学者报道的病例中,女性稍高于男性,陈小良等[86]报道的多原发性肿瘤4137例中,男1864例,女2273例,男女比为0.82∶1。孙海涛等[132]报道的184例MPNs中,78例为同时性多原发肿瘤,106例为异时性多原发肿瘤,男78例,女106例。奥婷等[113]报道了55例肺癌合并其他原发恶性肿瘤,男女比例为2.67∶1(男40例,女15例)。

多数研究报道[282-286],MPNs发病与年龄相关,年龄越大,发生率越高,50~60岁为高发年龄段,60岁以上人群比例达1/3,中位年龄为59岁(29~80岁);首次被诊断患有肿瘤的60~69岁患者,10年内患第二原发肿瘤的累积风险可达13%。

Luciani等[287]亦指出,患多原发肿瘤的风险随年龄增长而增加。Irimie等[223]报道,第二原发肿瘤的发病中位年龄为56.4岁,50岁以上者占79.4%($n=63$),发生年龄在S-MPNs和M-MPNs上无显著性差异,第二原发肿瘤发生与年龄显著性相关($r=0.99$)。梁智恒等[87]分析了中国中山市5369例多原发肿瘤,结果表明,35岁左右迅速上升,至75~79岁年龄组达高峰。张稚淳等[100]报道了中国120例多原发肿瘤,发病年龄为26~89岁,中位年龄58岁。

Lv等[121]开展的一项针对多原发肿瘤的临床回顾性研究结果显示,84.6%的同时性多原发肿瘤患者和71.7%的异时性多原发肿瘤患者年龄超过50岁,而在50岁以下的患者中,异时性多原发肿瘤患者多于同时性多原发肿瘤,提示在MPNs中,异时性多原发肿瘤患者可能较同时性多原发肿瘤患者更为年轻。但Lawnicz等[288]报道,同时性多原发胃肿瘤患者的确诊年龄较异时性MPNs平均小10岁左右。

肺癌合并MPCs的好发年龄为60~69岁。一项中国的研究指出[163],肺癌合并MPNs患者存在较大的年龄跨越,为28~86岁。奥婷等[113]报道了55例肺癌合并其他原发恶性肿瘤,以肺癌作为第一原发肿瘤16例,平均发病年龄为62.81岁,以其他肿瘤作为第一原发肿瘤39例,平均发病年龄为63.15岁。

值得注意的是，以乳腺癌为第一原发肿瘤，其年轻者发生第二原发肿瘤的风险增高。一项以年龄分组的研究中[289]，≥50岁的第一原发乳腺癌患者中，其再原发其他肿瘤的发病率要低于<50岁的乳腺癌患者。一份Meta分析指出，女性患者在患第一原发乳腺癌后，其患第二原发肿瘤的概率较普通人群高17%，而年轻女性的MPNs的患病率还在继续升高[181]。Motuzyuk等[290]亦报道，乳腺癌MPNs患者平均年龄仅46.6岁，明显低于其他MPNs。

对侧乳腺癌发生风险与第一原发乳腺癌年龄相关。一项对于瑞典77875例女性乳腺癌患者研究发现[291]，对侧乳腺癌累积发生风险在<50岁确诊乳腺癌患者中为23%，在50~59岁确诊患者中为17%，在>60岁确诊患者中仅为12%。因此，年龄的增加对于对侧乳腺癌的发生可能是一个保护性因素。

多数学者报道[292-293]，多原发结直肠内癌与单发结直肠癌在年龄、性别上无显著差异；但Chiang等[294]认为，同时性多原发结直肠内癌男女比例较单发结直肠癌高，男性更易发生异时性多原发结直肠内癌。

研究显示[295]，男性和老年患者发病率更高。性别方面，男性发病率高于女性[296]；年龄方面，同时性多原发结直肠内癌平均发病年龄较孤立性结直肠癌高[297]。

第三节 发病因素

目前，多原发肿瘤的真正发病因素尚不十分清楚，但一般认为，第二原发肿瘤、第三原发肿瘤等与第一原发肿瘤基本相同，即多种致癌因素长期作用的结果。

从现有文献报道来看[298-307]，多原发肿瘤的发病因素主要包括环境因素、生活方式（如吸烟、酗酒、肥胖等）、内分泌因素、家族遗传因素、免疫因素、治疗因素（如放射治疗、化学治疗等）、年龄因素等。

有研究表明[308-312]，高龄、男性、高血压、肝硬化为同时性多原发结直肠内癌的独立危险因素，合并有这些因素的患者为同时性多原发结直肠内癌的高风险人群。

第一章 总 论

一、环境因素

(一) 辐射

与单原发肿瘤一样，辐射亦可增加多原发肿瘤发生风险。日本对长崎原子弹爆炸地区的幸存患者进行了流行病学调查，其结果证实核辐射在一定程度上可增加第二原发肿瘤发生风险[313]。一项评估乌克兰乳腺多原发肿瘤的研究发现[290]，多原发肿瘤与切尔诺贝利核电站灾难造成的核辐射污染明显相关。

值得一提的是，紫外线可诱导 DNA 产生嘧啶聚二体，长期暴露于紫外线亦会导致部分恶性肿瘤的发生，如皮肤癌、皮肤黑色素瘤。

(二) 化学物质

接触有机化合物(如多环芳香烃、亚硝胺)、化学烟雾(如氯乙烯、甲醛)、生产性粉尘和废气(如二氧化硫、石棉、重金属粉尘)、烷基化物(如芥子气)等均可增加白血病、淋巴瘤等肿瘤的发病风险。

(三) 微生物感染

微生物感染包括病毒、细菌、寄生虫等，全球约 15.6% 的恶性肿瘤由乙型和丙型肝炎病毒(HBV、HCV)、人乳头状瘤病毒(HPV)、EB 病毒(EBV)、人类疱疹病毒(HHV)、人类嗜 T 淋巴细胞病毒 I (HTLV-I)、人类免疫缺陷病毒(HIV)、幽门螺杆菌(HP)、血吸虫或肝吸虫等微生物感染所致[314]。

人乳头状瘤病毒除增加宫颈癌、肛门癌、外阴癌等肿瘤的发生风险外，HPV-16/18 还与鼻咽癌、食管癌、喉癌等的发生密切相关。Neumann 等[315]的研究发现，HPV 相关的肿瘤发生多原发肿瘤的风险增加。Huang 等[316]报道，HPV 感染可增加宫颈癌、鼻咽癌和食管癌等的发生风险。

目前的研究已经证明 EB 病毒感染与鼻咽癌、Burkitt's 淋巴瘤发生有明确的相关性，Ghislaine 等[317]报道，在第一原发肿瘤为头颈鳞癌的 8947 例患者中，发生了 167 例第二原发肿瘤，头颈部鳞癌患者发生第二原发肿瘤为 NHL 的风险是无肿瘤病史者的 3.06 倍，作者认为可能与 EB 病毒感染有关。Ohno 等[318]报道了 2 例同时性肺腺癌合并弥漫大 B 细胞淋巴瘤患者，两例患者均有高滴度 EB 病毒 IgG。

Nakamura 等[273]的研究发现，当发生幽门螺杆菌感染时，其患胃癌、胃黏膜相关淋巴瘤、胰腺癌的发生风险随之增加,作者推测胃癌与胃黏膜相关淋巴瘤同时发生的原因可能为两者均与幽门螺杆菌感染有关。

二、家族遗传因素

遗传仅是一种倾向,即由于遗传或遗传性疾病所具有的 DNA 或染色体改变,增加了人体对病毒、化学致癌物质或物理性致癌因素的敏感性,亦影响了 DNA 分子的正常修复,进而促使肿瘤发生。

在一些特定情况下,多原发肿瘤发生的类型是高度特异性的,表明它们有共同的遗传背景。因此,常将此称为"遗传性癌症综合征",如遗传性乳腺癌、乳腺癌-卵巢癌、遗传性视网膜母细胞瘤、神经纤维瘤病、痣样基底细胞癌、利-弗劳梅尼(Li-Fraumeni)综合征、遗传性非息肉病性大肠癌(Lynch 综合征)、多发性内分泌腺瘤、Bloom 综合征、着色性干皮病等[319]。

家族遗传史一直被认为是 MPNs 发生的危险因素,同时性 MPNs 通常归因于已知和未知的遗传倾向[320]。有学者指出[321-323],遗传性癌症综合征本身就是第二原发肿瘤发生的一个危险因素,它们在第二原发肿瘤发生中起着重要作用。

家族性 MPNs 发生风险的增加可能是复杂的遗传结果,有学者认为[324],由于家族性肿瘤已经存在通过遗传获得的原始突变,不需要像散发性肿瘤积累更多的细胞突变即可导致肿瘤的发生,且这种遗传易感性存在于每一个细胞中,故家族性 MPNs 较散发性更加常见。

10%~15%的肿瘤与遗传性肿瘤综合征有关,这些综合征中有许多是常染色体显性遗传,携带该基因的人有 50%的概率将其遗传给孩子。在肿瘤幸存者中发现,种系突变预示着特定第二原发肿瘤发生的风险增加。研究表明[325-326],有肿瘤家族史的人群,其患原发肿瘤甚至多原发肿瘤的概率增高。Magid 等[182]报道,在参与研究的多原发肿瘤患者中,约 22.3%的患者有家族史。

乳腺癌合并卵巢癌患者一般有家族聚集现象,通常是由染色体显性基因突变导致[327],如易感基因 BRAC1 和 BRCA2,BRAC1 和 BRCA2 携带者的乳腺癌风险随着被诊断为乳腺癌的一级和二级亲属的数量增加而增加[328]。

有研究发现[329],乳腺癌人群中具有肿瘤家族史者,发生 MPNs 的概率增加。一级亲属患乳腺癌的女性其发生乳腺癌概率较无家族史的高 2~3 倍[330]。

Reiner 等[331]报道，对侧乳腺癌 10 年累积风险在无家族史的乳腺癌患者中为 4.3%，在二级亲属罹患乳腺癌的患者中为 6%，在一级亲属罹患乳腺癌的患者中为 8.1%。若一级亲属在 40 岁以前发病，该风险上升至 13.5%；若一级亲属罹患双侧乳腺癌，该风险上升至 14.1%。

在一项对中国 2025 例多原发结直肠癌病例进行分析的报道中[46]，有恶性肿瘤家族史的比例为 13.1%。

附：多原发结直肠内癌与结直肠腺瘤、锯齿状息肉

已有研究证明[332-333]，多原发结直肠内癌与结直肠腺瘤之间有密切关系，结直肠癌至少 1/2 或接近 2/3 来源于良性腺瘤。结直肠腺瘤可单发或多发，多发腺瘤则可能同时性癌变或异时性癌变，成为多原发结直肠内癌。

颜登国等[334]分析了多原发结直肠内癌的临床病理特点，发现合并息肉的发生率为 40%，有息肉癌变者 10 例，占 25%，如果以息肉数目计算，息肉癌变率达 48.1%。Yang 等[295]报道，同时性多原发结直肠内癌患者中 34.1% 伴发腺瘤，而孤立性结直肠癌患者中这一比例仅为 19.1%。

近年来的研究发现[264]，在同时性多原发结直肠内癌中更常见的癌前病变是多发性无柄锯齿状腺瘤、增生性息肉。有研究者指出[335-336]，锯齿状息肉与同时性多原发结直肠内癌形成的风险相关，同时性多原发结直肠内癌更有可能是由多个无柄锯齿状腺瘤所引起。Drew 等[337]报道，同时性多原发结直肠内癌更多地具有锯齿状腺瘤形成的特征性分子，如 BRAF 突变体、微卫星高度不稳定性。

三、内分泌因素

乳腺、子宫内膜、卵巢均为雌激素效应器官，这些部位可因受长期雌激素作用而极可能发生多原发肿瘤。Soliman 等[338]认为，年轻女性、超重、未孕以及未绝经为同时性子宫内膜及卵巢双原发肿瘤好发的危险因素。王加璐等[339]报道，患乳腺癌的女性合并卵巢癌的概率是一般女性的 2 倍。

对于女性人群而言，围绝经期以及绝经后，卵巢功能出现衰退，孕激

素水平逐渐降低,则会增加患子宫内膜癌发生的风险。日本一项基于2002—2010年16.5万尸检数据表明[340],女性激素与多原发肿瘤的发生密切相关。Le BouEdec等[341]指出,高雌激素水平在乳腺癌继发子宫内膜癌中发挥着重要作用。

目前有研究指出[342-345],乳腺癌同时性或异时性发生妇科多原发肿瘤(如子宫内膜癌、卵巢癌)均与雌激素、雌激素受体的变化有关。叶岚等[346]认为,宫颈癌与乳腺癌由于存在共同雌孕激素受体,两者同时发生的风险更高。

值得一提的是,雌激素调节在甲状腺与乳腺多原发肿瘤发生中具有重要作用[347-355]。Li等[213]认为,乳腺癌患者中激素受体表达阳性为第二原发性甲状腺癌发生的危险因素。美国国家癌症研究所(National Cancer Institute,NCI)就女性甲状腺癌和乳腺癌之间的发病情况开展了研究[150],结果表明,女性患甲状腺癌后继发第二原发性乳腺癌的风险增加了0.67倍,而女性患乳腺癌后继发第二原发性甲状腺癌的风险增加了2倍。韩国一项队列研究证实[356],游离甲状腺素异常升高可增加患乳腺癌的风险。

四、治疗因素

多原发肿瘤发生与治疗相关的因素主要包括第一原发肿瘤放射治疗、化学治疗及内分泌治疗[357],Watanabe等[358]指出,对于异时性多原发肿瘤,一个不可忽略的因素为第一原发肿瘤的放射治疗与化学治疗的致癌作用。

有研究报道[359-360],携带高外显率基因,如RB(与视网膜母细胞瘤相关)或TP53(与Li-Fraumeni综合征相关)基因突变的患者接受放射治疗后,相关组织第二原发肿瘤(SPNs)的发生率很高。

表1-2 治疗相关性第二原发肿瘤遗传易感性[361-370]

外显率和风险类型	综合征	通路和(或)基因
高外显率基因	Li-Fraumeni综合征	TP53
放射治疗后SPNs风险升高	视网膜母细胞瘤	RB
	Gorlin综合征	PTCH
	多发性神经纤维瘤	NF1
	肾母细胞肿瘤	WT1
化学治疗后SPNs风险升高	Li-Fraumeni综合征	TP53

续表

外显率和风险类型	综合征	通路和(或)基因
低外显率基因		
放射治疗后 SPNs 风险升高	谷胱甘肽转移酶	GSTM1
	碱基切除修复	XRCC3
化学治疗后 SPNs 风险升高	谷胱甘肽转移酶	GSTP1
	错配修复	MLH1，MSH2
	双链断裂修复	RAD51
	碱基切除修复	XRCC1
	核酸切除修复	ERCC2

(一)放射治疗与第二原发肿瘤

一般而言，放射线可损伤细胞 DNA、激活原癌基因、使抑癌基因发生突变，从而导致肿瘤发生[371-373]。

尽管如今放射治疗技术有显著进步，且有剂量低、放射野小等优点，但其所产生的分散或次级的放射颗粒仍会增加多原发肿瘤发生的风险[374-375]。Marees 等[376]报道，轨道放射治疗可使患有遗传性视网膜母细胞瘤的患者第二原发肿瘤发生风险增加3倍。目前，第一原发肿瘤放射治疗后发生第二原发肿瘤的现象已被临床证实[377-378]。

美国国家癌症研究所为评估第一原发肿瘤接受放射治疗后发生第二原发恶性肿瘤的风险展开了一项队列研究[356]，结果表明，约8%的放射治疗患者有发生第二原发肿瘤的风险。Morton 等[379]的研究发现，大部分与放射治疗有关的第二原发肿瘤通常发生在放射治疗后10年，且随着时间的延长风险亦持续增高。Chaturvedi 等[327]认为，虽然子宫颈癌患者接受盆腔放射治疗后的第一个10年发生卵巢癌的风险似乎有所降低，但放射治疗后超过30年者风险会增加。

第一原发肿瘤放射治疗后，女性发生第二原发肿瘤的风险高于男性，年轻患者(青春期、青年期)接受放射治疗后发生第二原发肿瘤的风险较高[380]。但也有学者认为[381]，放射治疗不会明显增加≥50岁肿瘤患者的第二原发肿瘤发生风险，仅在一些特殊情况下，如接受高剂量胸部、淋巴结放射治疗且生存期超过10年的乳腺癌患者中，第二原发肿瘤如食管癌、软组织肉瘤和肺癌的发生率明显升高。

放射治疗所致的第二原发肿瘤通常发生于放射治疗野内或放射治疗野周围[382],尤其是脑、甲状腺、乳腺、皮肤、骨和软组织等部位。

放射治疗所致的第二原发肿瘤以实体瘤多见,主要包括食管癌、肺癌、胸壁软组织肉瘤等[383-392]。Kabat[393]通过病例对照研究发现,女性生殖系统肿瘤病史及其放射治疗史与其第二原发肿瘤肺癌的发生有显著相关性。

Diallo等[394]指出,离治疗部位越远,放射治疗导致第二多原发肿瘤发生的风险越低。Berrington de Gonzalez等[395]的研究发现,接受每次1~5Gy的分次照射的患者第二原发肿瘤发生率较累积剂量15~50Gy的患者要低。

1. 第一原发肿瘤霍奇金淋巴瘤放射治疗后

第二原发肿瘤已被认为是霍奇金淋巴瘤放射治疗后最为严重的远期并发症,并成为导致霍奇金淋巴瘤已治愈患者的主要死因之一,且部分抵消了放射治疗所带来的生存获益[396]。Morton等[379]报道,霍奇金淋巴瘤放射治疗后发生第二原发肿瘤每1Gy的相对危险度,胃癌为0.09($95\% CI = 0.04 \sim 0.21$),肺癌为0.15($95\% CI = 0.06 \sim 0.39$),乳腺癌为0.15($95\% CI = 0.04 \sim 0.73$)。

放射治疗是霍奇金淋巴瘤患者发生第二原发肿瘤乳腺癌的主要危险因素[397-399],有研究报道[400-402],接受40Gy胸部照射剂量的霍奇金淋巴瘤儿童女性患者发生乳腺癌风险较未接受放射治疗患者增加11倍,接受>5Gy放射治疗剂量的霍奇金淋巴瘤女性患者发生乳腺癌风险较<5Gy放射治疗剂量的患者增加2.7倍,与月经初潮间隔6个月时间内接受放射治疗发生乳腺癌风险增加5.52倍。Moskowitz等[272]的研究发现,儿童时期的霍奇金淋巴瘤长期生存者,低剂量(中位14Gy)照射大体积(全肺野)的患者较高剂量(中位40Gy)斗篷野的患者,有更高的第二原发乳腺癌发病率,标准化发病率比分别为43.6%、24.2%。

儿童霍奇金淋巴瘤胸部放射治疗结束8~10年后乳腺癌的患病风险开始升高。有研究发现[403-404],霍奇金淋巴瘤放射治疗后发生第二原发肿瘤乳腺癌的高危因素是年龄,年龄<30岁是乳腺癌发生的最大危险因素,40~45岁的乳腺癌累积发病率为13%~20%。

2. 第一原发肿瘤头颈部肿瘤放射治疗后

Chuang等[382]报道,在头颈部肿瘤患者中,曾接受放射治疗的患者多原发肿瘤的发生率明显高于接受单纯手术治疗的患者。Hashibe等[405]在口腔癌病例研究中发现，口腔肿瘤采用放射治疗、手术治疗及放射治疗联合手术切除发生 MPNs 相对风险分别为 2.35（95% CI = 1.19～4.62）、1.71（95% CI = 0.92～3.19）、2.11（95% CI = 1.09～4.11），结果表明，经放射治疗后发生第二原发肿瘤的风险明显高于单独手术者，且多发生在照射野内。

有研究报道[406]，在头部、颈部和胸部肿瘤放射治疗后，第二原发肿瘤甲状腺癌的风险明显升高，放射治疗剂量与甲状腺癌之间存在线性指数关系，风险峰值发生在 15～20Gy 的放射剂量时，剂量超过 30Gy 风险大大降低。

3. 第一原发肿瘤乳腺癌放射治疗后

较多的研究报道[407-410]，乳腺癌患者接受术后放射治疗后患第二原发肿瘤的风险增加，乳腺癌放射治疗区域的器官已成为第二原发肿瘤的高发部位。Grantzau 等[216]在一篇基于 52 万例乳腺癌患者的荟萃分析中报道，放射治疗显著增加了乳腺癌患者发生第二原发肿瘤的概率，且第二原发肿瘤发病率随时间推移逐渐增加，在乳腺癌确诊后 10～15 年达到高峰，与放射治疗相关的第二原发肿瘤以肺癌、食管癌、甲状腺癌和软组织肿瘤多见。

有研究报道[411-412]，乳腺癌放射治疗后，第二原发肿瘤主要在肺部，且放射治疗患者的第二原发肺癌发病风险是非放射治疗患者的 10 倍，第二原发肺癌的发生风险与放射剂量呈线性相关。

4. 其他第一原发肿瘤放射治疗后

Tucker 等[413]的研究发现，小细胞肺癌患者发生第二原发肿瘤的整体风险是一般人群的 3.5 倍，有胸部放射治疗史的小细胞肺癌患者发生第二原发肿瘤肺癌的风险是一般人群的 13 倍，无放射治疗史的风险是一般人群的 7 倍。

第一原发肿瘤直肠癌放射治疗后，第二原发肿瘤主要分布在胃肠道、前列腺、膀胱、输尿管等[414]。

第一原发肿瘤前列腺癌放射治疗后，可发生第二原发肿瘤，如直肠癌、宫颈癌、食管癌、肝癌、肺癌、膀胱癌，以及血液系统恶性肿瘤[280]。

（二）化学治疗与第二原发肿瘤

许多细胞毒药物，尤其是烷化剂、拓扑异构酶Ⅱ抑制剂和抗代谢药物,可导致 DNA-蛋白质交联和(或)引起 DNA 链断裂、细胞转化、突变、染色体畸变等[415-416],长期接受细胞毒药物治疗的肿瘤患者可发生第二原发肿瘤[417-418]。Wei 等[187]的研究表明,细胞药物如蒽环类、烷化剂、紫杉醇类本身对机体即有一定的致癌作用,使得第一原发肿瘤化学治疗患者发生多原发肿瘤的风险增加。

有研究报道[419-422],拓扑异构酶抑制剂Ⅱ可导致染色体 11q23 上混合系白血病(mixed lineage leukemia,MLL)基因易位,继而增加白血病的发病风险,但该风险可在化学治疗结束后 10 年下降。

在与化学治疗相关的第二原发肿瘤中,报道较多的是急性髓系白血病(acute myeloid leukemia,AML)[423-427],除白血病外,肺癌、胃肠道癌、膀胱癌及软组织肉瘤等亦有报道[428-434]。

Leleu 等[435]报道,巨球蛋白血症患者使用氟达拉滨、硫唑嘌呤治疗后,有较高的急性白血病发生率。Liu 等[436]回顾性分析了 9 例慢性髓细胞性白血病的双原发恶性肿瘤患者,7 例是在多年综合抗肿瘤治疗后发生慢性髓细胞性白血病,认为化学治疗很可能是发生第二肿瘤的原因。

化学治疗相关性白血病通常发生在第一原发肿瘤治疗后的 10 年内,随后风险逐渐降低[437]。

1. 第一原发肿瘤乳腺癌化学治疗后

Grantzau 等[216]的研究表明,与未接受放射治疗的乳腺癌妇女相比,接受放射治疗的乳腺癌妇女第二原发癌的风险显著增加,而接受化学治疗的患者风险更高。

化学治疗可增加乳腺癌患者发生白血病的风险[438]。早在 1990 年,Curtis 等[439]就发现第一原发肿瘤乳腺癌患者化学治疗后更易发生第二原发肿瘤白血病,作者随访了 13734 例患者,其中 24 例患者发生急性白血病,较正常人群的发生率(2.1/万)明显提高。

乳腺癌患者单用环磷酰胺治疗后发生急性白血病的相对风险显著升高,卵巢癌患者使用含有紫杉类药物的化学治疗后引起急性髓系白血病亦有报道[440]。Shenolikar 等[441]的研究发现,卵巢癌、乳腺癌患者化学治疗后白血病发病率的增加与 DNA 损伤方案使用的持续时间有关。Hughes 等[442]通过观察发现,第一原发肿瘤乳腺癌化学治疗患者的宫颈原位癌发生概率也增加,认为是乳腺癌患者化学治疗中联合使用烷化剂促使了宫颈原位癌的发生。

2. 第一原发肿瘤淋巴血液肿瘤化学治疗后

Van Eggermond 等[443]的研究表明,第一原发肿瘤淋巴瘤化学治疗后第二原发肿瘤的发生率增高。有研究者认为[444-446],血液系统肿瘤患者造血干细胞移植(hematopoietic stem cell transplant,HSCT)后,通常免疫功能下降,易感染致瘤病毒,发生第二原发肿瘤的风险增加。Friedman 等[447]指出,血液系统肿瘤患者HSCT后再发第二原发肿瘤(如乳腺癌)的风险与使用全身照射(total body irradiation,TBI)相关,尤其是年轻患者。

(三) 内分泌治疗与第二原发肿瘤

三苯氧胺(他莫昔芬)是雌激素受体阳性乳腺癌患者内分泌治疗的主要药物,可使乳腺癌复发率降低约40%,死亡率降低30%,对侧相关乳腺癌发生风险减少40%。

然而,较多的文献报道[448-457],三苯氧胺可使子宫内膜细胞增殖、增生并向恶性转化,使长期使用的乳腺癌患者患第二原发肿瘤子宫内膜癌的风险大大增加。有研究报道[215],应用三苯氧胺超过2年的女性较未使用者患子宫内膜癌的危险性增加2.3倍,在用药后的8~9年中,患子宫内膜癌的风险增加2~4倍。Angurana 等[64]在对超过4000例乳腺癌患者的随访中发现,应用三苯氧胺患者发生子宫内膜癌的风险是不应用此药的4倍。

Ricceri 等[458]认为,除子宫内膜癌外,长期乳腺癌内分泌治疗患者还可能增加第二原发肿瘤胃癌、结肠癌和卵巢癌的发生风险。

(四) 其他治疗与第二原发肿瘤

Tarella 等[459]认为,大剂量利妥昔单抗联合自体干细胞移植治疗淋巴瘤已被证实是第二原发肿瘤发生的一个可能的危险因素。Zhou 等[460]研究报道,利妥昔单抗会导致急性髓系白血病。

多发性骨髓瘤患者使用高剂量来那度胺维持治疗后,急性白血病的风险增加[461]。

在一项涵盖23项临床试验的荟萃分析中[462],恶性肿瘤患者使用粒细胞集落刺激因子(granulocyte colony stimulating factor,G-CSF)后,发生急性白血病的绝对风险上升0.41%。

五、不良生活方式

一般而言,持续吸烟、饮酒,以及咀嚼槟榔、进食亚硝胺类食物等不良生活方式，在一定程度上可能导致多原发肿瘤的发生。有研究报道[463-464]，不良生活方式，如吸烟、肥胖、饮酒均会增加对侧乳腺癌的发生率。

(一) 吸烟与酗酒

MPNs 好发于第一原发肿瘤的病变部位或成对器官及同一管道器官系统，当消化道和呼吸道分别接受共同的吸烟、饮酒等致癌因素刺激时，均可能使 MPNs 的发生风险增加。因此，食管癌常常与口咽喉部肿瘤同时性发生[465-466]。在男性人群中，多原发消化道肿瘤、呼吸道肿瘤、胰腺癌、膀胱癌等均与吸烟相关[467-468]。在绝对风险方面，烟草和酒精相关的多原发肿瘤约占 35%[437]。

León 等[469]的研究结果表明，第一原发肿瘤位于非烟酒刺激部位较烟酒刺激部位多原发肿瘤的发生率明显降低。Chuang 等[470]认为，口腔癌、下咽癌易并发食管癌提示了烟酒刺激等共同的致病因素是多原发肿瘤的发生机制。Katada 等[471]的研究发现，吸烟、饮酒的食管癌鳞癌患者发生第二原发肿瘤如头颈部鳞癌的风险增加。

1. 吸烟

有较多的研究报道[472-476]，吸烟不仅可促进第一原发肿瘤的发生，还可能是第二原发肿瘤发生的因素。Park 等[477]的研究发现，持续吸烟的肿瘤患者，发生第二原发肿瘤如膀胱癌、结直肠癌的风险增加，而第一原发肿瘤确诊后戒烟，则可能降低第二原发肿瘤的发生风险。日本一项研究亦发现[472]，与不吸烟组肿瘤患者比较，吸烟组肿瘤患者的第二原发肿瘤发生风险增加了 59%。Romaszko-Wojtowicz 等[126]的研究表明，与持续吸烟的肿瘤患者相比，第一原发肿瘤确诊后戒烟患者的第二原发肿瘤发生时间可推迟约 5 年（$P=0.005$），生存期可延长 7.18 年（$P=0.004$）。

对于吸烟人群而言，上呼吸道（鼻、咽、喉）和下呼吸道（气管、支气管）等部位长期受到烟草中致癌物质的刺激，极有可能导致呼吸系统内的器官发生恶变，出现多原发肿瘤[478-479]。Garces 等[473]报道，有吸烟史的头颈部肿瘤患者发生多原发肿瘤的概率增加。

吸烟对肺癌的影响最大，吸烟患者更易发生包括肺癌在内的多原发肿瘤。Aredo 等[480]指出，吸烟是第一原发肿瘤肺癌患者发生第二原发肿瘤肺癌的危险因素，在男性患者中尤为明显，可能与暴露于吸烟等肺癌相关危险因素中的男性更多见有关[481]。

多项研究发现[482-486]，继续吸烟的肺癌患者发生第二原发肿瘤肺癌的风险较不吸烟的患者明显增加。Rice等[485]报道，15%的接受过全肺切除术的Ⅰ期非小细胞肺癌患者发生了第二原发肿瘤，第二原发肿瘤肺癌中有56%的患者吸烟，而从未吸烟的患者均未发生第二原发肿瘤肺癌。另外，Wang等[486]比较了16例同时性多原发肺癌与451例单原发肺癌，结果显示，多原发肺癌吸烟量较单发肺癌大。

有研究发现[458]，患有乳腺癌的女性患第二原发肿瘤的风险与吸烟状况呈正相关。Wood等[437]的研究表明，初发乳腺癌，戒烟后可推迟MPNs的患病时间。

一项前瞻性研究显示[337]，当前的吸烟状况和累计吸烟年数与同时性多原发结直肠癌的风险增加有关，且与当前继续吸烟比较，戒烟可降低发生同时性多原发结直肠癌的风险。

2. 饮酒

Dashti等[487]指出，饮酒后结肠中高浓度的乙醇代谢产物乙醛具有致癌作用，乙醛可影响DNA的合成和修复，改变谷胱甘肽的结构和功能，并增加结肠黏膜的增生，且乙醇可能通过改变甲基转移而具有致癌作用。

Pajares等[488]的观察发现，以每周平均酒精摄入量乘以饮酒年数计算的累计酒精摄入量，当超过9800g时，则为同时性多原发结直肠内癌的危险因素。研究表明[489-490]，中度至大量饮酒可增加患口腔癌、咽癌、食管癌、胃癌、喉癌、结肠直肠癌、中枢神经系统癌、胰腺癌、乳腺癌和前列腺癌等的风险。

研究发现[491]，高酒精度是头颈部癌发生第二原发肿瘤的危险因素。研究显示[492-493]，年龄大的食管癌患者较年龄较小的食管癌患者更易发生多原发肿瘤，男性食管癌患者较女性食管癌患者更易发生多原发肿瘤，推测其原因可能与男性患者具有饮酒史比例较女性患者高有关。Baba等[75]报道，第二多原发肿瘤食管癌患者较单发食管癌有明显的饮酒史。

(二) 肥胖或超重

目前研究表明，肥胖与多种肿瘤发生风险的增加有关，包括绝经后乳腺癌、子宫内膜癌、结直肠癌、食管癌、胆囊癌、肾癌、胰腺癌和甲状腺癌等[494]。Miyazaki等[495]指出，体重、体重指数(body mass index，BMI)及布林克曼指数较高者易发生多原发肿瘤。有研究报道[496-497]，糖尿病或糖耐量异常、肥胖女性易发生子宫内膜癌、结直肠癌。

在普通人群中，已经确定肥胖与绝经后乳腺癌有关[498]。Calle 等[499]报道了参与美国癌症协会癌症预防Ⅱ期调查的 90 万名以上的人群，统计分析结果表明，体重指数大于 $40kg/m^2$ 和小于 $25kg/m^2$ 的死亡相对风险在女性为 1.52（95% CI = 1.13 ~ 2.05），男性为 1.62（95% CI = 1.40 ~ 1.87），超重或肥胖与食管癌、结直肠癌、肝癌、胆囊癌、胰腺癌、肾癌的死亡率显著相关，女性患者死于乳腺癌、子宫癌、宫颈癌和卵巢癌的风险随着体重指数升高而增加。

Park 等[477]的研究发现，女性肥胖肿瘤患者再患乳腺癌、子宫内膜癌的风险较非肥胖肿瘤患者增加，且减肥后发生第二原发肿瘤风险有下降趋势。一项评估初次诊断乳腺癌时体重与第二原发肿瘤风险之间关联强度的荟萃分析显示[500]，体重指数每增加 $5kg/m^2$，对侧乳腺和子宫内膜第二原发肿瘤的风险显著增加。

六、年龄因素

近年来，随着肿瘤多学科诊疗技术的快速发展，第一原发肿瘤治疗疗效不断提高，老年肿瘤患者不断增多，MPNs 患者数量亦明显较前增加[501]，即长期生存的第一原发肿瘤患者再发第二原发肿瘤的风险高于普通人群。

较多的研究报道[502-504]，年龄与多原发肿瘤的发生率呈正相关，高龄是多原发肿瘤发病的独立危险因素，随着年龄增大，大部分肿瘤发生率亦随之增加。

Luciani 等[287]报道，65 岁以上的高龄肿瘤患者发生 MPNs 的风险较年轻肿瘤患者高。Soerjomataram 等[505]报道，超过 60 岁的肿瘤患者约有 1/3 发生多原发肿瘤。Amer[506]的研究显示，多原发肿瘤的好发年龄为 60 ~ 69 岁。Chuang 等[507]报道，<56 岁的年龄组较 >75 岁的年龄组头颈部肿瘤作为第二原发肿瘤的发生率更高。

有学者分析其原因[508]，可能是因为生存时间延长，致癌因子作用不断累积；免疫系统退化，功能下降，无法及时、有效地清除机体内出现的异常细胞；衰老的细胞对致癌因子的耐受性降低。

但亦有学者认为，年轻患者更易发生多原发肿瘤。James 等[509]的研究发现，<40 岁的喉癌患者发生多原发肿瘤的可能性相对较大，作者推测其

原因可能是年轻患者对肿瘤的治疗更加耐受，可获得较长的生存期，发生多原发肿瘤的机会亦增加。

一项以年龄为分组因素的研究中，≥50岁的乳腺癌患者中再次患其他原发肿瘤的标准化发病比率（standardized incidence ratio，SIR）明显低于＜50岁的乳腺癌患者，提示在老年乳腺癌患者中，发生第二原发肿瘤的概率要低于年轻乳腺癌患者[289]。鞠卫东等[510]报道了经手术及病理证实的45例甲状腺与乳腺多原发肿瘤患者，＞40岁的甲状腺肿瘤、＞50岁的乳腺肿瘤发生第二原发肿瘤的风险性较大，且发生间隔时间越长，对应部位第二原发肿瘤恶性的风险性更大。西班牙一项基于5897例乳腺癌患者流行病研究发现[511]，乳腺癌患者发生第二原发肿瘤的标准化发病比率是1.96%，年轻患者第二原发肿瘤以卵巢癌多见，＞50岁患者以子宫内膜癌多见。

第四节 发病机制

一、相关理论学说

目前，多原发肿瘤的发病机制仍不十分明确。有学者提出了"区域癌变"（field cancerization，FC）、"单克隆起源"（monoclonal origin，MO）、"癌症的二次打击"（"two-hit" hypothesis，THH）、"多中心起源"等理论。一般认为，多原发肿瘤并非由单个细胞DNA突变引起，而是涉及受同一致癌物质刺激的一个广泛区域范围的细胞，包括同一暴露器官及不同暴露器官，在接受同一致癌物质刺激的同时或异时发生DNA结构及功能的改变，从而产生不同的癌变过程[512-514]。

值得一提的是，解剖学研究表明，双侧乳腺组织及其皮肤之间原本并无相通的淋巴管，只有当肿瘤细胞转移过程中堵塞了淋巴管，才可能使得淋巴液及其中的转移癌细胞逆行至对侧乳腺组织甚至对侧腋窝形成转移病灶，故乳腺癌细胞实际上很少能从一侧乳腺转移到另一侧乳腺[515]。一般认为，第一原发性乳腺癌与对侧第二原发性乳腺癌所处内分泌和暴露环境大致相同，对单侧乳腺起作用的致癌因素亦可能导致另一侧乳腺癌变而发生双侧原发性乳腺癌。

(一)"区域癌变"学说

1953年，Slaughter等[254]对783例口腔鳞癌患者的手术标本进行了回顾性分析，发现几乎在所有患者的标本中距肿瘤组织远近不等的部位均存在不同程度的非典型增生上皮，11.2%（88/783）的病例存在相互独立的多中心肿瘤病灶，认为口腔多原发肿瘤由多灶的癌前病变在共同的致癌因素作用下独立发展而来，于是提出了"区域癌变学说"。

目前，"区域癌变学说"已被多位研究者所证实[516-526]，且存在于多个系统和器官中，如头颈部（口腔、咽部和喉）、肺、食管、外阴、宫颈、结直肠、乳腺、膀胱和皮肤等，是当今最广为学者接受的多原发肿瘤发病理论。

根据该理论，在前一阶段出现的较为广泛的DNA损伤，各肿瘤细胞可能存在部分相同的基因突变；在后期的进一步癌变过程中，多原发肿瘤的各个肿瘤细胞之间可发生不同的基因突变，表现出具有自身特异性的基因表型。

Brown等[527]指出，胃肠道为食物通道、肺为呼吸通道、泌尿道则为排泄废物通道，它们分别接受食物、空气中的共同致癌因素的慢性刺激。因此作者认为，消化道、呼吸道、泌尿道第一原发肿瘤发生后可同时性或异时性发生第二原发肿瘤。

目前多数学者认为[528]，长期暴露于烟、酒等致癌因素的上呼吸道和消化道黏膜易在本系统内发生多个原发肿瘤或多个部位的癌前病变，从而在第一原发肿瘤发生后的不同时期发生第二原发肿瘤。

食管作为一个运送食物的空腔脏器，从近端至远端所受外界环境刺激因素相同，故当一处黏膜上皮细胞DNA的结构及功能发生改变从而产生癌变时，其他部位亦易因同样的致癌因素出现癌变，从而形成多原发食管癌（multiple primary esophageal carcinoma，MPEC）[529]。Hori等[238]在食管鳞癌患者中，对口腔、下咽和食管进行碘染色观察时，发现黏膜存在散在多发碘染不着色区域的病例。

食管癌的形成通常需经过食管上皮发生单纯增生→轻度不典型增生→重度不典型增生→原位癌→浸润癌的多个复杂演变过程[530-533]。有研究发现[534]，食管原发癌灶相邻组织中出现不典型增生及原位癌的发生率高达30%以上。

（二）"多中心起源"学说

肿瘤多中心起源学说即肿瘤在早期阶段呈多中心发生，随着病程的不断进展，邻近的小病灶逐渐融合在一起，成为较大的单个病灶。有学者认为[535-537]，胃内多原发癌属于多中心起源，早期胃癌中的多原发癌的发生率较高，占14%~30%，而进展期仅占2.29%。

有研究表明[538-541]，同时性多原发结直肠内癌为多中心起源，在许多同时性多原发结直肠内癌患者中，同一患者的肿瘤细胞具有不同的MSI（微卫星不稳定）状态、p53突变和KRAS突变模式，表明每个肿瘤可能是由不同的分子事件驱动并独立形成。

Wang等[542]的研究发现，在25%的同时性多原发结直肠内癌患者中发现核糖体蛋白L22（RPL22）中的热点突变（K15fs），相对于单一原发肿瘤而言，RPL22突变在同时性多原发结直肠内癌中可能更聚集。

（三）"广泛迁徙"学说

广泛迁徙学说主要是指已经癌变的细胞，可迁移到不同的器官或组织，并在不同的组织或器官中呈现出不同的病理学表现。

有学者认为[543-544]，癌变的祖细胞可经过上皮内的迁移，迁移到相对较远的区域，形成新的肿瘤病灶，由此可导致多原发肿瘤的发生。Scholes等[545]指出，多原发肿瘤通常具有同源性，只是在后期分化中呈现出不同的病理学形态。

根据目前通用的多原发肿瘤诊断标准，癌性祖细胞在迁移分化后形成病理类型不同的肿瘤，方可认为是多原发肿瘤，如迁移后分化形成的新发肿瘤病理类型与第一原发肿瘤相似，无法排除是否为浸润或转移所致，则不可明确诊断为多原发肿瘤。

（四）"细胞转化"学说

胚胎发育中的神经嵴细胞，具有潜在的多向分化能力，保留着异源性组织，可向神经胶质、周围神经节细胞、表皮黑色素细胞、嗜铬细胞和神经膜细胞，以及交感-副交感神经节、脊神经节的成神经细胞分化[546]。

神经系统多原发肿瘤（multiple primary neoplasma of nervous system，NS-MPNs）的发生机制，曾被解释为邂逅、依附[547]。周怀伟等[548]认为，NS-MPNs是在不同组织、不同胚层间的相互转化或化生的结果。

有研究报道[549]，施万细胞、脑脊膜瘤细胞、神经纤维瘤细胞和神经上皮肿瘤细胞，均具有黑色素生成能力，可与黑色素细胞（melanocyte）相互转化。

有学者认为[550]，NS-MPNs由神经嵴起源的组织发生，部分属于先天性肿瘤与胚胎发育有关；部分属于遗传性肿瘤疾病，与染色体、基因异常有关，临床表现为 von Recklinghausen 病和 von Hippel – Lindau 病[551]。

神经纤维瘤病又称为 von Recklinghausen 病，属于家族性显性遗传病，常与颅内神经鞘瘤，尤其双侧神经鞘瘤、脑膜瘤、胶质瘤、结节性硬化病、皮下多发性脂肪瘤、色素痣、黑色素瘤、肾上腺嗜铬细胞瘤同时性发生；胶质母细胞瘤患者亦可同时性发生血管母细胞瘤，临床表现为 von Hippel – Lindau 病。

颅内脑膜瘤，尤其是多发性脑膜瘤，可与胶质瘤、垂体腺瘤、神经纤维瘤病同时发生。Witzig 等[552]报道 1 例 51 岁女性，左侧大脑半球凸面多发性脑膜瘤与同侧听神经复发性施万细胞瘤同时发生；Pomeroy 等[553]报道了 1 例颅后窝脑膜瘤与脊神经根施万细胞瘤同时发生的患者。

二、遗传性癌症综合征

前已述及，某些遗传性癌症综合征易发生多原发肿瘤，如遗传性乳腺癌 – 卵巢癌综合征、林奇综合征（Lynch syndrome，LS）、利 – 弗劳梅尼（Li – Fraumeni）综合征、家族性腺瘤性息肉病等；另外，Bloom 综合征、着色性干皮病是与 DNA 修复有关的罕见疾病，亦可导致白血病、淋巴瘤、皮肤肿瘤、软组织肉瘤等多原发肿瘤的发生。

据报道[508]，有 5%~10% 的多原发肿瘤可出现在先天性肿瘤易感人群中。

遗传易感性被认为与霍奇金淋巴瘤患者发生第二原发肿瘤乳腺癌相关，有研究报道[554]，位于 6q21 染色体 PRDM1 和 ATG5 之间的两个非编码单核苷酸多态性 rs4946728 和 rs1040411 与儿童霍奇金淋巴瘤接受放射治疗发生第二肿瘤相关，而 FGFR2 的变异 rs1219648 可增加放射治疗发生第二原发肿瘤乳腺癌的风险。

表 1 – 3　常见遗传性癌症综合征之基因改变

名词	基因改变
视网膜母细胞瘤	位于染色体 13q14 的 RB1 基因胚系突变
遗传性乳腺 – 卵巢癌综合征	乳腺癌易感基因 1（breast cancer susceptibility gene 1，BRAC1）；或乳腺癌易感基因 2（breast cancer susceptibility gene 2，BRCA2）突变

续表

名词	基因改变
多发性错构瘤综合征	磷酸酶张力蛋白同源物（phosphatase and tensinhomolog，PTEN）突变
利-弗劳梅尼（Li-Fraumeni）综合征	p53 突变
检查点激酶2（checkpoint kinase 2，CHEK2）综合征	CHEK2 的 51、52 位点突变
家族性非典型多发性葡萄胎黑色素瘤综合征	周期蛋白依赖性激酶抑制剂 2A（cyclin dependent kinase inhibitor 2A，CDKN2A）突变
Lynch 综合征	由至少 5 种不同错配修复（mismatch repair，MMR）基因的遗传突变引起，包括：mutL 同源物 1（mutL homolog 1，MLH1）、mutS 同源物 2（mutS homolog 2，MSH2）、mutS 同源物 6（mutS homolog 6，MSH6）和 PMS1 同源物 2 错配修复系统组件（PMS1 homolog 2，mismatch repair system component，PMS2）
家族性腺瘤性息肉病	WNT 信号通路的腺瘤性结肠息肉病调节因子（adenomatous polyposis coli，APC）突变
mutY DNA 糖基化酶（mutY DNA glycosylase，MUTYH）相关性息肉病	MUTYH 的种系双等位基因突变
遗传性弥漫性胃癌	编码 E-钙黏蛋白的钙黏蛋白 1（cadherin 1，CDH1）突变
von Hippel-Lindau（VHL）综合征（又称希佩尔-林道综合征）	3 号染色体短臂上 VHL 抑癌基因的种系突变

（一）视网膜母细胞瘤

视网膜母细胞瘤是一种罕见的小儿眼部肿瘤，与位于染色体 13q14 的 RB1 基因胚系突变有关，这些儿童癌症幸存者易继发放射相关性肉瘤、白血病、黑色素瘤等第二原发肿瘤。

视网膜母细胞瘤患者的发病年龄一般很小，随着年龄增长，第二原发肿瘤逐渐升高至 60~62 岁，包括骨和软组织肉瘤、黑色素瘤、癌和脑肿瘤等[555]。Kleinerman 等[556]的研究报道，1852 例视网膜母细胞瘤患者中有视网膜母细胞瘤家族史的患者50年内发生第二原发肿瘤的累积风险率为47%,高于无肿瘤家族史者(38%)。

(二) Li-Fraumeni 综合征

李-佛美尼综合征(Li-Fraumeni syndrome,LFS)与位于染色体17q13的p53基因胚系突变有关,具有多原发肿瘤的发生倾向,通常表现为乳腺癌、肉瘤、白血病、脑肿瘤、肾上腺皮质癌等多原发肿瘤发生的风险增加[557]。

三、主要基因异常

目前,多数学者认为多原发肿瘤的发生与原癌基因扩增、抑癌基因突变、错配修复基因缺陷等有关。近年来,有很多突变基因在不同肿瘤中被发现,如p73、p16、p21、p53、PTEN、BRAC1、BRCA2、ALDH2、PLCE1、rs2274223、HER2、Bcl-2、bax、mdm2、mdm4、MUC1、Rho家族和NF-κB p65等,某个或某几个基因突变既可导致第一原发肿瘤发生,亦可增加多原发肿瘤发生的风险[558-559]。Imyanitov等[560]指出,患对侧乳腺癌的高风险与癌相关基因的突变、致癌因素的持续存在等因素密切相关。

(一) MMR 缺失

1. Lynch 综合征

Lynch 综合征(Lynch syndrome,LS)又称遗传性非息肉性结直肠肿瘤综合征(hereditary nonpolyposis colorectal cancer,HNPCC),是由DNA错配修复基因(mismatch repair,MMR)突变引起的常染色体显性遗传性疾病,DNA错配修复基因有MSH2、MSH6、MLH1、PMS1、PMS2,若有1个或1个以上发生突变,则可能发生Lynch综合征[561-564]。

Lynch综合征的关键特征是加速致癌作用,一个微小的结肠腺瘤可以在2~3年的时间内形成结肠癌,而散发性结肠癌需要6~10年[565]。Lynch综合征患者一生中患结直肠癌的可能性为50%~80%,54%~61%的患者会发生第二原发肿瘤,15%~23%的患者会发生三原发或更多的原发肿瘤[566-567]。

Lynch综合征的临床特点是除肠道肿瘤外还表现为多种肠外同时性或异时性肿瘤,以子宫内膜癌最常见,其他有卵巢癌、胃癌、肝癌、胰腺癌等。Lancaster等[568]报道,年龄<50岁、同时性或异时性发生子宫内膜癌

与结直肠癌的女性患者中20%~25%为Lynch综合征。

有研究发现[569-570],20%的Lynch综合征患者在子宫内膜癌诊断后10年内发生结直肠癌,48%在20年内发生;12%的患者在结直肠癌诊断后10年内发生子宫内膜癌,24%在20年内发生。

微卫星不稳定性(microsatellite instability,MSI)是指由DNA复制错误引起的简单重复序列的增加或丢失,有研究报道[571-572],有肿瘤家族史者发生多原发肿瘤的概率高于无肿瘤家族史者,可能与MMR或染色体显性基因突变等有关。

有研究表明[573],MMR基因缺失者有患结直肠癌外的第二原发肿瘤的额外风险,包括肾、膀胱、小肠、胃、肝胆、前列腺、子宫内膜、乳腺和卵巢等部位的肿瘤。在一项关于胃多原发肿瘤的研究中发现[574],年龄>60岁或高度微卫星不稳定(microsatellite instability-high,MSI-H)状态的患者多原发肿瘤发生率较高。Miyoshi等[575]的研究发现,MSI在多原发胃癌中的出现频率高于单发胃癌,提示MSI在多原发胃癌的发展中可能起着重要作用。

2. MMR与结直肠内多原发肿瘤

一项Meta分析结果显示[576],MSI可增加散发性结直肠癌患者发生多原发肿瘤的概率。

同时性多原发结直肠内癌是一种与MSI高患病率(约35%)相关的独特疾病,在同时性多原发结直肠内癌患者中,MSI最常见的机制是MutL蛋白同系物1(MutL Homolog 1,MLH1)表达缺失,这种缺失最常见的原因是MLH1启动子甲基化过度表达[577]。通常情况下,微卫星高度不稳定性肿瘤淋巴细胞浸润较高,可引起机体更强的免疫反应[578]。

有研究显示[336],同时性多原发结直肠内癌患者的MSI阳性率高于单发结直肠癌患者。董锐增等[579]对散发性多原发结直肠内癌MSI的研究表明,在38例异时性多原发肿瘤患者中MSI阳性占39.5%,而散发性非多原发肿瘤MSI阳性率为5.7%。年龄<40岁的异时性多原发肿瘤患者,肿瘤组织MSI阳性率为62.5%,年龄>40岁为32.7%。提示在异时性多原发结直肠肿瘤患者中,肿瘤组织MSI阳性率明显高于单一原发结直肠肿瘤患者。Shitoh等[580]随访了272例结直肠癌术后患者,中位随访期74个月,17例发生异时性多原发结直肠癌,MSI阳性患者和MSI阴性患者,异时性多原发结直肠癌发生率分别为15.3%和3%,有显著性差异($P<0.001$)。

Lawes 等[581]亦报道,高度 MSI 发生率在多原发结直肠内癌中较高,占 52%,单发结直肠癌占 13.5%($P<0.01$)。在任延律等[582]报道的 38 例多原发结直肠内癌中,21 例 MLH1 表达阴性,6 例 MSH2 表达阴性,3 例二者皆阴性,MMR 表达阴性率为 47%。

3. MMR 与妇科多原发肿瘤

Tiwari 等[583]研究发现,Lynch 综合征患者不仅患有结肠癌,同时易并发其他多原发恶性肿瘤,如卵巢癌、胃癌和膀胱癌等。可能由于 MMR 基因突变导致 DNA 序列错误,而在全身多器官发生突变,导致多部位肿瘤发生。

Millar 等[584]在 40 例子宫内膜癌合并结直肠癌双原发肿瘤患者中发现,MMR 突变率为 18%。Schmeler 等[585]对证实 MMR 基因突变的女性随访发现,61 例行预防性子宫/双附件切除的患者中妇科恶性肿瘤发病率为 0,而保留子宫及双附件的 210 例女性患者中 69 例(33%)确诊为子宫内膜癌。

(二)BRAC1、BRCA2 基因突变

乳腺癌易感基因(BRCA1/2)是一种抑癌基因,广泛参与 DNA 损伤修复、细胞周期调控、表观遗传学修饰等多个过程,对于维护基因组稳定性具有十分重要的作用[586];BRCA 基因缺失或变异均会导致染色体不稳定,进而诱发正常细胞癌变。Chan 等[285]报道,在多原发肿瘤有害突变中,约有 3/4 的基因突变是 BRAC1/2 和错配修复基因突变。

较多的研究表明[320,587],BRAC1/2 基因突变的乳腺癌患者可能发生罹患对侧乳腺癌和卵巢癌的高家族风险。Hemminki 等[588]报道,约有 10% 的乳腺癌患者为遗传基因突变引起;BRAC1/2、BACH1 及 RAD51 等基因突变均可导致乳腺癌的发生[589-591]。Offit[592]报道,BRAC1、BRCA2 基因突变的女性发生乳腺癌的风险可达 80%。相关研究发现[223,593],携带 BRAC1/BRCA2 突变的乳腺癌患者的第二原发肿瘤发病率显著增加。

1. BRAC1、BRCA2 基因突变与对侧第二原发性乳腺癌

BRCA 基因突变被认为会增加对侧乳腺癌发生风险,Valencia 等[594]报道,携带 BRCA 基因突变的乳腺癌患者 25 年后对侧乳腺癌累积风险为 47.4%,其中 BRAC1 基因突变者对侧乳腺癌风险较 BRCA2 基因突变者高 1.6 倍。Narod 等[595]报道,有乳腺癌家族史或 BRAC1、BRCA2 基因突变的女性患者患对侧乳腺癌的风险增加,在 BRAC1 或 BRCA2 突变携带者中

增加到3%。

BRCA基因突变对于对侧乳腺癌发生风险的影响与首发乳腺癌年龄呈负相关。Graser等[596]对携带BRCA基因突变的乳腺癌者进行随访发现，若首发乳腺癌年龄<40岁，25年后约62.9%的患者发生对侧乳腺癌；若首发乳腺癌年龄>50岁，该比例下降为19.6%。荷兰学者对6294名发病年龄<50岁的乳腺癌患者进行中位12.5年的随访也得出了类似结果[597]。

2. 遗传性乳腺癌-卵巢癌综合征

遗传性乳腺癌-卵巢癌综合征(hereditary breast-ovarian cancer syndrome，HBOC)的发生主要与BRAC1、BRCA2基因发生突变密切相关[93,319]。Varol等[304]的研究发现，BRAC1和BRCA2作为乳腺癌和卵巢癌的易感基因，与乳腺癌和卵巢癌发生存在明显相关性，BRAC1和BRCA2除增加乳腺癌、卵巢癌的发生风险外，还会增加其他部位原发性肿瘤发生的风险。

有研究报道[36,598]，在绝经前(<45岁)患乳腺癌的妇女患卵巢癌风险更高，因BRAC1和BRCA2突变通常会在年轻时导致乳腺癌，从而增加这两种肿瘤异时性发生的风险。Fishman等[599]指出，乳腺、卵巢相关的多原发肿瘤患者中57%的患者存在BRAC1/2突变。一项Meta分析显示[599]，BRCA1/2基因突变的第一原发肿瘤乳腺癌患者同时性发生卵巢癌的发病率为2.6%~42.1%。Baker等[600]报道，BRCA基因突变的第一原发肿瘤卵巢癌患者再发第二原发肿瘤乳腺癌的概率为2%~6%，8.9%的BRCA突变携带卵巢癌患者在中位随访50.2个月后发生乳腺癌。

(三)PTEN基因突变

磷酸酯酶与张力蛋白同源物(phosphatase and tensin homolog，PTEN)定位于染色体10q23.3，由9个外显子组成，编码由403个氨基酸组成的蛋白质，具有磷酸酶活性，通过抑制PI3K/AKT信号通路而阻止肿瘤发生[601]。

Cowden综合征(Cowden's syndrome)又称多发性错构瘤综合征，为一种显性遗传病，主要由PTEN基因突变所致，常合并甲状腺癌、乳腺癌和子宫内膜癌等异时性多原发肿瘤[602-605]。

何晓乐等[606]研究指出，老年患者消化道MPNs的发生可能与PTEN蛋白低表达有关。

(四)其他基因突变

Park 等[607]对 1385 例多原发肿瘤患者和 9626 例单发肿瘤患者进行对照分析,使用 SNP 检测了 188 个肿瘤易感基因,从中发现 rs578776 和 rs11249433 基因位点与多原发恶性肿瘤有关,差异具有统计学意义。

Vogt 等[608]指出,miR-34a、miR-34b/c 失活可能导致多种肿瘤发生,如结直肠癌、胰腺癌、乳腺癌、卵巢癌、尿路上皮癌、肾癌和软组织恶性肿瘤。

Behrens 等[609]报道,与一般人群相比,6q13-14、9p21、TP53 是霍奇金淋巴瘤发生第二原发肿瘤乳腺癌患者的高频率杂合性缺失位点,其微卫星改变频率增加 4.2 倍。

已发现的与头颈部恶性肿瘤密切相关的原癌基因有 ras、c-myc、Bcl-2、c-abl 等,抑癌基因有 p53、Rb、p16、p21 等。Jin 等[610]的研究发现,在 p53 相关基因中,包括 p53、p73、p14ARF、mdm2 以及 mdm4 在内的高危基因型可能与头颈部鳞癌患者多原发肿瘤发生的风险增加有关。Zhang 等[611]报道,p53 和 p73 基因的共同变异可增加头颈部鳞癌患者多原发肿瘤的发生。

某些不同器官的肿瘤具有相同基因突变,如非小细胞肺癌与结肠癌均存在 v-raf 鼠类肉瘤滤过性病毒致癌基因同源体 B1(v-raf murine sarcoma viral oncogene homolog B1,BRAF)基因突变[612]。

HER-2 基因扩增可见于乳腺癌、胃癌等[613-614],HER-2 蛋白过表达在肠型胃癌中占 16%,在乳腺癌中占 30%[615]。

细胞周期检测点激酶 2 基因(cell cycle-checkpoint kinase 2 gene,CHEK2)突变与乳腺癌、前列腺癌的易感性有关,女性中若发生 CHEK2 基因突变,则可能增加乳腺癌和甲状腺癌同时性发生的风险[616]。Siolek 等[617]对 468 例甲状腺乳头状癌患者和 468 例健康人群进行对照研究发现,甲状腺癌患者 CHEK2 基因突变更明显(15.6% vs 6.0%,$P<0.001$),在 11 例甲状腺癌伴乳腺癌多原发肿瘤的患者中有 7 例存在 CHEK2 突变(63%,$P<0.001$)。

LKB1 基因突变是 Peutz-Jegher's 综合征(PJS)的致病基因,有研究报道[618-619],约 20% 的宫颈癌、30% 的非小细胞肺癌的发生与 LKB1 基因突变有显著的相关性。

第一章 总 论

不同组织学类型的甲状腺癌，其起源有一定差异，其乳头状癌（PTC）起源于滤泡上皮细胞肿瘤，根据分化程度分为滤泡状癌（FC）、乳头状癌和未分化癌；起源于滤泡旁细胞肿瘤即髓样癌（MTC），甲状腺胸腺样分化癌则起源于异位胸腺或后鳃体残留物[620]。Shiroko 等[621]认为，MTC、FC 起源于相同的干细胞。但 Volantc 等[622]在 MTC、FC 的肿瘤中发现有不同的 RET 基因重排、LOA 及 X-染色体的失活，提示这两种肿瘤的起源是不同的。Rossi 等[623]亦在 3 例 MTC、PTC 病例中，通过 RET 和 BRAF 基因分析证实这两种肿瘤有不同基因突变。

无论是同时性还是异时性发生，乳腺癌与甲状腺癌在基因突变方面均存在一定的相关性。Ikeda 等[624]的研究发现，PARP4 基因是原发性甲状腺癌和乳腺癌的易感基因，PARP4 蛋白的过表达已被证实是乳腺癌预后的保护因素。有研究报道[625-626]，有丝分裂相关 LncRNA（MANCR）是侵袭性乳腺癌的驱动者，其在甲状腺癌中表达上调。

Titze 等[627]研究发现，细胞周期蛋白 D1 和 p53 蛋白的过表达，与咽部和食管多原发肿瘤的发生高度相关。

APC、KRAS、p53 和 PIK3CA 等基因在结直肠癌中经常发生突变，并被证明通过调节参与增殖、分化和凋亡的驱动途径来促进肿瘤发生；且在同时性多原发结直肠内癌中也常发生突变，且多数突变位点与单发结直肠癌不同[543]。一项前瞻性队列研究结果显示[628]，与单原发结直肠癌比较，同时性多原发结直肠内癌在 BRAF 中的突变频率更高、MSI 更高。Leggett 等[629]的研究证明，染色体不稳定、MSI 和基因甲基化是同时性多原发直肠内癌的易感因素；同时性结直肠内癌通常 MSI 高，MSI 高而 CpG 岛甲基化阴性的结肠癌通常出现在近端结肠中，约占同期结肠癌的 10%；染色体不稳定阳性状态（导致肿瘤抑制基因失活）约占 60%。

有研究表明[630-633]，多原发结直肠内癌较单原发结直肠癌更频繁发生 17 号染色体和 p53 基因座数目和结构的畸变。Asakawa 等[634]的研究发现，同时性多原发结直肠内癌 p53 基因突变率较散发性结直肠内癌低。Koness 等[538]报道了 15 例同时性结直肠内癌患者的基因检查结果，12 例为 p53 突变，9 例为 Kras 突变，各有 1 例 2 个肿瘤均为 p53 或 Kras 基因突变，认为多原发结直肠内癌 p53 和 Kras 突变不一致表明肿瘤病灶发生的独立性。

参考文献

[1] Soerjomataram I, Coebergh JW. Epidemiology of Multiple Primary Cancers[J]. CA Cancer J Clin, 1977, 27(4): 233-240.

[2] Yagi Y, Kanemasa Y, Sasaki Y, et al. Synchronous multiple primary tumors in patients with malignant lymphoma: a retrospective study[J]. BMC Cancer, 2022, 22(1): 1-10.

[3] 陈双双, 马锐. 多原发癌的研究进展[J]. 癌症进展, 2019, 17(8): 883-886.

[4] 周剑烽, 王铁君. 异时性鼻咽癌、背部皮肤隆突性纤维肉瘤和外耳道癌三重癌一例[J]. 实用肿瘤杂志, 2021, 36(4): 358-362.

[5] Shin DW, Cho B, Kim SY, et al. Management of cancer survivors in clinical and public health perspectives: current status and future challenges in Korea[J]. J Korean Med Sci, 2013, 28(5): 651-657.

[6] Moertel CG, Doekerty MB, Baggenstoss AH. Multiple primary malignant neoplasms Ⅱ tumors of different tissues or organs[J]. Cancer, 1961, 14(2): 231-237.

[7] IARC/ENCR/IACR Working Group. International rules for multiple primary cancers[J]. Asian Pacific J Cancer Prev, 2005, 6(1): 104-106.

[8] Molina-Montes E, Requena M, Sanchez-Cantalejo E, et al. Risk of second cancers cancer after a first primary breast cancer: a systematic review and meta-analysis[J]. Gynecol Oncol, 2015, 136(1): 158-171.

[9] Nagasawa S, Onda M, Sasajima K, et al. Multiple primary malignant neoplasms in patients with esophageal cancer[J]. Dis Esophagus, 2000, 13(3): 226-230.

[10] International rules for multiple primary cancers (ICD-O third edition)[J]. Eur J Cancer Prev, 2005, 14(4): 307-308.

[11] 陈舒兰. 多原发恶性肿瘤的确定及编码[J]. 中国病案, 2017, 18(8): 36-39.

[12] 徐佩佩, 孔令非. 双侧乳腺癌的研究进展[J]. 临床与实验病理学杂志, 2020, 36(5): 557-559.

[13] 魏晓玲, 洪英极, 王林硕, 等. 潮汕地区原发性双侧乳腺癌癌灶间相关性分析[J]. 汕头大学医学院学报, 2018, 31(4): 234-238.

[14] Martini N, Melamed MR. Multiple primary lung cancers[J]. J Thorac Cardiovasc Surg, 1975, 9(4): 606-612.

[15] 韩连奎, 高树庚, 谭锋维, 等. 同时性多原发肺癌的诊治体会及处理策略新进展[J]. 中国肺癌杂志, 2018, 21(3): 180-184.

[16] Ishikawa Y, Nakayama H, Ito H, et al. Surgical treatment for synchronous primary lung adenocarcinomas[J]. Ann Thorac Surg, 2014, 98(6): 1983-1988.

[17] 陈亚男,滑炎卿.多原发肺癌HRCT影像特点及其临床意义的研究进展[J].国际医学放射学杂志,2018,41(2):175-179.

[18] 郑琴,孙依萍,蔡蓉,等.肺内同时性多原发癌的临床诊断与治疗[J].中国呼吸与危重监护杂志,2012,11(6):550-553.

[19] Engeland A, Bjorge T, Haldorsen T, et al. Use of multiple primary cancers to indicate associations between smoking and cancer incidence: an analysis of 500,000 cancer cases diagnosed in Norway during 1953-1993[J]. Int J Cancer, 1997, 70(4): 401-407.

[20] Levi F, Randimbison L, Te VC, et al. Multiple primary cancers in the Vaud Cancer Registry, Switzerland, 1974-1989[J]. Br J Cancer, 1993, 67(2): 391-395.

[21] Storm HH, Jensen OM, Ewertz M, et al. A summary: multiple primary cancers in Denmark, 1943-1980[J]. Natl Cancer Inst Monogr, 1985, 68(6): 411-430.

[22] Lee HP. Multiple primary cancers in Singapore 1968—1978[J]. Ann Acad Med Singapore, 1984, 13(2): 206-210.

[23] Copur MS, Manapuram S. Multiple primary tumors over a lifetime[J]. Oncology(Williston Park), 2019, 33(7): 629384-629392.

[24] Demandante CG, Troyer DA, Miles TP. Multiple primary malignant neoplasms: case report and a comprehensive review of the literature[J]. Am J Clin Oncol, 2003, 26(1): 79-83.

[25] Mariotto AB, Rowland JH, Ries LA, et al. Multiple cancer prevalence: A growing challenge in long-term survivorship[J]. Cancer Epidemiol Biomarkers Prevv, 2007, 16(3): 566-571.

[26] Berrington DA, Curtis RE, Kry SF, et al. Proportion of second cancers attributable to radiotherapy treatment in adults: a cohort study in the US SEER cancer registries[J]. Lancet Oncol, 2011, 12(4): 353-360.

[27] Rosso S, De Angelis R, Ciccolallo L, et al. Multiple tumours in survival estimates[J]. Eur J Cancer, 2009, 45(6): 1080-1094.

[28] Utada M, Ohno Y, Hori M, et al. Incidence of multiple primary cancers and interval between first and second primary cancers[J]. Cancer Sci, 2014, 105(7): 890-896.

[29] Lee J, Park S, Kim S, et al. Characteristics and survival of breast cancer patients with multiple synchronous or metachronous primary cancers[J]. Yonsei Med J, 2015, 56(5): 1213-1220.

[30] Fu JJ, Huang ZW, Lin YH, et al. Clinical analysis of 39 cases of multiple primary colorectal carcinoma[J]. Journal of Southern Medical University, 2013, 33(4): 578-581.

[31] 朱莉菲,薛鹏,王理伟.65例多原发癌的临床回顾性研究[J].复旦学报(医学版),2010,37(5):591-593.

[32] Li W, Zhan Y, Li G. Double cancers: a clinical analysis of 156 cases[J]. Zhonghua Zhong Liu Za Zhi, 1996, 18(4): 296-298.

[33] Wang H, Hou J, Zhang G, et al. Clinical characteristics and prognostic analysis of multiple primary malignant neoplasms in patients with lung cancer[J]. Cancer Gene Ther, 2019, 26(11-12): 419-426.

[34] Jiao F, Yao LJ, Zhou J, et al. Clinical features of multiple primary malignancies: a retrospective analysis of 72 Chinese patients[J]. Asian Pac J Cancer Prev, 2014, 15(1): 331-334.

[35] 郑希希, 贾勇圣, 史业辉, 等. 乳腺癌多原发癌的临床病理特征及预后分析[J]. 中国肿瘤临床, 2017, 44(5): 219-223.

[36] 师弘, 王伟, 贺新, 等. 多原发乳腺癌的临床流行病学特征——82例患者的回顾性研究[J]. 现代肿瘤医学, 2018, 26(20): 3307-3310.

[37] Chen SC, Liu CJ, Hu YW, et al. Second primary malignancy risk among patients with gastric cancer: a nation-wide population-based study in Taiwan[J]. Gastric Cancer, 2016, 19(2): 490-497.

[38] 潘源, 王家仓, 梁寒, 等. 消化系统原发恶性肿瘤116例临床分析[J]. 中华肿瘤杂志, 2002, 24(2): 191-193.

[39] 李威, 詹友庆, 李国辉. 双原发癌156例临床分析[J]. 中华肿瘤杂志, 1996, 18(4): 58-60.

[40] 刘复生, 秦德兴, 王奇璐. 多原发癌瘤172例临床病理分析[J]. 中华肿瘤杂志, 1979, 1(2): 113-119.

[41] 张正伟, 张盛, 曾贵林, 等. 123例多原发癌的临床分析[J]. 四川生理科学杂志, 2016, 38(4): 204-206.

[42] 耿振英, 焦顺昌, 王甦, 等. 106例多原发癌的临床回顾性研究[J]. 世界最新医学信息文摘, 2017, 17(12): 1-2, 19.

[43] Xu LL, Gu KS. Clinical retrospective analysis of cases with multiple primary malignant neoplasms[J]. Genet Mol Res, 2014, 13(4): 9271-9284.

[44] 钟海鸣, 陈景胜, 吴昱冶, 等. 多原发癌86例临床分析[J]. 广东医学院学报, 2009, 27(4): 433-434.

[45] 何建军. 双侧原发性乳腺癌2942例荟萃分析[J]. 中国现代医生, 2010, 48(5): 8-10.

[46] 何建军. 中国人2025例多原发结直肠癌荟萃分析[J]. 中华胃肠外科杂志, 2006, 9(3): 225-229.

[47] Centers for Disease Prevention. Cancer survivors - United States, 2007[J]. MMWR Morb Mortal Wkly Rep, 2011, 60(9): 269-272.

[48] Hayat MJ, Howlader N, Reichman ME, et al. Cancer statistics, trends, and multiple primary cancer analyses from the surveillance, epidemiology, and end results (SEER) program[J]. Oncologist, 2007, 12(1): 20-37.

[49] Miller KD, Nogueira L, Mariotto AB, et al. Cancer treatment and survivorship statistics, 2019[J]. CA Cancer J Clin, 2019, 69(5): 363-385.

[50] Marioao AB, Rowland JH, Ries LA, et al. Multiple cancer prevalence: a growing challenge in long-term survivorship[J]. Cancer Epidemiol Biomarkers Prev, 2007, 16(3): 566-571.

[51] Patrascu T, Doran H, Catrina E, et al. Synchronous tumors of the gastrointestinal tract[J]. Chirurqia(Bucur), 2010, 105(1): 93-96.

[52] Andrea L, Lodovico B. Multiple primary malignancies. Semin Oncol, 2004, 31(3): 264-273.

[53] Siegel RL, Miller KD, Fuchs HE, et al. Cancer statistics, 2021[J]. CA Cancer J Clin, 2021, 71(1): 7-33.

[54] Tanjak P, Suktitipat B, Vorasan N, et al. Risks and cancer associations of metachronous and synchronous multiple primary cancers: a 25-year retrospective study[J]. BMC Cancer, 2021, 21(1): 1045-1056.

[55] Ward ZJ, Grover S, Scott AM, et. al. The role and contribution of treatment and imaging modalities in global cervical cancer management: survival estimates from a simulation-based analysis[J]. Lancet Oncol, 2020, 21(8): 1077-1088.

[56] Feller A, Matthes KL, Bordoni A, et al. The relative risk of second primary cancers in Switzerland: a population based retrospective cohort study[J]. BMC Cancer, 2020, 20(1): 51-62.

[57] Kong Y, Li J, Lin H, et al. Landscapes of synchronous multiple primary cancers detected by next-generation se-quencing[J]. FEBS Open Bio, 2022, 12(11): 1996-2005.

[58] Li RM, Zhang Y, Ma BQ, et al. Survival analysis of second primary malignancies after cervical cancer using a competing risk model: implications for prevention and surveillance[J]. Ann Translat Med, 2021, 9(3): 239-246.

[59] Qiao B, Hsieh MC, Wu XC, et al. Multiple primary cancers in the United States[J]. J Registry Manag, 2020, 47(2): 60-66.

[60] Sert F, Caner A, Haydaroglu A. Trends in the incidence and overall survival of multiple primary cancers in Turkey[J]. J BUON, 2020, 25(2): 1230-1236.

[61] Ye Y, Otahal P, Wills KE, et al. Temporal trends in the risk of second primary cancers among survivors of adult-onset cancers, 1980 through 2013: an Australian population-based study[J]. Cancer, 2018, 124(8): 1808-1818.

[62] Falini ECB. Multiple primary cancer incidence in Italy[J]. Eur J Cancer, 2001, 37(18): 2449-2456.

[63] Izmajlowicz B, Kornafel J, Blaszczyk J. Multiple neoplasms among cervical cancer patients in the material of the lower silesian cancer registry[J]. Adv Clin Exp Med, 2014, 23(3):

433-440.

[64] Angurana SL, Kapoor R, Kumar P, et al. Quadruple malignancy in a single patient: a case report and comprehensive review of literature[J]. J Cancer Res Ther, 2010, 6(2): 230-232.

[65] Demandante CG, Troyer DA, Miles TP. Multiple primary malignant neoplasms: case report and a comprehensive review of the literature[J]. Am J Clin Oncol, 2003, 26(1): 79-83.

[66] Molina-Montes E, Requena M, Sánchez-Cantalejo E, et al. Risk of second cancers cancer after a first primary breast cancer: a systematic review and meta-analysis[J]. Gynecol Oncol, 2015, 136(1): 158-171.

[67] Ye Y, Neil AL, Wills KE, et al. Temporal trends in the risk of developing multiple primary cancers: a systematic review[J]. BMC Cancer, 2016, 16(1): 849-858.

[68] Kim SW, Kong KA, Kim DY, et al. Multiple primary cancers involving lung cancer at a single tertiary hospital: clinical features and prognosis[J]. Thorac Cancer, 2015, 6(2): 159-165.

[69] Travis LB. The epidemiology of second primary cancers[J]. Cancer Epidemiol Biomarkers Prevv, 2006, 15(11): 2020-2026.

[70] Kaneko S, Yamaguchi N. Epidemiological analysis of site relationships of synchronous and metachronous multiple primary cancers in the National Cancer Center, Japan, 1962-1996[J]. Jpn J Clin Oncol, 1999, 29(2): 96-105.

[71] Friedman DL, Whitto J, Leisenring W, et al. Subsequent neoplasms in 5-year survivors of childhood cancer: the Childhood Cancer Survivor Study[J]. J Natl Cancer Inst, 2010, 102(14): 1083-1095.

[72] Sankila R, Pukkala E, Teppo L. Risk of subsequent malignant neoplasms among 470,000 cancer patients in Finland, 1953-1991[J]. Int J Cancer, 1995, 60(4): 464-470.

[73] Donin NM, Kwan L, Lenis AT, et al. Second primary lung cancer in United States Cancer Survivors, 1992—2008[J]. Cancer Causes Control, 2019, 30(5): 465-475.

[74] Amikura K, Ehara K, Kawashima Y. The risk of developing multiple primary cancers among long-term survivors five years or more after stomach carcinoma resection[J]. Tohoku J Exp Med, 2020, 250(1): 31-41.

[75] Baba Y, Yoshida N, Kinoshita K, et al. Clinical and prognostic features of patients with esophageal cancer and multiple primary cancers[J]. Ann Surg, 2018, 267(3): 478-483.

[76] Si L, Feng Y, Wang Y, et al. Clinical and pathological characteristics of multiple primary malignant neoplasms cases[J]. Int J Clin Pract, 2021, 75(11): e14663-e14672.

[77] Chang CC, Chung YH, Liou CB, et al. Influence of Residential Environment and Lifestyle on Multiple Primary Malignancies in Taiwan[J]. Asian Pac J Cancer Prev, 2015, 16(8):

3533-3538.

[78] Halamkova J, Kazda T, Pehalova L, et al. Second primary malignancies in colorectal cancer patients[J]. Sci Rep, 2021, 11(1): 2759-2766.

[79] De Luca A, Frusone F, Vergine M, et al. Breast cancer and multiple primary malignant tumors: case report and review of the literature[J]. In Vivo, 2019, 33(4): 1313-1324.

[80] Chateau CS, Stokkel MP. Second primary tumors involving non-small cell lung cancer: prevalence and its influence on survival[J]. Chest, 2005, 127(4): 1152-1158.

[81] Lin FW, Yeh MH, Lin CL, et al. Association between breast cancer and second primary lung cancer among the female population in taiwan: a nationwide population-based cohort study[J]. Cancers (Basel), 2022, 14(12): 2977-2981.

[82] Zhai C, Cai Y, Lou F, et al. Multiple primary malignant tumors: A clinical analysis of 15 321 patients with malignancies at a singlecenter in China[J]. J Cancer, 2018, 9(16): 2795-2801.

[83] Zheng R, Li H, Ye Y, et at. Clinicopathological features and prognostic analysis of 77 patients with multiple primary cancers[J]. J BUON, 2020, 25(4): 2110-2116.

[84] Lee GD, Kim YH, Kim JB, et al. Esophageal cancer associated with multiple primary cancers: Surgical approaches and long-term survival[J]. Ann Surg Oncol, 2013, 20(13): 4260-4266.

[85] Natsugoe S, Matsumoto M, Okumura H, et al. Multiple primary carcinomas with esophageal squamous cell cancer: Clinicopathologic outcome[J]. World J Surg, 2005, 29(1): 46-49.

[86] 陈小良, 雷林, 郭春美, 等. 深圳市多原发恶性肿瘤流行病学特征分析[J]. 中国慢性病预防与控制, 2023, 31(5): 393-396.

[87] 梁智恒, 李柱明, 刘宁, 等.1970—2019年广东省中山市多原发恶性肿瘤发病分析[J]. 中国肿瘤, 2023, 32(4): 265-270.

[88] 陈颖, 赵明芳, 曲秀娟, 等.30例多原发癌回顾性分析[J]. 中国医科大学学报, 2012, 41(4): 340-342.

[89] 杨建光, 李晓霞, 孔凡民. 多原发癌临床特征分析[J]. 现代肿瘤医学, 2011, 19(12): 2551-2553.

[90] 张献文, 江浩, 汪庚明, 等. 食管-口底异时性四重多原发癌1例并文献复习[J]. 肿瘤防治研究, 2017, 44(7): 509-512.

[91] Kilciksiz S, Gokce T, Baloglu A, et al. Characteristics of synchronous-and metachronous-type multiple primary neoplasms: a study of hospital-based cancer registry in Turkey[J]. Clin Genitourin Cancer, 2007, 5(7): 438-445.

[92] Pacheco-Figueiredo L, Antunes L, Bento MJ, et al. Evaluation of the frequency of and survival from second primary cancers in North Portugal: a population-based study[J]. Eur J

Cancer Prev, 2013, 22(6): 599 – 606.

[93] Noh SK, Yoon JY, Ryoo UN, et al. A case report of quadruple cancer in a single patient including the breast, rectum, ovary, and endometrium[J]. J Gynecol Oncol, 2008, 19(19), 265 – 269.

[94] Sprogel P, Karkov JN. Multiple primary cancer. Presence of more than 4 primary cancers[J]. Ugeskr Laeger, 1990, 153(1): 27 – 39.

[95] Xin DY. A report of 5 cases of multiple primary cancer[J]. Zhonghua Yi Xue Za Zhi, 1982, 62(8): 485 – 486.

[96] Zhao J, Tan Y, Wu Y, et al. A rare case of eight multiple primary malignant neoplasms in a female patient: A case report and review of the literature[J]. Oncol Lett, 2015, 9(2): 587 – 590.

[97] Arakawa K, Hata K, Yamamoto Y, et al. Nine primary malignant neoplasms involving the esophagus, stomach, colon, rectum, prostate, and external ear canal – without microsatellite instability: a case report[J]. BMC Cancer, 2018, 18(1): 24 – 29.

[98] Powell S, Tarchand G, Rector T, et al. Synchronous and metachronous malignancies: analysis of the Minneapolis Veterans Affairs (VA) tumor registry[J]. Cancer Causes Control, 2013, 24(8): 1565 – 1573.

[99] Arpaci E, Tokluoglu S, Yetigyigit T, et al. Multiple primary malignancies – a retrospective analysis at a single center in Turkey[J]. Asian Pac J Cancer Prev, 2013, 14(21): 769 – 773.

[100] 张稚淳，贾梦冉，丁皓，等. 120例多原发肿瘤临床分析[J]. 肿瘤防治研究，2019, 46(2): 153 – 158.

[101] Seegobin K, Staggs E, Khawaja R, et al. Pilot study on the occurrence of multiple cancers following cancer – related therapy at the University of Florida, Jacksonville (2011 – 2016)[J]. J Investig Med, 2018, 66(7): 1050 – 1054.

[102] Jemal A, Bray F, Center MM, et al. Global cancer statistics[J]. CA Cancer J Clin, 2011, 61(2): 69 – 90.

[103] Kim BK, Oh SJ, Song JY, et at. Clinical characteristics and prognosis associated with multiple primary cancers in breast cancer patients[J]. J Breast Cancer, 2018, 21(1): 62 – 69.

[104] 肖彩宏，吴万垠. 重复癌151例临床分析[J]. 中国医学创新，2012, 9(29): 118 – 119.

[105] Panosetti E, Luboinski B, Mamelle G, et al. Multiple synchronous and metachronous cancers of the upper aerodigestive tract: a nine – year study[J]. Laryngoscope, 1989, 99(12): 1267 – 1273.

[106] Liu Z, Liu C, Guo W, et al. Clinical analysis of 152 cases of multiple primary malignant

tumors in 15,398 patients with malignant tumors[J]. PLoS One, 2015, 10(5): e0125754-e0125766.

[107] 王帆, 郭瑞嵩, 韩海鱼, 等. 多原发癌384例临床分析[J]. 实用医技杂志, 2009, 16(12): 960-961.

[108] 刘爱蕙, 吴玉梅. 乳腺癌合并妇科原发癌23例临床分析[J]. 中国妇幼保健, 2012, 27(19): 2932-2933.

[109] Tabuchi T, Ito Y, Ioka A, et al. Incidence of metachronous second primary cancers in Osaka, Japan: update of analyses using population-based cancer registry data[J]. Cancer Sci, 2012, 103(6): 1111-1119.

[110] Brown AP, Chen J, Hitchcock YJ, et al. The risk of second primary malignancies up to three decades after the treatment of differentiated thyroid cancer[J]. J Clin Endocrinol Metab, 2008, 93(2): 504-515.

[111] Rosso S, Terracini L, Ricceri F, et al. Multiple primary tumours: incidence estimation in the presence of competing risks[J]. Popul Health Metr, 2009, 7(1): 5468-5477.

[112] 王成峰, 邵永孚, 兰忠民. 乳腺癌与多原发恶性肿瘤[J]. 中国肿瘤临床, 2000, 27(5): 349-351.

[113] 奥婷, 孙军平, 张明月, 等. 肺癌合并其他原发恶性肿瘤55例发病特点分析[J]. 解放军医学院学报, 2016, 37(3): 226-228.

[114] Duchateau CS, Stokkel MP. Second primary tumors involving non-small cell lung cancer: prevalence and its influence on survival[J]. Chest, 2005, 127(4): 1152-1158.

[115] Curtis RE, Freedman DM, Ron E, et al. New malignancies among cancer survivors. SEER cancer registries, 1973—2000[M]. MD: National Cancer Institute, 2006.

[116] Jena A, Patnayak R, Lakshmi AY, et al. Multiple primary cancers: an enigma[J]. South Asian J Cancer, 2016, 5(1): 29-32.

[117] 吕佳铭, 熊华才, 吴波, 等. 138例首发于消化系统的多原发癌临床分析[J]. 中华肿瘤杂志, 2018, 40(2): 147-150.

[118] Coyte A, Morrison DS, Mcloone P. Second primary cancer risk-the impact of applying different definitions of multiple primaries: results from a retrospective population-based cancer registry study[J]. BMC Cancer, 2014, 14(1): 272-280.

[119] Pan SY, Huang CP, Chen WC. Synchronous/metachronous multiple primary malignancies: review of associated risk factors[J]. Diagnostics(Basel), 2022, 12(8): 1940-1953.

[120] 张真, 蔡昌豪, 吴本俨. 141例多原发恶性肿瘤的临床分析[J]. 中华老年多器官疾病杂志, 2008, 7(2): 128-131.

[121] Lv M, Zhang X, Shen Y, et al. Clinical analysis and prognosis of synchronous and metachronous multiple primary malignant tumors[J]. Medicine(Baltimore), 2017, 96(17): e6799-e6805.

[122] 陈武军,龙裔宁.800例消化系统恶性肿瘤多重癌发生率的回顾性调查[J].中国现代医生,2012,50(17):6-7.

[123] Babacan NA, Aksoy S, Cetin B, et al. Multiple primary malignant neoplasms: multi-center results from Turkey[J]. J BUON, 2012, 17(4): 770-775.

[124] Corso G, Veronesi P, Santomauro GI, et al. Multiple primary non-breast tumors in breast cancer survivors[J]. J Cancer Res Clin Oncol, 2018, 144(3): 979-986.

[125] Stefano R, Roberta A, Laura C, et al. Multiple tumours in survival estimates[J]. Eur J Cancer, 2009, 45(6): 1080-1094.

[126] Romaszko W, Buciński A, Doboszyńska A. Impact of smoking on multiple primary cancers survival: a retrospective analysis[J]. Clin Exp Med, 2018, 18(3): 391-397.

[127] Wittekind C, Klimpfinger M, Hermanek P, et al. Multiple simultaneous gastric carcinomas[J]. Br J Cancer, 1997, 76(12): 1604-1609.

[128] Giardiello C, Angelone G, Iodice G, et al. Diagnosis, therapy, and follow up in synchronous colorectal cancer of the colon[J]. G Chir, 2001, 22(11): 122-124.

[129] Gursel B, Meydan D, Ozbek N, et al. Multiple primary malignant neoplasms from the black sea region of Turkey[J]. J Int Med Res, 2011, 39(2): 667-674.

[130] 沈秋丹,袁慕知,韩迎利,等.血液系统肿瘤相关多原发恶性肿瘤10例临床分析[J].交通医学,2016,30(3):245-247.

[131] 贺舜,刘勇,刘晓,等.食管鳞癌相关原发恶性肿瘤的临床特点分析[J].中华医学杂志,2015,95(35):2868-2870.

[132] 孙海涛,王南,刘艺,等.184例多原发恶性肿瘤临床特征及其预后分析[J].现代肿瘤医学,2023,31(8):1530-1535.

[133] 王松,刘正,王贵玉,等.多原发癌的研究现状[J].肿瘤研究与临床,2018,30(9):645-648.

[134] 文珍,张彦秋,吴蓉,等.首发为食管鳞癌的多原发癌患者临床特征及生存分析[J].中国应用生理学杂志,2021,37(4):407-414.

[135] 董莉莉,牛艳洁,潘峰,等.第二原发癌为肺癌的多原发癌患者临床分析[J].临床与病理杂志,2017,37(4):724-728.

[136] Naik A, Bhandari V, Saadvik RY, et al. Incidence of second primary malignant neoplasm in Malwa region of central India[J]. J Cancer Res Ther, 2018, 14(5): 999-1004.

[137] Haraguchi S, Koizumi K, Hioki M, et al. Hereditary factors in multiple primary malignancies associated with lung cancer[J]. Surg Today, 2007, 37(5): 375-378.

[138] Fujita S, Masago K, Takeshita J, et al. Multiple primary malignancies in patients with non-small cell lung cancer[J]. Intern Med, 2015, 54(3): 325-331.

[139] Zhang S, Xu Z, Dong G, et al. Analysis of clinical characteristics of lung cancer combined with multiple primary malignancies in other organs[J]. Chinese Journal of Lung Cancer,

2021,24(1):7-12.

[140] 柯金,胡喜梅,周水阳,等.结肠癌合并多发性骨髓瘤1例报道[J].实用肿瘤杂志,2014,29(1):96-97.

[141] 王艳峰,王菀菀,段轶鋆,等.恶性肿瘤继发恶性血液病类型分析[J].中华临床医师杂志,2015,9(21):3859-3864.

[142] 徐新运,章宜芬,吴鸿雁,等.甲状腺原发性乳头状癌合并鳞状细胞癌的临床病理分析[J].东南大学学报,2007,26(3):215.

[143] 张功亮,郭广秀,王建,等.胸内原发性甲状腺乳头状癌伴存鳞状细胞癌1例[J].临床与实验病理杂志,2007,23(5):635.

[144] 吴义春,吴强,吴继峰,等.甲状腺乳头状癌合并髓样癌1例[J].临床与实验病理杂志,2007,23(1):115.

[145] 宋光耀,席峥,高志安,等.甲状腺髓样癌合并乳头状癌1例[J].中国误诊学杂志,2004,4(6):958.

[146] 张丽华,石群立,马恒辉,等.原发性甲状腺滤泡型乳头状癌伴鳞状细胞癌[J].医学研究学报,2000,13(4):277-278.

[147] 杜国防,曲桂玉.两种病理类型甲状腺癌并存1例[J].潍坊医学院学报.1999,21(2):114.

[148] Nielsen SM, White MG, Hong S, et al. The Breast-Thyroid Cancer Link: A Systematic Review and Meta-analysis[J]. Cancer Epidemiol Biomarkers Prevv, 2016, 25(2): 231-238.

[149] Kuo JH, Chabot JA, Lee JA. Breast cancer in thyroid cancer survivors: An analysis of the Surveillance, Epidemiology, and End Results-9 data base[J]. Surgery, 2016, 159(1): 23-29.

[150] Vanfossen VL, Wilhelm SM, Eaton JL, et al. Association of thyroid, breast and renal cell cancer: a population-based study of the prevalence of second malignancies[J]. Ann Surg Oncol, 2013, 20(4): 1341-1347.

[151] Rajoria S, Suriano R, Shanmugam A, et al. Metastatic phenotype is regulated by estrogen in thyroid cells[J]. Thyroid, 2010, 20(1): 33-41.

[152] Gan SJ, Dahlstrom KR, Peck BW, et al. Incidence and pattern of second primary malignancies in patients with index oropharyngeal cancers versus index nonoropharyngeal head and neck cancers[J]. Cancer, 2013, 119(14): 2593-2601.

[153] Morris LGT, Sikora AG, Hayes RB, et al. Anatomic sites at elevated risk of second primary cancer after an index head and neck cancer[J]. Cancer Causes Control, 2011, 22(5): 671-679.

[154] Morris LGT, Sikora AG, Patel SG, et al. Second primary cancers after an index head and neck cancer: subsite-specific trends in the era of human papillomavirus-associated

oropharyngeal cancer[J]. J Clin Oncol, 2011, 29(6): 739-746.

[155] Yamamoto E, Shibuya H, Yoshimura R, et al. Site specific dependency of second primary cancer in early stage head and neck squamous cell carcinoma[J]. Cancer, 2002, 94(7): 2007-2014.

[156] Chen PT, Lu CH, Kuan-Der L, et al. The incidence and risk of developing a second primary esophageal cancer in patients with oral and pharyngeal carcinoma: a population-based study in Taiwan over a 25 year period[J]. BMC Cancer, 2009, 9(1): 373-375.

[157] Michael T, Milano MD, Carl R, et al. Second primary lung cancer after head and neck squamous cell cancer: Population - based study of risk factors[J]. Head Neck, 2012, 34(12): 1782-1788.

[158] Raghavan UF, Quraishi SF, Bradley PJ. Multiple primary tumors in patients diagnosed with hypopharyngeal cancer[J]. Otolaryngol Head Neck Surg, 2003, 128(3): 419-425.

[159] 田慎之, 陈福进, 曾宗渊, 等. 喉鳞状细胞癌多原发癌81例临床报道[J]. 中华耳鼻咽喉头颈外科杂志, 2006, 41(10): 767-772.

[160] Zhou YQ, Li XM, Gao CM, et al. Clinical analysis of 71 cases of multiple primary cancers in head and neck squamous carcinomas[J]. Zhonghua Er Bi Yan Hou Ke Za Zhi, 2004, 39(4): 232-236.

[161] Beyreuther H. Multiplicitat von Carcinomon bei einem Fal Von Sog. "Schneeberger" Lungenkrebs Mit Tuberkulose[J]. Virchows Arch Pathol Anat Physiol Klin Med, 1924, 250(1): 230-243.

[162] 陈克终, 王迅, 杨帆, 等. 不同影像学表现的多原发肺癌的临床特点及诊疗效果分析[J]. 中华外科杂志, 2015, 53(10): 731-736.

[163] 侯晶晶, 王慧娟, 张国伟, 等. 多原发肺癌的诊断与治疗[J]. 中国肺癌杂志, 2015, 17(12): 764-769.

[164] Shan S, She J, Xue ZQ, et al. Clinical characteristics and survival of lung cancer patients associated with multiple primary malignancies[J]. PLoS One, 2017, 12(9): e0185485.

[165] Jiang L, He J, Shi X, et al. Prognosis of synchronous and metachronous multiple primary lung cancers: Systematic review and meta-analysis[J]. Lung Cancer, 2015, 87(3): 303-310.

[166] Suh YJ, Lee HJ, Sung P, et al. A Novel Algorithm to Differentiate Between Multiple Primary Lung Cancers and Intrapulmonary Metastasis in Multiple Lung Cancers With Multiple Pulmonary Sites of Involvement[J]. J Thorac Oncol, 2020, 15(2): 203-215.

[167] Creach KM, Bradley JD, Mahasittiwat P, et al. Stereotactic body radiation therapy in the treatment of multiple primary lung cancers[J]. Radiother Oncol, 2012, 104(1): 19-22.

[168] Xue X, Liu Y, Pan L, et al. Diagnosis of multiple primary lung cancer: A systematic review[J]. J Int Med Res, 2013, 41(6): 1779-1787.

[169] 郭海法，毛锋，张辉，等．同时性多原发肺癌的预后及生存相关因素研究［J］．中国肺癌杂志，2017，20（1）：21－27．

[170] 王亚龙，王永岗．多原发肺癌研究现状和展望［J］．中华肿瘤防治杂志，2019，26（9）：670－674．

[171] Yuan L, Liu LX, Che GW. The advancement of predictive diagnosis and molecular mechanism in multiple primary lung cancer[J]. Chin J Cancer, 2010, 29(5): 575－578.

[172] 张琦，谢国明，陈科，等．同时性多原发肺癌患者生存状况及其影响因素分析［J］．浙江医学，2019，41（15）：1655－1656，1659．

[173] 李营，金波，施建新，等．41例可手术多原发肺癌临床分析［J］．中国癌症杂志，2014，23（9）：700－706．

[174] 易胜中，张德超，王永岗，等．肺癌和肺外器官恶性肿瘤组成的多原发癌281例临床分析［J］．癌症，2006，25（6）：731－735．

[175] 李连弟，张思维，鲁凤珠，等．中国恶性肿瘤死亡谱及分类构成特征研究［J］．中华肿瘤杂志，1997，19（5）：323－325．

[176] 刘丽，衡伟．EML4－ALK融合基因阳性肺腺癌合并淋巴瘤1例并文献复习［J］．中国肺癌杂志，2015，18（2）：89－91．

[177] 李辉，王伟，尚立群，等．肺癌与多原发癌［J］．中国肺癌杂志，2002，5（3）：211－213．

[178] Grundmann RT, Meyer F. Second primary malignancy among cancer survivors － epidemiology, prognosis and clinical relevance [J]. Zentralbl Chir, 2012, 137 (6): 565－574.

[179] Shibahara Y, Sugawara Y, Miki Y, et al. Analysis of multiple primary cancer autopsy cases associated with breast cancer: 2002－2010[J]. Pathol Int, 2016, 66(12): 695－700.

[180] Weir HK, Johnson CJ, Thompson TD. The effect of multiple primary rules on population－based cancer survival[J]. Cancer Causes Control, 2013, 24(6): 1231－1242.

[181] Jin YK, Hong SS. Metachronous Double Primary Cancer after Treatment of Breast Cancer [J]. Cancer Res Treat, 2014, 47(1): 64－71.

[182] Magid A. Multiple neoplasms, single primaries, and patient survival[J]. Cancer Manag Res, 2014, 6(5): 119－134.

[183] Jobsen JJ, vander Palen J, Ong F, et al. Bilateral breast cancer, synchronous and metachronous: differences and outcome[J]. Breast Cancer Res Treat, 2015, 153（2）: 277－283.

[184] 张慧，山长平．双侧原发性乳腺癌高危因素的研究进展［J］．山东医药，2016，56（13）：99－101．

[185] Ayhan A, Bmer T, Tuneer ZS, et al. Synchronous primary malignancies of the female

genital tract[J]. Eur J Obstet Gynecol Reprod Biol，1992，45(1)：63－66.

[186] Chirila DN，Turdeanu NA，Constantea NA，et al. Multiple malignant tumors[J]. Chirurgia (Bucur)，2013，108(4)：498－502.

[187] Wei JL. Survival and chemotherapy－related risk of second primary malignancy in breast cancer patients：a SEER－based study[J]. Int J Clin Oncol，2019，24(8)：934－940.

[188] Howe HL，Weinstein R，Alvi R，et al. Women multiple primary breast cancers diagnosed with in a five year period，1994—1998[J]. Breast Cancer Res Treat，2005，90(3)：223－232.

[189] 范黎，于钊，任军，等. 61例多原发癌的病种分布和预后分析[J]. 医学争鸣，2002，23(1)：95－96.

[190] Evans HS，Lewis CM，Robinson D，et al. Incidence of multiple primary cancers in a cohort of women diagnosed with breast cancer in southeast England[J]. Br J Cancer，2001，84(3)：435－440.

[191] 杨韵，王宁霞. 合并第二原发癌的乳腺癌患者的病理特征及预后[J]. 暨南大学学报（自然科学与医学版），2018，39(2)：127－130，148.

[192] Soerjomataram I，Louwman WJ，Vandersangen MJ，et al. Increased risk of second malignancies after in situ breast carcinoma in a population－based registry[J]. Br J Cancer，2006，95(3)：393－397.

[193] Ozturk A，Alco G，Sarsenov D，et al. Synchronous and metachronous bilateral breast cancer：a long－term experience[J]. J BUON，2018，23(6)：1591－1600.

[194] Ozer E，Canda T，Kuyucuodlu F. p53 mutations in bilateral breast carcinoma. Correlation with Ki－67 expression and the mean nuclear volume[J]. Cancer Lett，1998，122(1－2)：101－106.

[195] Demirci U，Buğdayci F，Cakir A，et al. Bilateral breast cancer in a survivor of acute lymphoblastic leukemia：a case report[J]. Med Oncol，2010，27(2)：481－483.

[196] Lee KD，Chen SC，Chan CH，et al. Increased risk for second primary malignancies in women with breast cancer diagnosed at young age：a population－based study in Taiwan[J]. Cancer Epidemiol Biomarkers Prevv，2008，17(10)：2647－2655.

[197] 吕淑贞，李艳萍，吕大鹏，等. 31例原发性双侧乳腺癌患者的临床特征分析[J]. 癌症进展，2018，16(4)：452－454.

[198] 沈霖，王惠. 国内486例双侧原发性乳腺癌的临床特点分析[J]. 湖南师范大学学报（医学版），2018，15(1)：58－61.

[199] 王维娜，陈海霞，张银华，等. 双侧原发性乳腺癌90例临床病理及预后分析[J]. 临床与实验病理学杂志，2022，38(1)：9－14.

[200] Huang L，Liu Q，Lang GT，et al. Concordance of hormone receptor satus and BRAC1/2 mutation among women with synchronous bilateral breast cancer[J]. Front Oncol，2020，10

(27): 1-7.

[201] Anwar SL, Prabowo D, Avanti WS, et al. Characteristics and the associated risk factors of the development of bilateral breast cancers: a case-control study[J]. Ann Med Surg, 2020, 60(11): 285-296.

[202] Reinr AS, Lynch CF, Sisti JS, et al. Hormone receptor status of a first primary breast cancer predicts contralateral breast cancer risk in the WECARE study population[J]. Breast Cancer Res, 2017, 19(1): 83-92.

[203] 陈学燕，李利亚，万冬桂，等. 双侧原发性乳腺癌两侧肿瘤病灶的差异性分析[J]. 浙江医学，2020，42(1): 39-43.

[204] Kramer I, Schaapveld M, Oldenburg HSA, et al. The Influence of Adjuvant Systemic Regimens on Contralateral Breast Cancer Risk and Receptor Subtype[J]. J Natl Cancer Inst, 2019, 111(7): 709-718.

[205] Kurian AW, Mcclure LA, John EM, et al. Second primary breast cancer occurrence according to hormone receptor status[J]. J Natl Cancer Inst, 2009, 101(15): 1058-1065.

[206] 康虹，刘新兰. 双侧原发性乳腺癌临床病理特征分析[J]. 宁夏医学杂志，2017，39(1): 67-69.

[207] 徐晓玥，杨为戈，朱玮，等. 25例原发性双侧乳腺癌（BPBC）临床分析[J]. 复旦学报（医学版），2014，41(5): 651-657.

[208] 田青青，刘杰，袁静萍，等. 双侧原发性乳腺癌13例临床病理分析[J]. 诊断病理学杂志，2016，23(5): 324-327.

[209] Ramin C, Withrow DR, Davis Lynn BC, et al. Risk of contralateral breast cancer according to first breast cancer characteristics among women in the USA, 1992-2016[J]. Breast Cancer Res, 2021, 23(1): 24-31.

[210] Rasool M, Naseer MI, Zaigham K, et al. Comparative Study of Alterations in Tri-iodothyronine(T3) and Thyroxine(T4) Hormone Levels in Breast and Ovarian Cancer[J]. Pak J Med Sci, 2014, 30(6): 1356-1360.

[211] Hall LC, Salazar EP, Kane SR, et al. Effects of thyroid hormones on human breast cancer cell proliferation[J]. J Steroid Biochem Mol Biol, 2008, 109(1-2): 57-66.

[212] Joseph KR, Edirimanne S, Eslick GD. The association between breast cancer and thyroid cancer: a meta-analysis[J]. Breast Cancer Res Treat, 2015, 152(1): 173-181.

[213] Li S, Yang J, Shen Y, et al. Clinicopathological features, survival and risk in breast cancer survivors with thyroid cancer: an analysis of the SEER data base[J]. BMC Public Health, 2019, 19(1): 1592-1598.

[214] 王成锋，赵平，白晓枫，等. 乳腺癌合并多原发恶性肿瘤的临床特点[J]. 中华医学杂志，2002，82(18): 1229-1231.

[215] 刘晨, 吴龙, 蒋宏传, 等. 乳腺癌术后并发妇科生殖道恶性肿瘤的高危因素分析[J]. 首都医科大学学报, 2017, 38(1): 92-96.

[216] Grantzau T, Overgaard J. Risk of second non-breast cancer among patients treated with and without postoperative radiotherapy for primary breast cancer: A systematic review and meta-analysis of population-based studies including 522, 739 patients[J]. Radiother Oncol, 2016, 121(3): 402-413.

[217] Grantzau T, Thomsen MS, Vaeth M, et al. Risk of second primary lung cancer in women after radiotherapy for breast cancer[J]. Radiother Oncol, 2014, 111(3): 366-373.

[218] Lu Y, Segelman J, Nordgren A, et al. Increased risk of colorectal cancer inpatients diagnosed with breast cancer in women[J]. Cancer Epidemiol, 2016, 41(7): 57-62.

[219] Levi F, Randimbison L, Blanc-Moya R, et al. High constant incidence of second primary colorectal cancer[J]. Int J Cancer, 2013, 132(7): 1679-82.

[220] Ueno M, Muto T, Oya M, et al. Multiple primary Cancer, all experience at the Cancer Institute Hospital with special reference to colorectal cancer[J]. International Journal of Clinical Oneology, 2003, 8(3): 162-167.

[221] Cheng HY, Chu CH, Chang WH, et al. Clinical analysis of multiple primary malignancies in the digestive system: a hospital-based study[J]. World J Gastmenterot, 2005, 11(27): 4215-4219.

[222] 徐玲玲, 顾康生. 170例多原发恶性肿瘤的临床分析[J]. 安徽医科大学学报, 2011, 46(12): 1318-1321.

[223] Irimie A, Achimas-Cadariu P, Burz C, et al. Multiple primary malignancies - epidemiological analysis at a single tertiary institution[J]. J Gastrointestin Liver Dis, 2010, 19(1): 69-73.

[224] Matsubara T, Yamada K, Nakagawa A. Risk of second primary malignancy after esophagectomy for squamous cell carcinoma ofthe thoracic esophagus[J]. J Clin Oncol, 2003, 21(23): 4336-41.

[225] 张立力, 张振书. 胃肠道多原发恶性肿瘤35例分析[J]. 中华内科杂志, 1999, 38(2): 88-90.

[226] 张培趁, 程骏, 余作黔, 等. 48例胃肠道多原发性肿瘤的临床分析[J]. 浙江临床医学, 2005, 7(1): 15-16.

[227] 苏若瑟, 王其山. 食管与胃相对同时性双原发癌32例临床分析[J]. 中国内镜杂志, 2004, 10(3): 67-68.

[228] 宋丽杰, 吴华星, 付丽娜, 等. 同时性食管多原发癌99例内镜检查分析[J]. 实用肿瘤学杂志, 2008, 22(3): 244-245.

[229] Wang R, Wang MJ, Yang JI, et al. Upper gastrointestinal endoscopy detection of synchronous multiple primary cancers in esophagus and stomach: single center experience

from China[J]. Gastroenterol Res Pract, 2012, 2012(3): 1-4.

[230] Bai Y, Zou DW, Li ZS, et al. Clinical presentation, endoscopic feature streatment and prognosis of synchronous upper gastrointestinal malignancies[J]. J Dig Dis, 2012, 13(1): 19-23.

[231] Agaimy A, Wunsh PH, Sobin LH, et al. Occurrence of other malignancies in patients with gastrointesitnal stromal tumors[J]. Semin Diagn Pathol, 2006, 23(2): 120-129.

[232] Liszka L, Zielinska-Pajak E, Pajk J, et al. Coexistence of gastrointestinal stromal tumors with other neoplasms[J]. J Gastroenterol, 2007, 42(8): 641-649.

[233] Zhao L, Zhang XM, Sun G, et al. The value of lugol chromoendoscopy in diagnosis of multiple primary esophageal carcinoma[J]. Chin J Gastroenterol Hepatol, 2017, 26(5): 534-535.

[234] He S, Liu Y, Liu X, et al. Clinical characteristics of multiple primary cancer associated with esophageal squamous carcinomas[J]. Nat Med J China, 2015, 95(35): 2868-2870.

[235] Koide N, Komatsu D, Hiraga R, et al. Esophageal cancer associated with other primary cancers - historical comparison of clinicopathologic features in 359 esophageal cancer patients[J]. Hepatogastroenterology, 2010, 57(99-100): 513-518.

[236] Chuang, SC, Hashibe, M, Scelo, G, et al. Risk of second primary cancer among esophageal cancer patients: a pooled analysis of 13 cancer registries[J]. Cancer Epidemiol Biomarkers Prevg, 2008, 17(6): 1543-1549.

[237] Gaddam S, Mathur SC, Singh M, et al. Novel probe-based confocal laser endoscroscopy criteria and interobserver agreement for the detection of dysplasia in Barrett's esophagus[J]. Am J Gastroenterol, 2011, 106(11): 1961-1969.

[238] Hori K, Okada H, Kawahara Y, et al. Lugol-voiding lesions are an important risk factor for a second primary squamous cell carcinoma in patients with esophageal cancer or head and neck cancer[J]. Am J Gastroenterol, 2011, 106(5): 858-866.

[239] Otowa Y, Nakamura T, Takiguchi G, et al. Safety and benefit of curative surgical resection for esophageal squamous cell cancer associated with multiple primary cancers[J]. Eur J Surg Oncol, 2016, 42(3): 407-411.

[240] Li QW, Zhu YJ, Zhang WW, et al. Chemoradiotherapy for Synchronous Multiple Primary Cancers with Esophageal Squamous Cell Carcinoma: a Case control Study[J]. J Cancer, 2017, 8(4): 563-569.

[241] Lo OS, Law S, Wei WI, et al. Esophageal cancers with synchronous or antecedent head and neck cancers: a more formidable challenge?[J]. Ann Surg Oncol, 2008, 15(6): 1750-1756.

[242] 章国芬, 蒋锡初, 常建华, 等. 胸段食管癌淋巴结转移特点及意义[J]. 河南肿瘤学

杂志，2003，16(1)：25-26.

[243] Li M, Lin ZX. Characteristics and prognostic factors of synchronous multiple primary esophageal carcinoma：A report of 52 cases[J]. Thorac Cancer, 2014, 5(1)：25-30.

[244] 付尚志，李万平. 多原发癌的诊断与治疗[J]. 临床军医杂志，2011，39(3)：595-596.

[245] SchneiderU, Zwahlen D, Ross D, et al. Estimation of radiation-induced cancer from three-dimensional dose distributions：Concept of organ equivalent dose[J]. Int J Radiat Oncol Biol Phys, 2005, 61(5)：1510-1515.

[246] Kry SF, Salehpour M, Followill DS, et al. The calculated risk of fatal secondary malignancies from intensity-modulated radiation therapy[J]. Int J Radiat Oncol Biol Phys, 2005, 62(4)：1195-1203.

[247] 孙洁，李学良. 食管早癌及癌前病变伴食管外原发肿瘤的临床分析[J]. 胃肠病学和肝病学杂志，2017，26(8)：894-897.

[248] 洪明，陈锦辉，陈金坝. 从食管癌多癌灶及壁内外播散探讨手术范围[J]. 中国肿瘤临床与康复，2003，10(1)：72-74.

[249] Lee JS, Ahn JY, Choi KD, et al. Synchronous second primary cancers in patients with squamous esophageal cancer：clinical features and survival outcome[J]. Korean J Intern Med, 2016, 31(2)：253-259.

[250] Urabe Y, Hiyama T, Tanaka S, et al. Metachronous multiple esophageal squamous cell carcinomas and Lugol-voiding lesions after endoscopic mucosal resection[J]. Endoscopy, 2009, 41(4)：304-309.

[251] 李麦冬，胡长路. 多原发癌176例临床分析[J]. 安徽医药，2017，21(12)：2222-2224.

[252] Shirai K, Tamaki Y, Kitamoto Y, et al. Prognosis was not deteriorated by multiple primary cancers in esophageal cancer patients treated by radiotherapy[J]. J Radiat Res, 2013, 54(4)：706-711.

[253] Strong MS, Incze J, Vaughan CW. Field cancerization in the aerodigestive tractits etiology, manifestation, and significance[J]. J Otolaryngol, 1984, 13(1)：1-6.

[254] Slaughter DP, Southwick HW, Smejkal W. Field cancerization in oral stratified squamous epithelium, clinical implications of multicentric origin[J]. Cancer, 1953, 6(5)：963-968.

[255] Yamamoto M, Yamanaka T, Baba H, et al. The postoperative recurrence and the occurrence of second primary carcinomas in patients with early gastric carcinoma[J]. J Surg Oncol, 2008, 97(3)：231-235.

[256] Ikeda Y, Saku M, Kawanaka H, et al. Features of second primary cancer in patients with gastric cancer[J]. Oncology, 2003, 5(2)：113-117.

[257] 项武,林芳英,陈坚. 37例胃多原发癌的临床病理特征和诊治分析[J]. 中国医疗前沿,2009,3(19):20-21.

[258] 李小毅,钟定荣,陈思,等. 胃癌合并其他器官原发癌103例分析[J]. 中国普外基础与临床杂志,2012,19(1):43-47.

[259] Fernández-Ruiz M, Guerra-Vales JM, Castelbón-Fernández FJ, et al. Multiple primary malignancies in Spanish patients with hepatocellular carcinoma: analysis of a hospital-based tumor registry[J]. J Gastroenterol Hepatol, 2009, 24(8): 1424-1430.

[260] 赵岩,李勇,胡宝山,等. 回顾性总结56例肝细胞癌合并肝外原发恶性肿瘤[J]. 介入放射学杂志,2015,24(1):34-37.

[261] Papadopoulos V, Michalooulos A, Basdan ISG, et al. Synchronous and metachronous colorectal carcinoma[J]. Tech Coloproctol, 2004, 8(1): 97-100.

[262] He WB, Zheng CJ, Wang YH, et al. Prognosis of synchronous colorectal carcinoma compared to solitary colorectal carcinoma: a matched pair analysis[J]. Eur J Gastroenterol Hepatol, 2019, 31(12): 1489-1495.

[263] Tomio Arai, Motoji Sawabe, Kaiyo Takubo, et al. Multiple colorectal cancers in the elderly: a retrospective study of both surgical and autopsy cases[J]. J Gastroenterol, 2001, 36(11): 748-752.

[264] Lam AK, Chan SS. Synchronous colorectal cancer: clinical, pathological and molecular implications[J]. World J Gastroenterol, 2014, 20(22): 6815-6820.

[265] Ikeda Y, Saku M, Kawanaka H, et al. Distribution of synchronous and metachronous multiple colorectal cancers[J]. Hepatogastroenterology, 2004, 51(56): 443-446.

[266] Lee JW, Kim JW, Kim NK. Clinical characteristics of colorectal cancer patients with a second primary cancer[J]. Ann Coloproctol, 2014, 30(1): 18-22.

[267] Brennan P, Scelo G, Hemminki K, et al. Second primary cancers among 109000 cases of non-Hodgkin's Lymphoma[J]. Br J Cancer, 2005, 93(1): 159-166.

[268] 秦燕,冯奉仪,石远凯. 淋巴瘤与多原发肿瘤的关系[J]. 北京医学,2009,31(9):520-522.

[269] Schaapveld M, Aleman BMP, Vaneggermond AM, et al. Second Cancer Risk Up to 40 Years after Treatment for Hodgkin's Lymphoma[J]. N Engl J Med, 2015, 373(26): 2499-2511.

[270] Hill DA, Gilbert E, Dores GM, et al. Breast cancer risk following radiotherapy for Hodgkin lymphoma: modification by other risk factors[J]. Blood, 2005, 106(10): 3358-3365.

[271] Sud A, Thomsen H, Sundquist K, et al. Risk of Second Cancer in Hodgkin's Lymphoma Survivors and Influence of Family History[J]. J Clin Oncol, 2017, 35(14): 1584-1590.

[272] Moskowitz CS, Chou JF, Wolden SL, et al. Breast Cancer After Chest Radiation Therapy for Childhood Cancer[J]. J Clin Oncol, 2014, 32(21): 2217-2223.

[273] Nakamura K, Omagari J, Kunitake N, et al. Non – Hodgkin's lymphoma and coexisting primary cancers: a retrospective clinical analysis of 10 patients[J]. Am J Clin Oncol, 1999, 22(9): 283 – 285.

[274] 谢通,王之龙,王正航,等. 结直肠癌合并淋巴瘤病例诊疗分享[J]. 肿瘤综合治疗电子杂志,2023,9(2): 170 – 173.

[275] Barron BA, Localio SA. A statistical note on the association of colorectal cancer and lymphoma[J]. Am J Epidemiol, 1976, 104(5): 517 – 522.

[276] Pineda M, Castellsague E, Musulen E, et al. Non – Hodgkin lymphoma related to hereditary nonpolyposis colorectal cancer in a patient with a novel heterozygous complex deletion in the MSH2 gene[J]. Genes Chromosomes Cancer, 2008, 47(4): 326 – 332.

[277] Rosty C, Briere J, Cellier C, et al. Association of a duodenal follicular lymphoma and hereditary nonpolyposis colorectal cancer[J]. Mod Pathol, 2000, 13(5): 586 – 590.

[278] Kataoka J, Nitta T, Oota M, et al. Collision Tumor Comprising Primary Malignant Lymphoma and Adenocarcinoma in the Ascendin Colon[J]. Case Rep Gastroenterol, 2021, 15(1): 379 – 388.

[279] Joung JY, Lim J, Oh CM, et al. Risk of second primary cancer among prostate cancer patients in korea: a population – based cohort study[J]. PLoS One, 2015, 10(10): e0140693.

[280] Fan CY, Huang WY, Lin CS, et al. Risk of second primary malignancies among patients with prostate cancer: a population – based cohort study[J]. PLoS One, 2017, 12(4): e0175217.

[281] 叶天仪,姚洪文,吴令英,等. 34例子宫内膜癌合并结直肠癌双原发癌的临床特征及其与Lynch综合征关系分析[J]. 中国肿瘤临床,2015,42(8): 432 – 436.

[282] Etiz D, Metcalfe E, Akcay M. Multiple primary malignant neoplasms: A 10 – year experience at a single institution from Turkey[J]. J Cancer Res Ther, 2017, 13(1): 16 – 20.

[283] Boice JD Jr, Kleinerman RA, Flannery JT, et al. Multiple primary cancers in Connecticut, 1935 – 1982[J]. Yale J Biol Med, 1986, 59(5): 533 – 545.

[284] Cavazos TB, Kachuri L, Graff RE, et al. Assessment of genetic susceptibility to multiple primary cancers through whole – exome sequencing in two large multi – ancestry studies[J]. BMC Med, 2022, 20(1): 332 – 341.

[285] Chan GHJ, Ong PY, Low JJH, et al. Clinical genetic testing outcome with multi – gene panel in Asian patients with multiple primary cancers[J]. Oncotarget, 2018, 9(55): 30649 – 30660.

[286] Murphy CC, Gerber DE, Pruittsl P. Revalence of prior cancer a – Mong persons newly diagnosed with cancer: An initial report from the survey Uance, epidemiology, and end

results program[J]. JAMA Oncol, 2018, 4(6): 832-836.

[287] Luciani A, Ascione G, Marussi D, et al. Clinical analysis of multiple primary malignancies in the elderly[J]. Med Oncol, 2009, 26(1): 27-31.

[288] Lawniczak M, Gawin A, Jaroszewicz-Heigelmann H, et al. Synchronous and metachronous neoplasms in gastric cancer patients: a 23-year study[J]. World J Gastroenterol, 2014, 20(23): 7480-7487.

[289] Rubino C, De Vathaire F, Diallo I, et al. Increased risk of second cancers following breast cancer: role of the initial treatment[J]. Breast Cancer Res Treat, 2000, 61(3): 183-195.

[290] Motuzyuk I, Sydorchuk O, Kovtun N, et al. Analysis of Trends and Factors in Breast Multiple Primary Malignant Neoplasms [J]. Breast Cancer (Auckl), 2018, 12: 1178223418759959.

[291] NarodSA, Kharazmi E, Fallah M, et al. The risk of contralateral breast cancer in daughters of women with and without breast cancer[J]. Clin Genet, 2016, 89(3): 332-335.

[292] 张常华, 何裕隆, 詹文华, 等. 结直肠多原发癌患者的临床分析[J]. 中华胃肠外科杂志, 2005, 8(1): 38-40.

[293] Wang HZ, Huang XF, Wang Y, et al. Clinical features, diagnosis, treatment and prognosis of multiple primary colorectal carcinoma[J]. World J Gastroenterol, 2004, 10(14): 2136-2139.

[294] Chiang JM, Yeh CY, Changchien CR, et al. Clinical features of second other site primary cancers among sporadic colorectal cancer patients a hospital based study of 3,722 cases [J]. Hepatogastroenterology, 2004, 51(59): 1341-1344.

[295] Yang J, Peng JY. Synchronous colorectal cancers: a review of clinical features, diagnosis, treatment, and prognosis[J]. Dig Surg, 2011, 28(5-6): 379-385.

[296] Samadder NJ, Curtin K, Wong J, et al. Epidemiology and familial risk of synchronous and metachronous colorectal cancer: a population-based study in Utah[J]. Clin Gastroenterol Hepatol, 2014, 12(12): 2078-2084.

[297] Lee BC, Yu CS, Kim J, et al. Clinicopathological features andsurgical options for synchronous colorectal cancer[J]. Medicine, 2017, 96(9): e6224.

[298] Girard N, Deshpande C, Azzoli CG, et al. Use of epidermal growth factor receptor/Kirsten rat sarcoma 2 viral oncogene homolog mutation testing to define clonal relationships among multiple lung adenocarcinomas: comparison with clinical guidelines[J]. Chest, 2010, 137(1): 46-52.

[299] Arai J, Tsuchiya T, Oikawa M, et al. Clinical and molecular analysis of synchronous double lung cancers[J]. Lung cancer(Amsterdam, Netherlands), 2012, 77(2): 281-287.

[300] Freedman ND, Abnet CC, Caporaso NE, et al. Impact of changing US cigarette smoking patterns on incident cancer: risks of 20 smoking-related cancers among the women and men of the NIH-AARP cohort[J]. Int J Epidemiol, 2016, 45(3): 846-856.

[301] Spratt JS, Jr M, Hoag MG. Incidence of multiple primary cancers per man-year of follow up: 20-year review from the Ellis Fischel State Cancer Hospital[J]. Ann Surg, 1966, 164(5): 775-784.

[302] Haas JF, Kittelmann B, Mehnert WH, et al. Risk of leukaemia in ovarian tumour and breast cancer patients following treatment by cyclophosphamide[J]. Br J Cancer, 1987, 55(2): 213-218.

[303] Yamamoto S, Yoshimura K, Ri S, et al. The risk of multiple primary malignancies with colorectal carcinoma[J]. Dis Colon Rectum, 2006, 49(10 Suppl): s30-s36.

[304] Varol U, Kucukzeybek Y, Alacacioglu A, et al. BRCA genes: BRCA 1 and BRCA 2 [J]. J BUON, 2018, 23(4): 862-866.

[305] 陈洪兴, 周桂娥, 杨云利. 多原发癌的研究进展[J]. 中国肿瘤临床与康复, 2009, 16(5): 452-454.

[306] Thomas GA. Solid cancers after therapeutic radiation-can we predict which patients are most at risk?[J]. Clin Oncol, 2004, 16(6): 429-434.

[307] Travis LB, Demark Wahnefried W, Allan JM, et al. Aetiology, genetics and prevention of secondary neoplasms in adult cancer survivors[J]. Nat Rev Clin Oncol, 2013, 10(5): 289-301.

[308] Dubey AK, Gupta U, Jain S. Breast cancer statistics and prediction methodology: a systematic review and analysis[J]. Asian Pac J Cancer Prev, 2015, 16(10): 4237-4245.

[309] Jégu J, Colonna M, Daubisse-Marliac L, et al. The effect of patient characteristics on second primary cancer risk in France[J]. BMC Cancer, 2014, 14(1): 1-14.

[310] Quilon JM, Day S, Lasker JC. Synchronous tumors: Hodgkin disease presenting in mesenteric lymphnodes from a right hemicolectomy for colon carcinoma[J]. South Med J, 2004, 97(11): 1133-1135.

[311] Kato T, Alonso S, Muto Y, et al. Clinical characteristics of synchronous colorectal cancers in Japan[J]. World J Surg Oncol, 2016, 14(1): 272.

[312] Chin CC, Kuo YH. Synchronous colorectal carcinoma: predisposing factors and characteristics[J]. Colorectal Dis, 2019, 21(4): 432-440.

[313] Nakashima M, Kondo H, Miura S, et al. Incidence of multiple primary cancers in Nagasaki atomic bomb survivors: association with radiation exposure[J]. Cancer Sci, 2008, 99(1): 87-92.

[314] Pisani P, Parkin DM, Mufioz N, et al. Cancer and infection: estimates of the attributable

fraction in 1990[J]. Cancer Epidemiol Biomarkers Prev, 1997, 6(6): 387 - 400.

[315] Neumann F, Jagu J, Mougin C, et al. Risk of second primary cancer after a first potentially - human papilloma virus - related cancer: A population - based study[J]. Prev Med, 2016, 90: 52 - 58.

[316] Huang WB, Chan JY, Liu DL. Human papillomavirus and World Health Organization type Ⅲ nasopharyngeal carcinoma: Multicenter study from an endemic area in Southern China [J]. Cancer, 2017, 124(3): 530 - 536.

[317] Ghislaine S, Paolo B, Marilys C, et al. Second primary cancers in patients with nasopharyngeal carcinoma: a pooled analysis of 13 cancer registries[J]. Cancer Causes Control, 2007, 18(3): 269 - 278.

[318] Ohno Z, Tamaki H, Ohsuga T, et al. Primary lung cancer complicated by malignant lymphoma in two cases of epstein - barr virus infection[J]. Case Rep Oncol, 2012, 5(2): 367 - 372.

[319] Cybulski C, Nazarali S, Narod SA. Multiple primary cancers as a guide to heritability[J]. Int J Cancer, 2014, 135(8): 1756 - 1763.

[320] Nyqvist J. Metachronous and synchronous occurrence of 5 primary malignancies in a female patient between 1997 and 2013: a case report with germline and somatic genetic analysis [J]. Case Rep Oncol, 2017, 10(3): 1006 - 1012.

[321] Ravis LB, Rabkin CS, Brown LM, et al. Cancer Survivorship - Genetic Susceptibility and Second Primary Cancers: Research Strategies and Recommendations[J]. J Natl Cancer Inst, 2006, 98(1): 15 - 25.

[322] 付文静, 李吉林, 郭二涛, 等. 1011例食管/贲门双原发癌(双源癌)患者的家族史、临床病理及生存期分析[J]. 河南大学学报(医学版), 2012, 31(3): 206 - 209.

[323] 李永丽, 张立玮, 丁国瑾, 等. 单发及双原发癌食管鳞癌CDH1基因甲基化的研究[J]. 实用医学杂志, 2011, 27(24): 4411 - 4413.

[324] Wen D, Shan B, Wang S, et al. Apositive family history of esophageal/gastric cardia cancer with gastric cardia adenocarcinom a is associated with a younger age at onset and more likely with another synchronous esophageal/gastric cardia cancer in a Chinese high - risk area[J]. Eur J Med Genet, 2010, 53(5): 250 - 255.

[325] Simpkins F, Zahurak M, Armstrong D, et al. Ovarian malignancy in breast cancer patients with an adnexal mass[J]. Obstet Gynecol, 2005, 105(3): 507 - 513.

[326] Zheng G, Hemminki A, Försti A, et al. Second Primary cancer after female breast cancer: Familial risks and cause of death[J]. Cancer Med, 2019, 8(1): 400 - 407.

[327] Chaturvedi AK, Engels EA, Gilbert ES, et al. Second cancers among 104,760 survivors of cervical cancer: evaluation of long - term risk[J]. J Natl Cancer Inst, 2007, 99(21): 1634 - 1643.

[328] Kuchenbaecker KB. Risks of breast, ovarian, and contralateral breast cancer for BRCAL and BRCA2 mutation carriers[J]. JAMA, 2017, 317(23): 2402-2416.

[329] Bouchardy C, Benhamou S, Fioretta G, et al. Risk of second breast cancer according to estrogen receptor status and family history[J]. Breast Cancer Res Treat, 2011, 127(1): 233-241.

[330] Hopper JL. Genetic epidemiology of female breast cancer[J]. Semin Cancer Biol, 2001, 11(5): 367-374.

[331] Reiner AS, Sisti J, John EM, et al. Breast Cancer Family History and Contralateral Breast Cancer Risk in Young Women: An Update From the Women's Environmental Cancer and Radiation Epidemiology Study[J]. J Clin Oncol, 2018, 36(15): 1513-1520.

[332] Winawer SJ, Zauser AG, Ho MN, et al. Prevention of colorectal cancer by colonoscopic polypectomy. The national polyp study workgroup[J]. N Engl J Med, 1993, 329(27): 1977-1981.

[333] 郑杰. 结直肠息肉和结直肠癌[J]. 中华病理学杂志, 2005, 34(1): 4-5.

[334] 颜登国, 张汝一, 甄运寰, 等. 多原发大肠癌的临床病理特点(附40例报告)[J]. 中华临床医学实践杂志, 2005, 24(1): 11-12.

[335] Ng SC, Ching JY, Chan VC, et al. Association between serrated polyps and the risk of synchronous advanced colorectal neoplasia in average-risk individuals[J]. Aliment Pharmacol Ther, 2015, 41(1): 108-115.

[336] Hu H, Chang DT, Nikiforova MN, et al. Clinicopathologic features of synchronous colorectal carcinoma: a distinct subset arising from multiple sessile serrated adenomasand associated with high levels of microsatellite instability and favorable prognosis[J]. Am J Surg Pathol, 2013, 37(11): 1660-1670.

[337] Drew DA, Nishihara R, Lochhead P, et al. Aprospective study of smoking and risk of synchronous colorectal cancers[J]. Am J Gastroenterol, 2017, 112(3): 493-501.

[338] Soliman PT, Slomovitz BM, Broaddus RR, et al. Synchronous primary cancers of the endometrium and ovary: a single institution review of 84 cases[J]. Gynecol Oncol, 2004, 94(2): 456-462.

[339] 王加璐, 赵隽, 张颖. 雌激素受体与乳腺癌、子宫内膜癌及卵巢癌关系的研究及争议[J]. 中国实用医药, 2008, 3(24): 191-192.

[340] Miki Y, Sugawara Y, Shibahara Y, et al. Multiple primary cancers associated with endometrial and ovarian cancers: An analysis based upon the Japan Autopsy Annual Database from 2002 to 2010[J]. J Obstet Gynaecol Res, 2019, 45(5): 1012-1018.

[341] Le BouEdec G, Kauffmann P, Richard JF, et al. Association of breast cancer and cancer of the uterus 34 case reports[J]. Rev Fr Gynecol Obstet, 1993, 88(3): 136-141.

[342] Sommer S, Fuqu A, Sa W. Estrogen receptor and breast cancer[J]. Semin Cancer Biol,

2001, 11(5), 339-352.

[343] Wik E, Raeder MB, Krakstad C, et al. Lack of estrogen receptor-a is associated with epithelial-mesenchy maltransition and pi3k alterations in endometrial carcinoma[J]. Clin Cancer Res, 2013, 19(5): 1094-1051.

[344] Aust S, Bachmayr-Heyda A, Pateisky P, et al. Role of trap 1 and estrogen receptor alpha in patients with ovarian cancer-a study of the ovcad consortium[J]. Mol Cancer, 2012, 11(1): 1-10

[345] Network TC. Comprehensive molecular portraits of human breast tumours[J]. Nature, 2012, 490(7418): 61-70.

[346] 叶岚, 艾毅钦, 吴星娆, 等. 宫颈癌合并乳腺癌7例临床分析[J]. 实用妇产科杂志, 2016, 32(3): 229-232.

[347] 黄剑波, 汲广岩, 邢雷, 等. 合并原发性甲亢的乳腺癌患者围术期及化疗期间甲状腺危象的防治[J]. 重庆医学, 2012, 41(27): 2873-2874.

[348] 谢天红, 姜松伍, 邱志武. 乳腺癌患者再发甲状腺癌9例临床分析[J]. 肿瘤学杂志, 2011, 17(6): 471-472.

[349] 运新伟, 高明. 甲状腺与乳腺多原发肿瘤的临床特征分析[J]. 中华内分泌外科杂志, 2012, 6(1): 28-31.

[350] Vannucchi G, De Leo S, Perrino M, et al. Impact of estrogen and progesterone receptor expression on the clinical and molecular features of papillary thyroid cancer[J]. Eur J Endocrinol, 2015, 173(1): 29-36.

[351] 张楠, 李国萍, 孙瑞梅, 等. 甲状腺及生殖系统多原发癌临床分析[J]. 昆明医科大学学报, 2014, 35(3): 32-35.

[352] 殷德涛, 唐艺峰, 王勇飞, 等. 甲状腺及乳腺多原发癌的临床分析[J]. 中华内分泌外科杂志, 2014, (2): 109-111.

[353] 郑美珠, 郑刚, 左文述, 等. 乳腺和甲状腺及胸骨多原发恶性肿瘤一例诊疗启示[J]. 中华肿瘤防治杂志, 2013, 20(1): 156.

[354] 许泽艳, 杨志贤, 廖承德, 等. 合并甲状腺癌的多原发性癌的临床及病理特征分析[J]. 中国肿瘤临床, 2018, (18): 163-165.

[355] 赖兴建, 张波. 甲状腺及乳腺多原发癌临床及超声特征[J]. 协和医学杂志, 2014, 5(1): 22-25.

[356] Kim EY, Chang Y, Lee KH, et al. Serum concentration of thyroid hormones in abnormal and euthyroid ranges and breast cancer risk: A cohort study[J]. Int J Cancer, 2019, 145(12): 3257-3266.

[357] van Denbelt-Duseboutmsc AW, Berthempalemanmd PD, Scg BM, et al. Roles of Radiation Dose and Chemotherapy in the Etiology of Stomach Cancer as a Second Malignancy[J]. Int J Radiat Oncol Biol Phys, 2009, 75(5): 1420-1429.

[358] Watanabe S. Epidemiology of multiple primary cancer[J]. Gan To Kagaku Ryoho, 1990, 17(5): 967 - 973.

[359] Wong FL, Boice JD, Abramson DH. Cancer Incidence After Retinoblastoma[J]. JAMA, 2008, 278: 1263 - 1267.

[360] Kleinerman RA, Tucker MA, Tarone RE, et al. Risk of New Cancers After Radiotherapy in Long - Term Survivors of Retinoblastoma: An Extended Follow - Up[J]. J Clin Oncol, 2005, 23(10): 2272 - 2279.

[361] Bhatia S. Role of Genetic Susceptibility in Development of Treatment - Related Adverse Outcomes in Cancer Survivors[J]. Cancer Epidemiol Biomarkers Prev, 2011, 20(10): 2048 - 2067.

[362] Wallin JL, Tai AN, Misra S, et al. Sinonasal carcinoma after irradiation for medulloblastoma in nevoid basal cell carcinoma syndrome[J]. Am J Otolaryngol, 2007, 28(5): 360 - 362.

[363] Sharif S, Ferner R, Birch JM, et al. Second Primary Tumors in Neurofibromatosis 1 Patients Treated for Optic Glioma: Substantial Risks After Radiotherapy[J]. J Clin Oncol, 2006, 24(16): 2570 - 2575.

[364] Bassal M, Mertens AC, Taylor L, et al. Risk of Selected Subsequent Carcinomas in Survivors of Childhood Cancer: A Report From the Childhood Cancer Survivor Study[J]. J Clin Oncol, 2006, 24(3): 476 - 483.

[365] Breslow NE, Lange JM, Friedman DL, et al. Secondary malignant neoplasms after Wilms tumor: An international collaborative study[J]. Int J Cancer, 2010, 127(3): 657 - 666.

[366] Henderson TO, Whitton J, Stovall M, et al. Secondary Sarcomas in Childhood Cancer Survivors: A Report From the Childhood Cancer Survivor Study[J]. J Natl Cancer Inst, 2007, 99(4): 300 - 308.

[367] Best T, Li D, Skol AD, et al. Variants at 6q21 implicate PRDM 1 in the etiology of therapy - induced second malignancies after Hodgkin's lymphoma[J]. Nat Med, 2011, 17(8): 941 - 943.

[368] Mudie NY, Swerdlow AJ, Higgins CD, et al. Risk of Second Malignancy After Non - Hodgkin'S Lymphoma: A British Cohort Study[J]. J Clin Oncol, 2006, 24(10): 1568 - 1574.

[369] Seedhouse C. The genotype distribution of the XRCC 1 gene indicates a role for base excision repair in the development of therapy - related acute myeloblastic leukemia[J]. Blood, 2002, 100(10): 3761 - 3766.

[370] Allan JM. Genetic variation in XPD predicts treatment outcome and risk of acute myeloid leukemia following chemotherapy[J]. Blood, 2004, 104(13): 3872 - 3877.

[371] Mahmood S, Vu K, Tai P, et al. Radiation-induced Second Malignancies[J]. Anticancer Res, 2015, 35(4): 2431-2434.

[372] Najafi M, Fardid R, Takhshid MA, et al. Radiation-Induced Oxidative Stress at Out-of-Field Lung Tissues after Pelvis Irradiation in Rats[J]. Cell J, 2016, 18(3): 340-345.

[373] Allan JM, Travis LB. Mechanisms of therapy-related carcinogenesis[J]. Nat Rev Cancer, 2005, 5(12): 943-955.

[374] Patil VM, Kapoor R, Chakraborty S, et al. Dosimetric risk estimates of radiation-induced malignancies after intensity modulated radiotherapy[J]. J Cancer Res Ther, 2010, 6(4): 442-448.

[375] Barazzuol L, Coppes RP, van Luijk P. Prevention and treatment of radiotherapy-induced side effects[J]. Mol Oncol, 2020, 14(7): 1538-1554.

[376] Marees T, Moll AC, Imhof SM, et al. Risk of Second Malignancies in Survivors of Retinoblastoma: More Than 40 Years of Follow-up[J]. J Natl Cancer Inst, 2008, 100(24): 1771-1779.

[377] Begg AC, Stewart FA, Vens C. Strategies to improve radiotherapy with targeted drugs[J]. Nat Rev Cancer, 2011, 11(4): 239-253.

[378] Warnakulasuriya KA, Robinson D, Evans H. Multiple primary tumours following head and neck cancer in Southern England during 1961-68[J]. Oral Pathol Med, 2003, 32(8): 443-449.

[379] Morton LM, Swerdlow AJ, Schaapveld M, et al. Current knowledge and future research directions in treatment-related second primary malignancies[J]. EJC Suppl, 2014, 12(1): 5-17.

[380] Preston DL, Ron E, Tokuoka S, et al. Solid cancer incidence in atomic bomb survivors: 1958-1998[J]. Radiat Res, 2007, 168(1): 1-64.

[381] Supramaniam R. New malignancies among cancer survivors: SEER cancer registries, 1973-2000[J]. J Epidemiol Community Health, 2013, 62(4): 375-376.

[382] Chuang SC, Hashibe M, Yu GP, et al. Radiotherapy for primary thyroid cancer as a risk factor for second primary cancers[J]. Cancer Lett, 2006, 238(1): 42-52.

[383] Brown LM, Chen BE, Pfeiffer RM, et al. Risk of second non-hematological malignancies among 376,825 breast cancer survivors[J]. Breast Cancer Res Treat, 2007, 106(3): 439-451.

[384] Schenke JG, Levinsky R, Ohel G. Multiple primary malignant neoplasms in breast cancer patients in Israel[J]. Cancer, 1984, 54(1): 145-152.

[385] Aleman BM, Van DEN, Belt-dusebout AW, et al. Long-term cause-specific mortality of patients treated for Hodgkin's disease[J]. J Clin Oncol, 2003, 21(18): 3388-3390.

[386] Yung L, Ljnch D. Hodgkin's lymphoma[J]. Lancet, 2003, 361(9361): 943-951.

[387] Bhatia S, Yasui Y, Robison LL, et al. High Risk of Subsequent Neoplasms Continues With Extended Follow-Up of Childhood Hodgkin'S Disease: Report From the Late Effects Study Group[J]. J Clin Oncol, 2003, 21(23): 4386-4394.

[388] Morton LM, Gilbert ES, Hall P, et al. Risk of treatment-related esophageal cancer among breast cancer survivors[J]. Ann Oncol, 2012, 23(12): 3081-3091.

[389] Dores GM, Metayer C, Curtis RE, et al. Second malignant neoplasms among long-term survivors of Hodgkin'S disease: a population-based evaluation over 25 years[J]. J Clin Oncol, 2002, 20(16): 3484-3494.

[390] Travis LB, Hill DA, Dores GM. Breast Cancer Following Radiotherapy and Chemotherapy Among Young Women With Hodgkin Disease[J]. JAMA, 2003, 290(4): 465-475.

[391] Sigurdson AJ, Ronckers CM, Mertens AC, et al. Primary thyroid cancer after a first tumour in childhood(the Childhood Cancer Survivor Study): a nested case-control study [J]. Lancet, 2005, 365(9476): 2014-2023.

[392] Mph RAK, Mph SAS, Md EH, et al. Radiation Dose and Subsequent Risk for Stomach Cancer in Long-term Survivors of Cervical Cancer[J]. Int J Radiat Oncol Biol Phys, 2013, 86(5): 922-929.

[393] Kabat GC. Previous cancer and radiotherapy as risk factors for lung cancer in lifetime non-smokers[J]. Cancer Causes Control, 1993, 4(5): 489-495.

[394] Diallo I, Haddy N, Adjadj E, et al. Frequency distribution of second solid cancer locations in relation to the irradiated volume among 115 patients treated for childhood cancer[J]. Int J Radiat Oncol Biol Phys, 2009, 74(3): 876-883.

[395] Berrington de Gonzalez A, Gilbert E, Curtis R, et al. Second solid cancers after radiation therapy: a systematic review of the epidemiologic studies of the radiation dose-response relationship[J]. Int J Radiat Oncol Biol Phys, 2013, 86(2): 224-233.

[396] Morton LM, Dores GM, Curtis RE, et al. Stomach Cancer Risk After Treatment for Hodgkin's Lymphoma[J]. J Clin Oncol, 2013, 31(27): 3369-3377.

[397] Dmaae DM, Samyae-Badawy MF, Alphonse G, et al. Breast Cancer after Treatment of Hodgkin's Lymphoma: General Review[J]. Int J Radiat Oncol Biol Phys, 2008, 72(5): 1291-1297.

[398] Travis LB, Hill D, Dores GM, et al. Cumulative Absolute Breast Cancer Risk for Young Women Treated for Hodgkin Lymphoma[J]. J Natl Cancer Inst, 2005, 97(19): 1428-1437.

[399] Elkin EB, Klem ML, Gonzales AM, et al. Characteristics and Outcomes of Breast Cancer in Women With and Without a History of Radiation for Hodgkin'S Lymphoma: A Multi-Institutional, Matched Cohort Study[J]. J Clin Oncol, 2011, 29(18): 2466-2473.

[400] Inskip PD, Robison LL, Stovall M, et al. Radiation dose and breast cancer risk in the

childhood cancer survivor study[J]. J Clin Oncol, 2009, 27(24): 3901-3907.

[401] Debruin ML, Sparidans J, Vantveer MB, et al. Breast cancer risk in female survivors of Hodgkin's lymphoma: lower risk after smaller radiation volumes[J]. J Clin Oncol, 2009, 27(26): 4239-4246.

[402] Cooke R, Jones ME, Cunningham D, et al. Breast cancer risk following Hodgkin lymphoma radiotherapy in relation to menstrual and reproductive factors[J]. Br J Cancer, 2013, 108(11): 2399-2406.

[403] Swerdlow AJ, Cooke R, Bates A, et al. Breast Cancer Risk After Supradiaphragmatic Radiotherapy for Hodgkin'S Lymphoma in England and Wales: A National Cohort Study[J]. J Clin Oncol, 2012, 30(22): 2745-2752.

[404] Taylor AJ, Winter DL, Stiller CA, et al. Risk of breast cancer in female survivors of childhood Hodgkin's disease in Britain: A populmion-based study[J]. Int J Cancer, 2006, 120(2): 384-391.

[405] Hashibe M, Ritz B, Le AD, et al. Radiotherapy for oral cancer risk factor for second primary cancers[J]. Cancer Lett, 2005, 220(2): 185-195.

[406] Taylor AJ, Croft AP, Palace AM, et al. Risk of thyroid cancer in survivors of childhood cancer: Results from the British Childhood Cancer Survivor Study[J]. Int J Cancer, 2009, 125(10): 2400-2405.

[407] De Gonzalez AB, Curtis RE, Gilbert E, et al. Second solid cancers after radiotherapy for breast cancer in SEER cancer registries[J]. Br J Cancer, 2010, 102(1): 220-226.

[408] Schaapveld M, Visser O, Louwman MJ, et al. Risk of new primary non-breast cancers after breast cancer treatment: a Dutch population-based study[J]. J Clin Oncol, 2008, 26(8): 1239-1246.

[409] Salminen EK, Pukkala E, Kiel KD, et al. Impact of radiotherapy in the risk of esophageal cancer as subsequent Primary cancer after breast cancer[J]. Int J Radiat Oncol Biol Phys, 2006, 65(3): 699-704.

[410] Grantzau T, Mellemkj R, Lovergaard J. Second primary cancers after adjuvant radiotherapy in early breast cancer patients: a national population based study under the Danish Breast Cancer Cooperative Group(DBCG)[J]. Radiother Oncol, 2013, 106(1): 42-49.

[411] Huang YJ, Huang TW, Lin FH, et al. Radiation therapy for invasive breast cancer increases the risk of second primary lung cancer: a nation wide population-based cohort analysis[J]. J Thoracic Oncol, 2017, 12(5): 782-790.

[412] Andersson M, Jensen MB, Engholm G, et al. Risk of second primary canceramong patients with early operable breast cancer registered or randomised in Danish Breast Cancer cooperative Group(DBCG) protocols of the 77, 82 and 89 programmes during 1977-2001[J]. Acta Oncol, 2008, 47(4): 755-764.

[413] Tucker MA, Nevin M, Shaw EG, et al. Second Primary Cancers Related to Smoking and Treatment of Small-Cell Lung Cancer[J]. J Natl Cancer Inst, 1997, 89(23): 1782-1788.

[414] Birgisson H, Pahlman L, Gunnarsson U, et al. Occurrence of second cancers in patients treated with radiotherapy for rectal cancer[J]. J Clin Oncol, 2005, 23(25): 6126-6131.

[415] Travis LB, Gospodarowicz M, Curtis RE, et al. Lung cancer following chemotherapy and radiotherapy for hodgkin's disease[J]. J Natl Cancer Inst, 2002, 94(3): 182-192.

[416] Sill H, Olipitz W, Zebisch A, et al. Therapy-related myeloid neoplasms: pathobiology and clinical characteristics[J]. Br J Pharmacol, 2011, 162(4): 792-805.

[417] Rondeau V, Mathoulin-P Lissier S, Tanneau L, et al. Separate and combined analysis of successive dependent outcomes after breast-conservation surgery: Recurrence, metastases, second cancer and eath[J]. BMC Cancer, 2010, 10(1): 1-12.

[418] Oeffinger KC, Baxi SS, Moskowitz CS, et al. Solid tumor second primary neoplasms: who is at risk, what can we do? [J]. Semin Oncol, 2013, 40(6): 676-689.

[419] Leone G, Pagano L, Ben-Yehuda D, et al. Therapy-related leukemia and myelodysplasia: susceptibility and incidence[J]. Haematologica, 2007, 92(10): 1389-1398.

[420] Azarova AM, Lyu YL, Lin CP, et al. Roles of DNA topoi-somerase II isozymes in chemotherapy and secondary malignancies[J]. Proc Natl Acad Sci USA, 2007, 104(26): 11014-11019.

[421] Seedhouse C, Russell N. Advances in the understanding of susceptibility to treatment-related acute myeloid leukaemia[J]. Br J Haematol, 2007, 137(6): 513-529.

[422] Bhatia S. Therapy-Related Myelodysplasia and Acute Myeloid Leukemia[J]. Semin Oncol, 2013, 40(6): 666-675.

[423] 蔡耿喜, 卢绮思, 刘情, 等. 乳腺癌治疗相关性急性白血病九例临床分析并文献复习[J]. 中国全科医学, 2016, 19(6): 710-714.

[424] Matesich SMA, ShaPiro CL. Second cancers after breast cancer treatment[J]. Semin Oncol, 2003, 30(6): 740-748.

[425] Dong C, Chen L. Second malignancies after breast cancer: The impact of adjuvant therapy[J]. Mol Clin Oncol, 2014, 2(3): 331-336.

[426] Kwast AB, Liu L, Roukema JA, et al. Increased risks of third primary cancers of non-breast origin among women with bilateral breast cancer[J]. Br J Cancer, 2012, 107(3): 549-555.

[427] Howard RA, Gilbert ES, Chen BE, et al. Leukemia following breast cancer: An international population-based study of 376,825 womens[J]. Breast Cancer Res Treat, 2007, 105(3): 359-368.

[428] Swerdlow AJ, Higgins CD, Smith P, et al. Second Cancer Risk After Chemotherapy for Hodgkin'S Lymphoma: A Collaborative British Cohort Study[J]. J Clin Oncol, 2011, 29(31): 4096-4104.

[429] Andre M. Second cancers and late toxicities after treatment of aggressive non-Hodgkin lymphoma with the ACVBP regimen: a GELA cohort study on 2837 patients[J]. Blood, 2004, 103(4): 1222-1228.

[430] Casorelli I. Drug treatment in the development of mismatch repair defective acute leukemia and myelodysplastic syndrome[J]. DNA Repair (Amst), 2003, 2(5): 547-559.

[431] Seedhouse CH, Das-Gupta EP, Russell NH. Methylation of the hMLH 1 promoter and its association with microsatellite instability in acute myeloid leukemia[J]. Leukemia, 2003, 17(1): 83-88.

[432] Bermejo JL, Sundquist J, Hemminki K. Bladder cancer in cancer patients: population-based estimates from a large Swedish study[J]. Br J Cancer, 2009, 101(7): 1091-1099.

[433] Tara O, Henderso N, Preetha R, et al. Risk Factors Associated With Secondary Sarcomas in Childhood Cancer Survivors: A Report From the Childhood Cancer Survivor Study[J]. Int J Radiat Oncol Biol Phys, 2012, 84(1): 224-230.

[434] Kottage K, Mcfarlane J, Krasin MJ, et al. Secondary Colorectal Carcinoma After Childhood Cancer[J]. J Clin Oncol, 2012, 30(20): 2552-2558.

[435] Leleu X, Soumerai J, Roccaro A, et al. Increased Incidence of Transformation and Myelodysplasia/Acute Leukemia in Patients With Waldenstrom Macroglobulinemia Treated With Nucleoside Analogs[J]. J Clin Oncol, 2009, 27(2): 250-255.

[436] Liu C, Wang C, Du Z, et al. Clinical features and prognosis of duplex primary malignant neoplasms involving chronic myeloid leukemia[J]. Medicine (Baltimore), 2020, 99(44): e22904-e22909.

[437] Wood ME, Vogel V, Ng A, et al. Second malignant neoplasms: assessment and strategies for risk reduction[J]. J Clin Oncol, 2012, 30(30): 3734-3745.

[438] Kirova YM, Rycke YD, Gambotti L, et al. Second malignancies after breast cancer: the impact of different treatment modalities[J]. Br J Cancer, 2008, 98(5): 870-874.

[439] Curtis RE, Moloney WC, Ries LG, et al. Leukemia following chemotherapy for breast cancer[J]. Cancer Res, 1990, 50(9): 2741-2746.

[440] See HT, Thomas DA, Bueso-Ramos C, et al. Secondary leukemia after treatment with paclitaxel and carboplatin in a patient with recurrent ovarian cancer[J]. Int J Gynecol Cancer, 2006, 16(Suppl 1): 236-240.

[441] Shenolikar R, Durden E, Meyer N, et al. Incidence of secondary myelodysplastic syndrome (MDS) and acute myeloid leukemia (AML) in patients with ovarian or breast cancer in a

real-world setting in the United States[J]. Gynecol Oncol, 2018, 151(2): 190-195.

[442] Hughes KS, Schnaper LA, Bellon JR, et al. Lumpectomy plus tamoxifen with or without irradiationin women age 70 years or older with early breast cancer: long-term follow-up of calgb 9343[J]. J Clin Oncol, 2013, 31(19), 23-82.

[443] Van Eggermond AM, Schaapveld M, Lugtenburg PJ, et al. Risk of multiple primary malignancies following treatment of Hodgkin lymphoma[J]. Blood, 2014, 124(3): 319-327.

[444] Milligan DW, Ruizeelvira MC, Kolb HJ, et al. Secondary leukaemia and myelodysplasia after autografting for lymphoma: results from the EBMT[J]. Br J Haematol, 1999, 106(4): 1020-1026.

[445] Brown JR, Yeckes H, Friedberg JW, et al. Increasing Incidence of Late Second Malignancies After Conditioning With Cyclophosphamide and Total-Body Irradiation and Autologous Bone Marrow Transplantation for Non-Hodgkin'S Lymphoma[J]. Clin Oncol, 2005, 23(10): 2208-2222.

[446] Leisenring W, Friedman DL, Flowers MED, et al. Non-melanoma Skin and Mucosal Cancers After Hematopoietic Cell Transplantation[J]. Clin Oncol, 2006, 24(7): 1119-1126.

[447] Friedman DL, Rovo A, Leisenring W, et al. Increased risk of breast cancer among survivors of allogeneic hematopoietic cell transplantation: a report from the FHCRC and the EBMT-Late Effect Working Party[J]. Blood, 2008, 111(2): 939-944.

[448] Cuzick J, Powles T, Veronesi U, et al. Overview of the main outcomes in breast-cancer prevention trials[J]. Lancet, 2003, 361(9354): 296-211.

[449] 郭华. 乳腺癌术后服用三苯氧胺致子宫内膜病变的临床病理分析[J]. 深圳中西医结合杂志, 2016(5): 92-93.

[450] Dibi RP. Tamoxifen use and endometrial lesions: hysteroscopic, histological, and immunohistochemical findings in postmenopausal women with breast cancer[J]. Menopause, 2009, 16(2): 293-300.

[451] 李敏, 谢明. 多原发恶性肿瘤研究进展[J]. 中国癌症杂志, 2017, 27(2): 156-160.

[452] 李琳, 王淑珍, 张震宇, 等. 乳腺癌患者三苯氧胺治疗后妇科良性疾患的随访研究[J]. 中华医学杂志, 2010, 90(25): 1735-1738.

[453] 郭宏霞, 王淑珍, 崔秀平. 乳腺癌患者发生妇科肿瘤情况的随访研究[J]. 中国妇幼卫生杂志, 2013(4): 18-19.

[454] Deligdisch L, Kalir T, Cohen CJ, et al. Endometrial histopathology in 700 patients treated with tamoxifen for breast cancer[J]. Gynecol Oncol, 2000, 78(2): 181-186.

[455] Cuzick J, Sestak I, Baum M, et al. Effect of anastrozole and tamoxifen as adjuvant

treatment for early-stage breast cancer: 10-year analysis of the ATAC trial[J]. Lancet Oncol, 2010, 11(12): 1135-1141.

[456] Fisher B, Costantino JP, Redmond CK, et al. Endometrial cancer in tamoxifen-treated breast cancer patients: findings from the National Surgical Adjuvant Breast and Bowel Project(NSABP)B-14[J]. J Natl Cancer Inst, 1994, 86(7): 527-537.

[457] Jung H, Jung JK, Kim SB, et al. Comparative study on hysteron-scopic and histologic examinations of the endometrium in postmenopausal women taking tamoxifen[J]. J Menopausal Med, 2018, 24(2): 81-86.

[458] Ricceri F, Fasanelli F, Giraudo MT, et al. Risk of second primary malignancies in women with breast cancer: Results from the European prospective investigation into cancer and nutrition(EPIC)[J]. Int J Cancer, 2015, 137(4): 940-948.

[459] Tarella C, Passera R, Magni M, et al. Risk Factors for the Development of Secondary Malignancy After High-Dose Chemotherapy and Autograft, With or Without Rituximab: A 20-Year Retrospective Follow-Up Study in Patients With Lymphoma[J]. J Clin Oncol, 2011, 29(7): 814-824.

[460] Zhou Y, Tang G, Medeiros LJ, et al. Therapy-related myeloid neoplasms following fludarabine, cyclophosphamide, and rituximab(FCR) treatment in patients with chronic lymphocytic leukemia/small lymphocytic lymphoma[J]. Mod Pathol, 2012, 25(2): 237-245.

[461] Mccarthy PL, Owzr K, Hofmeister C. Lenalidomide after Stem-Cell Transplantation for Multiple Myeloma[J]. N Engl J Med, 2012, 366(19): 1770-1781.

[462] Lyamn GH, Dale DC, Wolff DA, et al. Acute Myeloid Leukemia or Myelodysplastic Syndrome in Randomized Controlled Clinical Trials of Cancer Chemotherapy With Granulocyte Colony-Stimulating Factor: A Systematic Review[J]. J Clin Oncol, 2010, 28(17): 2914-2924.

[463] Akdeniz D, Klaver MM, Smith CZA, et al. The impact of life style and reproductive factors on the risk of a second new primary cancer in the contralateral breast: a systematic review and meta-analysis[J]. Cancer Causes Control, 2020, 31(5): 403-416.

[464] Knight JA, Fan J, Malone KE, et al. Alcohol consumption and cigarette smoking in combination: A predictor of contralateral breast cancer risk in the WECARE study[J]. Int J Cancer, 2017, 141(5): 916-924.

[465] Shiels MS, Gibson T, Sampson J, et al. Cigarette smoking prior to first cancer and risk of second smoking-associated cancers among survivors of bladder, kidney, head and neck, and stage I lung cancers[J]. J Clin Oncol, 2014, 32(35): 3989-3995.

[466] Watanabe S, Kodama T, Shimosato Y, et al. Multiple primary cancers in 5456 autopsy cases in the national cancer center of Japan[J]. J Natl Cancer Inst, 1984, 72(5): 1021-

1027.

[467] He Y, Jing B, Li LS, et al. Changes in smoking behavior and subsequent mortality risk during a 35-year follow-up of a cohort in xi'an, China[J]. Am J Epidemiol, 2014, 179(9): 1060-1070.

[468] Clarke MA, Long BJ, Sherman ME, et al. A prospective clinical cohort study of women at increased risk for endometrial cancer[J]. Gynecol Oncol, 2020, 156(1): 169-177.

[469] León X, Quer M, Diez S, et al. Second neoplasm in patients with head and neck cancer[J]. Head Neck, 1999, 21(3): 204-210.

[470] Chuang S, Hashibe MG, Brewster D, et al. Risk of second primary cancer among esophageal cancer patients: a pooled analysis of 13 cancer registries[J]. Eur J Cancer Supplements, 2008, 6(10): 2390-2396.

[471] Katada C, Muto M, Nakayama M, et al. Risk of superficial squamous cell carcinoma developing in the head and neck region in patients with esophageal squamous cell carcinoma[J]. Laryngoscope, 2012, 122(6): 1291-1296.

[472] Tabuchi T, Ito Y, Ioka A, et al. Tobacco smoking and the risk of subsequent primary cancer among cancer survivors: a retrospective cohort study[J]. Ann Oncol, 2013, 24(10): 2699-2704.

[473] Garces YI, Schroeder DR, Nirelli LM, et al. Second primary tumors following tobacco dependence treatments among head and neck cancer patients[J]. American J Clin Oncol, 2007, 30(5): 531-539.

[474] Dok A, Johnson MM, Lee JJ, et al. Longitudinal study of smoking patterns in relation to the development of smoking-related secondary primary tumors in patients with upper aerodigestive tract malignancies[J]. Cancer, 2004, 101(12): 2837-2842.

[475] Tabuchi T, Ito Y, Ioka A, et al. Incidence of metachronous second primary cancers in Osaka, Japan: update of analyses using population-based cancer registry data[J]. Cancer Sci, 2012, 103(6): 1111-1120.

[476] Luis IV, Macedo R, Teixeira EA, et al. Clinical characteristics of patients with lung cancer and metachronous or synchronous tumours with other locations[J]. Rev Port Pneumol, 2010, 16(3): 391-405.

[477] Park SM, Li T, Wu S, et al. Risk of second primary cancer associated with prediagnostic smoking, alcohol, and obesity in women with keratinocyte carcinoma[J]. Cancer Epidemiol, 2017, 47(2): 106-113.

[478] Liu YY, Chen YM, Yen SH, et al. Multiple primary malignancies involving lung cancer-clinical characteristics and prognosis[J]. Lung Cancer, 2002, 35(2): 189-194.

[479] 陈万青, 张思维, 邹小农. 中国肺癌发病死亡的估计和流行趋势研究[J]. 中国肺癌杂志, 2010, 13(5): 488-493.

[480] Aredo JV, Luo SJ, Gardner RM, et al. Tobacco smoking and risk of second primary lung cancer[J]. J Thorac Oncol, 2021, 16(6): 968-979.

[481] Parente B, Queiroga H, Teixeira E, et al. Epidemiological study of lung cancer in Portugal(2000/2002)[J]. Rev Port Pneumol, 2007, 13(2): 255-265.

[482] Tohnson BE. Second Lung Cancers in Patients After Treatment for an Initial Lung Cancer[J]. J Natl Cancer Inst, 1998, 90(18): 1135-1145.

[483] Karp DD, Lee SJ, Shaw Wright GL, et al. A phase Ⅲ, intergroup, randomized, double-blind, chemoprevention trial of selenium(Se) supplementation in resected stage I non-small cell lung cancer(NSCLC)[J]. J Clin Oncol, 2010, 28(suppl 18): CRA7004.

[484] Dijkman BG, Schuurbiers OCJ, Vriens D, et al. The role of ^{18}F-FDG PET in the differentiation between lung metastases and synchronous second primary lung tumours[J]. Eur J Nucl Med Mol Imaging, 2010, 37(11): 2037-2047.

[485] Rice D, Kim HW, Sabichi A, et al. The risk of second primary tumors after resection of stage I non-small cell lung cancer[J]. Ann Thorac Surg, 2003, 76(4): 1001-1007.

[486] Wang X, Christiani DC, Mark EJ, et al. Carcinogen exposure, p53 alteration, and K-ras mutation in synchronous multiple primary lung carcinoma[J]. Cancer, 1999, 85(8): 1734-1739.

[487] Dashti SG, Buchanan DD, Jayasekara H, et al. Alcohol consumption and the risk of colorectal cancer for mismatch repair gene mutation carriers[J]. Cancer Epidemiol Biomarkers Prev, 2017, 26(3): 366-375.

[488] Pajares JA. Multiple primary colorectal cancer: individual or familial predisposition[J]. World J Gastrointest Oncol, 2015, 7(12): 434-444.

[489] De Menezes RF, Bergmann A, Thuler LC. Alcohol consumption and risk of cancer: a systematic literature review[J]. Asian Pac J Cancer Prev, 2013, 14(9): 4965-4972.

[490] Oppeltz RF, Jatoi I. Tobacco and the Escalating Global Cancer Burden[J]. J Clin Oncol, 2011, 2011(6): 1-8.

[491] Leoncini E, Vukovic V, Cadoni G, et al. Tumour stage and gender predict recurrence and second primary malignancies in head and neck cancer: a multicentre study within the INHANCE consortium[J]. Eur J Epidemiol, 2018, 33(12): 1205-1218.

[492] Hori K, Okada H, Kawahara Y, et al. Lugol-voiding lesions are an important risk factor for a second primary squamous cell carcinoma in patients with esophageal cancer or head and neck cancer[J]. Am J Gastroenterol, 2011, 106(5): 858-866.

[493] Morita M, Kumashiro R, Kubo N, et al. Alcohol drinking, cigarette smoking, and the development of squamous cell carcinoma of the esophagus: Epidemiology, clinical findings, and prevention[J]. Int J Clin Oncol, 2010, 15(2): 126-134.

[494] 俞斌, 黄煜庆, 曹君, 等. 合并乳腺癌的甲状腺癌152例临床病理学特征分析[J].

肿瘤学杂志, 2018, 24(4): 313-317.

[495] Miyazaki T, Tanaka N, Sano A, et al. Clinical significance of total colonoscopy for screening of colon lesions in patients with esophageal cancer[J]. Anticancer Res, 2013, 33(11): 5113-5117.

[496] Zhang ZH, Su PY, Hao JH, et al. The role of preexisting diabetes mellitus on incidence and mortality of endometrial cancer: a meta-analysis of prospective cohort studies[J]. Int J Gynecol Cancer, 2013, 23(2): 294-303.

[497] Deng L, Gui Z, Zhao L, et al. Diabetes mellitus and the incidence of colorectal cancer: an updated systematic review and meta-analysis[J]. Dig Dis Sci, 2012, 57(6): 1576-1585.

[498] Neuhouser ML, Aragaki AK, Prentice RL, et al. Overweight, Obesity, and Postmenopausal Invasive Breast Cancer Risk[J]. JAMA Oncol, 2015, 1(5): 611-621.

[499] Calle EE, Rodriguez C, Walker-Thurmond K, et al. Overweight, obesity, and mortality from cancer in a prospectively studied cohort of U.S. adults[J]. N Engl J Med, 2003, 348(17): 1625-1638.

[500] Druesne-Pecollo N. Excess body weight and second primary cancer risk after breast cancer: a systematic review and meta-analysis of prospective studies[J]. Breast Cancer Res Treat, 2012, 135(3): 647-654.

[501] Navarrete-Reyes AP, Soto-Perez-De-Celis E, Hurria A. Cancer and Aging: A Complex Biological Association[J]. Rev Invest Clin, 2016, 68(1): 17-24.

[502] Demandante CG, Troyer DA, Miles TP. Multiple primary malignant neoplasms: case report and a comprehensive review of the literature[J]. Am J Clin Oncol, 2003, 26(1): 79-91.

[503] Lee DH, Roh JL, Baek S, et al. Second cancer incidence, risk factor, and specific mortality in head and neck squamous cell carcinoma[J]. Otolaryngol Head Neck Surg, 2013, 149(4): 579-586.

[504] Youlden DR, Baade PD. The relative risk of second primary cancers in Queensland, Australia: a retrospective cohort study[J]. BMC Cancer, 2011, 11(1): 1-12.

[505] Soerjomataram I, Coebergh JW. Epidemiology of multiple primary cancers[J]. Methods Mol Biol, 2009, 471: 85-105.

[506] Amer MH. Multiple neoplasms, single primaries, and patient survival[J]. Cancer Manag Res, 2014, 6: 119-134.

[507] Chuang SC, Scelo G, Lee YC, et al. Risk of second primary cancer among patients with lung cancer for men and women: A pooled analysis of 13 cancer registries[J]. Int J Cancer, 2008, 123(10): 2390-2398.

[508] 孙俊杰, 李双庆. 多原发癌病因及发病机制的探索[J]. 中国全科医学, 2017, 20

(9): 1136-1141.

[509] James TA, Ronit K, Allan KT, et al. Second malignant neoplasms in patients under 40 years of age with laryngeal cancer[J]. Laryngoscope, 2001, 111(4): 563-567.

[510] 鞠卫东, 崔楠楠, 李文远, 等. 甲状腺与乳腺多原发肿瘤的临床特征分析[J]. 中国现代医生, 2014, 52(3): 32-33.

[511] Molina-Montes E, Pollan M, Payer T, et al. Risk of second primary cancer among women with breast cancer: a population-based study in Granada (Spain)[J]. Gynecol Oncol, 2013, 130(2): 340-345.

[512] Moore EK, Roylance R, Rosenthal AN. Breast cancer metastasising to the pelvis and abdomen: what the gynaecologist needs to know[J]. BJOG, 2012, 119(7): 788-797.

[513] Vrachnis N, Iavazzo C, Iliodromiti Z, et al. Diabetes mellitus and gynecologic cancer: molecular mechanisms, epidemiological, clinical and prognostic perspectives[J]. Arch Gynecol Obstet, 2016, 293(2): 239-247.

[514] Moorman PG, Havrilesky LJ, Gierisch JM, et al. Oral contraceptives and risk of ovarian cancer and breast cancer among high-risk women: a systematic review and meta-analysis[J]. J Clin Oncol, 2013, 31(33), 4188-4198.

[515] 徐露, 丁强, 陶爱娣, 等. 同时性双侧原发性乳腺癌10例临床分析[J]. 江苏医药, 2012, 38(19): 2258-2260.

[516] 魏子豪, 龚旺, 周敏, 等. 区域癌化的概念及其临床应用[J]. 中华口腔医学杂志, 2016, 51(9): 562-565.

[517] Chen Z, Li S, He Z, et al. Clinical analysis of 117 cases with synchronous multiple primary esophageal squamous cell carcinomas[J]. Korean J Intern Med, 2021, 36(6): 1356-1364.

[518] Lee YC, Wang HP, Wang CP, et al. Revisit of field cancerization in squamous cell carcinoma of upper aerodigestive tract: better risk assessment with epigenetic markers[J]. Cancer Prev Res(Phila), 2011, 4(12): 1982-1992.

[519] Mattavelli F, Pizzi N, Pennachioli E, et al. Neoplastic lymphangiosis of the upper aerodigestive tracts imulating field cancerization: histopathological analysis, surgical limits and literature review[J]. Tumori, 2012, 98(4): 1156-1172.

[520] Zeki SS, Me Donald SA, Graham T. Field cancerization in Barrett's esophagus[J]. Discov Med, 2011, 12(66): 371-379.

[521] Fortuna G, Mignogna MD. Oral field cancerization[J]. CMAJ, 2011, 183(14): 1622.

[522] Kato H, Nomura J, Matsumura Y, et al. A case of oral multiple primary cancer including spindle cell carcinoma[J]. J Maxillofac Oral Surg, 2010, 9(2): 213-217.

[523] van Rees BP, Cleton-Jansen AM, Cense HA, et al. Molecular evidence of field cancerization in a patient with 7 tumors of the aerodigestive tract[J]. Hum Pathol, 2000,

31(2): 269-271.

[524] Ono K, Sugio K, Uramoto H, et al. Discrimination of multiple primary lung cancers from intrapulmonary metastasis based on the expression of four cancer-related proteins[J]. Cancer, 2009, 115(15): 34489-34500.

[525] 娄诚,杜智,高英堂. 区域癌化的概念及其临床意义[J]. 国际肿瘤学杂志, 2007, 34(10): 747-750.

[526] Braakhuis BJ, Tabor MP, Kummer JA, et al. A genetic explanation of Slaughter's concept of field cancerization: evidence and clinical implications[J]. Cancer Res, 2003, 63(8): 1727-1730.

[527] Brown SR, Finan PJ, Hall NR, et al. Incidence of DNA replication errors in patients with multiple primary cancers[J]. Dis Colon Rectum, 1998, 41(6): 765-769.

[528] Hsieh WC, Chen YM, Perng RP. The temporal relationship of lung cancer and upper aerodigestive cancer[J]. J Clin Oncol, 1997, 27(2): 63-66.

[529] Baba Y, Ishimoto T, Kurashige J, et al. Epigenetic field cancerization in gastrointestinal cancers[J]. Cancer Lett, 2016, 375(2): 360-366.

[530] Kuwano H, Watanabe M, Sadanaga N, et al. Squamous epithelial dysplasia associated with squamous cell carcinoma of the esophagus[J]. Cancer Lett, 1993, 72(3): 141-147.

[531] Kuwano H, Matsuda H, Matsuoka H, et al. Intra-epithelial carcinoma concomitant with esophageal squamous cell carcinoma[J]. Cancer, 1987, 59(4): 783-787.

[532] Shimizu M, Ban S, Odze RD. Squamous Dysplasia and Other Precursor Lesions Related to Esophageal Squamous Cell Carcinoma[J]. Gastroenterol Clin North Am, 2007, 36(4): 797-811.

[533] Joseph-Incze CWV, Jr PLM, Stuarstrong BK, et al. Premalignant changes in normal appearing epithelium in patients with squamous cell carcinoma of the upper aerodigestive tract[J]. Am J Surg, 1982, 144(4): 401-405.

[534] Kuwano H, Ohno S, Matsuda H, et al. Serial histologic evaluation of multiple primary squamous cell carcinomas of the esophagus[J]. Cancer, 1988, 61(8): 1635-1638.

[535] 张文范,王梅先,阎瑞方,等. 多发性早期胃癌[J]. 中国医科大学学报, 1981, 10(5): 33-35.

[536] 张荫昌,白雅珍,张文范,等. 胃黏膜上皮不典型增生的病理及其演变的追踪观察[J]. 中华肿瘤学杂志, 1979, 1(1): 23-24.

[537] 严树柏. 12例多原发性胃癌临床病理分析[J]. 肿瘤防治杂志, 2000, 7(1): 109.

[538] Koness RJ, King TC, Schechter S, et al. Synchronous colon carcinomas: molecular-genetic evidence for multicentricity[J]. Ann Surg Oncol, 1996, 3(2): 136-143.

[539] Eguchi K, Yao T, Konomoto T, et al. Discordance of p53 mutations of synchronous colorectal carcinomas[J]. Modern Pathology, 2000, 13(2): 131-139.

[540] Bae JM, Cho NY, Kim TY. Clinicopathologic and molecular characteristics of synchronous colorectal cancers: heterogeneity of clinical outcome depending on microsatellite instability status of individual tumors[J]. Dis Colon Rectum, 2012, 55(2): 181-190.

[541] Arakawa K, Hata K, Nozawa H, et al. Molecular subtypes are frequently discordant between lesions in patients with synchronous colorectal cancer: molecular analysis of 59 patients[J]. Anticancer Res, 2019, 39(3): 1425-1432.

[542] Wang XF, Fang H, Cheng Y, et al. The molecularl and scape of synchronous colorectal cancer reveals genetic heterogeneity[J]. Carcinogenesis, 2018, 39(5): 708-718.

[543] Bedi GC, Westra WH, Gabrielson E, et al. Multiple head and neck tumors: Evidence for a common clonal origin[J]. Cancer Res, 1996, 56(11): 2484-2487.

[544] Califano J, van der Riet P, Westra W, et al. Genetic progression model for head and neck cancer: Implications for field cancerization[J]. Cancer Res, 1996, 56(11): 2488-2492.

[545] Scholes AG, Woolgar JA, Boyle MA, et al. Synchronous oral carcinomas: Independent or common clonal origin[J]. Cancer Res, 1998, 58(9): 2003-2006.

[546] Goodkin R, Zaias B, Michelsen WJ. Arteriovennus malformation and glioma. Coexistence or sequential[J]. J Neurosurg, 1990, 72(2): 798-805.

[547] Moertel CG. Multiple primary malignant neoplasms[J]. Cancer, 1977, 40(3): 1786-1998.

[548] 周怀伟, 孙同舟, 鲍民. 神经系统多原发肿瘤生物学特性分析[J]. 中国医科大学学报, 2004, 33(1): 88-89.

[549] Ellen EM. Neurotropic melanoma A case report and review of the literature[J]. J Neurol Oncol, 1992, 13(1): 165-188.

[550] 周怀伟. 亲神经性黑色素型肿瘤[J]. 中国肿瘤临床, 1995, 22(6): 400-402.

[551] 周怀伟. von Hippel-Lindau 病三例[J]. 中华病理杂志, 1993, 22(5): 298-299.

[552] Witzig TE, Timm M, Stenson M, et al. Induction of apoptosis in malignant B cells by phenylbutyrate or phenglacetate in combination with chemotherapeutic agents[J]. Clin Cancer Res, 2000, 6(2): 681-692.

[553] Pomeroy SL, Tamayo P, Gaasenbeek M, et al. Prediction of central nervous system embrgonal tumour outcome based on gene expression[J]. Nature, 2002, 415(1): 436-442.

[554] Ma YP, Vankeeuwen FE, Cooke R, et al. FGFR2 genotype and risk of radiation-associated breast cancer in Hodgkin lymphoma[J]. Blood, 2012, 119(4): 1029-1031.

[555] Yu CL, Tucker MA, Abramson DH, et al. Cause-Specific Mortality in Long-Term Survivors of Retinoblastoma[J]. J Natl Cancer Inst, 2009, 101(8): 581-591.

[556] Kleinerman RA, Yu CL, Little MP, et al. Variation of second cancer risk by family history

of retinoblastoma among long-term survivors[J]. J Clin Oncol, 2012, 30(9): 950-957.

[557] Metcalfe K, Gershman S, Lynch HT, et al. Predictors of contralateral breast cancer in BRAC1 and BRCA2 mutation carriers[J]. Br J Cancer, 2011, 104(9): 1384-1392.

[558] Martin A, Kanestsky P, Amirimani B, et al. Germline TP53 mutation in breast cancer families with multiple primary cancers: is TP53 a modifier of BRAC1[J]. J Med Genet, 2003, 40(4): e34.

[559] De Vivo I, Gertig DM, Nagase S, et al. Novel germline mutations in the PTEN tumour suppressor gene found in women with multiple cancers[J]. J Med Genet, 2000, 37(5): 336-341.

[560] Imyanitov EN, Kuligina ES. Systemic investigations into the molecular features of bilateral breast cancer for diagnostic purposes[J]. Expert Rev Mol Diagn, 2020, 20(1): 41-47.

[561] Bonadona V, Bonati B, Olschwang S, et al. Cancer risks associated with germline mutations in MLH1, MSH2, and MSH6 genes in Lynch syndrome[J]. JAMA, 2011, 305(22): 2304-2310.

[562] Lipkin SM, Wang V, Jacoby R, et al. MLH3: a DNA mismatch repair gene associated with mammalian microsatellite instability[J]. Nat Genet, 2000, 24(1): 27-35.

[563] Delachapelle A. The incidence of Lynch syndrome[J]. Familial Cancer, 2005, 4(3): 233-237.

[564] 李红梅, 李平. 多原发恶性肿瘤的病因和发病机制的探讨[J]. 华西医学, 2016, 31(5): 991-995.

[565] 李小会, 赵文婕, 刘变英. 林奇综合征诊疗进展[J]. 中华结直肠疾病电子杂志, 2016, 5(6): 513-518.

[566] Walsh MD, Cummings MC, Buchanan DD, et al. Molecular, pathologic, and clinical features of early onset endometrial cancer: identifying presumptive Lynch syndrome patients [J]. Clin Cancer Res, 2008, 14(6): 1692-1700.

[567] 文家治, 朱腾, 韩春晨, 等. 易感基因在林奇综合征相关结直肠癌、腺瘤筛查中应用研究[J]. 临床军医杂志, 2018, 46(8): 972-973.

[568] Lancaster JM, Powell CB, Kauff ND, et al. Society of Gynecologic Oncologists Education Committee statement on risk assessment for inherited gynecologic cancer predispositions[J]. Gynecol Oncol, 2007, 107(2): 159-162.

[569] Win AK, Lindor NM, Winship I, et al. Risks of colorectal and other cancers after endometrial cancer for women with Lynch syndrome[J]. J Natl Cancer Inst, 2013, 105(4): 274-279.

[570] Win AK, Lindor NM, Young JP, et al. Risks of primary extra-colonic cancers following colorectal cancer in Lynch syndrome[J]. J Natl Cancer Inst, 2012, 104(18): 1363-

1372.

[571] Orlow I, Park BJ, Mujumdar U, et al. DNA damage and repair capacity in patients with lung cancer: prediction of multiple primary tumors[J]. J Clin Oncol, 2008, 26(21): 3560-3566.

[572] Win AK, Young JP, Lindor NM, et al. Colorectal and other cancer risks for carriers and noncarriers from families with a DNA mismatch repair gene mutation: a prospective cohort study[J]. J Clin Oncol, 2012, 30(9): 958-964.

[573] Goecke T, Schulmann K, Engel C, et al. Genotype-Phenotype Comparison of German MLH1 and MSH2 Mutation Carriers Clinically Affected With Lynch Syndrome: A Report by the German HNPCC Consortium[J]. J Clin Oncol, 2006, 24(26): 4285-4292.

[574] Cho I, An JY, Kwon IG, et al. Risk factors for double primary malignancies and their clinical implications in patients with sporadic gastric cancer[J]. Eur J Surg Oncol, 2014, 40(3): 338-344.

[575] Miyoshi E, Hamma K, Hiyama T, et al. Microsatellite instability is a genetic marker for the development of multiple gastric cancers[J]. Int J Cancer, 2001, 95(6): 350-353.

[576] Kong P, Wu R, Lan Y, et al. Association between Mismatch-repair Genetic variation and the Risk of Multiple Primary Cancers: A Meta-Analysis[J]. J Cancer, 2017, 8(16): 3296-3308.

[577] Velayos FS, Lee SH, Qiu H, et al. The mechanism of microsatellite instability is different in synchronous and metachronous colorectal cancer[J]. J Gastrointest Surg, 2005, 9(3): 329-335.

[578] 董彩红, 吴利娟, 张广平, 等. 39例多原发性大肠癌的内镜及临床分析[J]. 中国内镜杂志, 2007, 13(8): 851-853.

[579] 董锐增, 蔡宏, 莫善兢, 等. 散发性多原发大肠癌微卫星不稳定研究[J]. 肿瘤学杂志, 2005, 11(5): 363-366.

[580] Shitoh K, Konish IF, Miyakura Y, et al. Microsatellite instability as a marker in predicting metachronous multiple colorectal carcinomas after surgery[J]. Dis Colon Rectum, 2002, 45(3): 329-333.

[581] Lawes DA, Pearson T, Sengupta S, et al. The role of MLH1, MSH2 and MSH6 in the development of multiple colorectal cancers[J]. Br J Cancer, 2005, 93(4): 472-477.

[582] 任延律, 张岂凡, 于志伟, 等. 大肠重复癌MMR、p53、Bax、PCNA表达及微卫星不稳定性研究[J]. 中华普通外科杂志, 2004, 19(1): 43-45.

[583] Tiwari AK, Roy HK, Lynch HT. Lynch syndrome in the 21st century: clinical perspectives [J]. QJM, 2016, 109(3): 151-158.

[584] Millar AL, Pal T, Madlensky L, et al. Mismatch repair gene defects contribute to the genetic basis of double primary cancers of the colorectum and endometrium[J]. Hum Mol

Genet, 1999, 8(5): 823-829.

[585] Schmeler KM, Lynch HT, Chen LM, et al. Prophylactic surgery to reduce the risk of gynecologic cancers in the Lynch syndrome[J]. N Engl J Med, 2006, 354(3): 261-269.

[586] Farmer H, Mccabe N, Lord, CJ, et al. Targeting the dna repair defect in brca mutant cells as a therapeutic strategy[J]. Nature, 2005, 434(7035), 917-921.

[587] Cheung M, Kadariya Y, Talarchek J, et al. Germline BAP1 mutation in a family with high incidence of multiple primary cancers and a potential gene-environment interaction[J]. Cancer Lett, 2015, 369(2): 261-265.

[588] Hemminki K, Forsti A, Lorenzo Bermejo J. Surveying germline genomic landscape of breast cancer[J]. Breast Cancer Res Treat, 2009, 113(3): 601-603.

[589] Antoniou A, Pharoah PD, Narod S, et al. Average risks of breast and ovarian cancer associated with BRAC1 or BRCA2 mutations detected in case series unselected for family history: A combined analysis of 22 studies[J]. Am J Hum Genet, 2003, 72(5): 1117-1130.

[590] Cantor SB, Bell DW, Ganesan S, et al. BACH 1, a novel helicase-like protein, interacts directly with BRAC1 and contributes to its DNA repair function[J]. Cell, 2001, 105(1): 149-160.

[591] Antoniou AC, Sinilnikova OM, Simard J, et al. RAD51 135G>C modifies breast cancer risk among BRCA2 mutation carriers: Results from a combined analysis of 19 studies[J]. Am J Hum Genet, 2007, 81(6): 1186-1200.

[592] Offit K. BRCA mutation frequency and penetrance: new data, old debate[J]. J Natl Cancer Inst, 2006, 98(23): 1675-1677.

[593] Molina-Montes E, Perez-Nevot B, Pollan M, et al. Cumulative risk of second primary contralateral breast cancer in BRAC1/BRCA2 mutation carriers with a first breast cancer: A systematic review and meta-analysis[J]. Breast, 2014, 23(6): 721-742.

[594] Valencia OM, Samuel SE, Viscusi RK, et al. The Role of Genetic Testing in Patients With Breast Cancer: A Review[J]. JAMA Surg, 2017, 152(6): 589-594.

[595] Narod SA. Bilateral breast cancers[J]. Nat Rev Clin Oncol, 2014, 11(3): 157-166.

[596] Graser MK, Engel C, Rhiem K, et al. Contralateral breast cancer risk in BRAC1 and BRCA2 mutation carriers[J]. J Clin Oncol, 2009, 27(35): 5887-5892.

[597] Vandenbroek AJ, Vantveer LJ, Hooning MJ, et al. Impact of Age at Primary Breast Cancer on Contralateral Breast Cancer Risk in BRAC1/2 Mutation Carriers[J]. J Clin Oncol, 2016, 34(5): 409-418.

[598] Mellemkjær L, Friis SH, Olsen J, et al. Risk of second cancer among women with breast cancer[J]. Int J Cancer, 2006, 118(9): 2285-2292.

[599] Fishman A, Dekel E, Chetrit A, et al. Patients with double primary tumors in the breast and ovary - clinical characteristics and brca 1 - 2 mutations status[J]. Gynecol Oncol, 2000, 79(1): 74 - 78.

[600] Baker B, Morcos B, Daoud F, et al. Histo - biological comparative analysis of bilateral breast cancer[J]. Med Oncol, 2013, 30(4): 711 - 720.

[601] Liu P, Cheng H, Roberts TM, et al. Targeting the phosphoinositide 3 - kinase pathway in cancer[J]. Nat Rev Drug Discov, 2009, 8(8): 627 - 644.

[602] Bubien V, Bonnet F, Brouste V, et al. High cumulative risks of cancer in patients with PTEN hamartoma tumour syndrome[J]. J Med Genet, 2013, 50(4): 255 - 263.

[603] Yoon TI, Kwak BS, Yi OV, et al. Age - related risk factorsassociated with primary contralateral breast cancer among younger women versus older women[J]. Breast Cancer Res Treat, 2019, 173(3): 657 - 665.

[604] Eng C. Will the real Cowden syndrome please stand up: revised diagnostic criteria[J]. J Med Genet, 2000, 37(11): 828 - 830.

[605] Liaw D, Marsh DJ, Li J, et al. Germline mutations of the PTEN gene in Cowden disease, an inherited breast and thyroid cancer syndrome[J]. Nat Genet, 1997, 16(1): 64 - 67.

[606] 何晓乐, 刘军, 王晓明, 等. 抑癌基因 PTEN 在老年人消化道多原发癌中的表达及其临床意义[J]. 临床医药实践, 2011, 20(10): 759 - 761.

[607] Park SL, Caberto CP, Lin Y, et al. Association of cancer susceptibility variants with risk of multiple primary cancers: the population architecture using genomics and epidemiology study[J]. Cancer Epidemiol Biomarkers Prev, 2014, 23(11): 2568 - 2578.

[608] Vogt M, Munding J, Grüner M, et al. Frequent concomitant inactivation of miR - 34a and miR - 34b/c by CpG methylation in colorectal, pancreatic, mammary, ovarian, urothelial, and renal cell carcinomas and soft tissue sarcomas[J]. Virchows Arch, 2011, 458(3): 313 - 322.

[609] Behrens C, Travis LB, Wistuba H, et al. Molecular changes in second primary lung and breast cancers after therapy for Hodgkin's disease[J]. Cancer Epidemiol Biomarkers Prev, 2000, 9(10): 1027 - 1035.

[610] Jin L, Sturgis EM, Zhang Y, et al. Genetic variants in p53 - related genes confer susceptibility to second primary malignancy in patients with index squamous cell carcinoma of head and neck[J]. Carcinogenesis, 2013, 34(7): 1551 - 1557.

[611] Zhang Y, Sturgis EM, Huang Z, et al. Genetic variants of the p53 and p73 genes jointly increase risk of second primary malignancies in patients after index squamous cell carcinoma of the head and neck[J]. Cancer, 2012, 118(2): 485 - 492.

[612] Lei J, Hsu J, Jen P, et al. KRAS, BRAF, and EGFR mutational analysis in ovarian, colon, and lung cancers by highly multiplex PCR/barcoded - magnetic - bead (BMB)

suspension – array assays[J]. Cancer Res, 2014, 74(Suppl 19): 4663.

[613] 闫振宇, 买春阳, 高鹏, 等. Her-2 在乳腺癌和胃癌中表达的临床意义[J]. 中国免疫学杂志, 2016, 32(6): 858-862.

[614] Blanter J, Zimmerman B, Tharakan S, et al. BRCA Mutation Association with Recurrence Score and Discordance in a Large Oncotype Data base[J]. Oncology, 2020, 98(4): 248-251.

[615] Huang D, Lu N, Fan Q, et al. HER2 status in gastric and gastroe – sophageal junction cancer assessed by local and central laboratories: Chinese results of the HER – EAGLE study[J]. PLoS One, 2013, 8(11): e80290-e80294.

[616] Cybulski C, Gbrski B, Huzarski T, et al. CHEK2 is a multiorgan cancer susceptibility gene[J]. Am J Hum Genet, 2004, 75(6): 1131-1135.

[617] Siołek M, Cybulski C, Gąsior – Perczak D, et al. CHEK2 mutations and the risk of papillary thyroid cancer[J]. Int J Cancer, 2015, 137(3): 548-552.

[618] Wingo SN, GaUardo TD, Akbay EA, et al. Somatic LKB1 mutations promote cervical cancer progression[J]. PLo Sone, 2009, 4(4): e5122-e5137.

[619] Sanchez – Cespedes M. A role for LKB1 gene in human cancer beyond the Peutz – Jeghers syndrome[J]. Oncogene, 2007, 26(57): 7825-7832.

[620] 陆鸣, 陈书媛, 周小鸽. 甲状腺呈胸腺样分化癌的临床病理特点[J]. 诊断病理杂志, 2008, 15(1): 37-39.

[621] Shoroko T, Yokoo N, Okomoto K, et al. Mixed Medullary – papillary carcinoma of the thyroid with lymph node metastases: report of a case[J]. Surg today, 2001, 31(4), 317-321.

[622] Volante M, Papotti M, Roth J, et al. Mixed medullary – follicular thyroid carcmoma: molecular evidence for a dual origin of tumor components[J]. Am J Pathol, 1999, 155(5): 1499-1509.

[623] Rossi S, Fugazzola L, De Pasquale L, et al. Medullary and papillary carcinoma of the thyroid gland occurring as a collision tumour: report of three cases with molecular analysis and review of the literature[J]. Endocr Relat Cancer, 2005, 12(2): 281-289.

[624] Ikeda Y, Kiyotani K, Yew PY, et al. Germline PARP4 mutations in patients with primary thyroid and breast cancers[J]. Endocr Relat Cancer, 2016, 23(3): 171-179.

[625] Track KM, Tye CE, Ghule PN, et al. Mitotically – Associated lncRNA (MANCR) Affects Genomic Stability and Cell Division in Aggressive Breast Cancer[J]. Mol Cancer Res, 2018, 16(4): 587-598.

[626] Lu W, Xu Y, Xu J, et al. Identification of differential expressed lncRNAs in human thyroid cancer by a genome – wide analyses[J]. Cancer Med, 2018, 7(8): 3935-3944.

[627] Titze IR, Schmidt SS, Titze MR. Phonation threshold pressure in aphysical model of the

vocal fold mucosa[J]. J Acoust Soc Am, 1995, 97(5): 3080-3084.

[628] Nosho K, Kure S, Irahhara N, et al. A prospective cohort study shows unique epigenetic, genetic, and prognostic features of synchronous colorectal cancers[J]. Gastroenterology, 2009, 137(5): 1609-1620.

[629] Leggett BA, Worthley DL. Synchronous colorectal cancer not just bad luck[J]. Gastroenterology, 2009, 137(5): 1559-1562.

[630] Taqawa Y, Nanashima A, Tsji T, et al. Importance of cytogenetic markers for multiple primary carcinomas in colorectal cancer: chromosome 17 and p53 locus translocation[J]. J Gastroenterol, 1998, 33(5): 670-677.

[631] Sawa IT, Nanashima A, Tsji T, et al. Instability of chromosome 17 and the p53 locus in non-familial colorectal cancer with multiple primary malignancies[J]. J Exp Clin Cancer Res, 2001, 20(3): 401-405.

[632] Sawa IT, Sasano O, Tsji T, et al. Numerical aberration of chromosome 17 is correlated with multiple primary cancer in colorectal carcinoma[J]. Nihon Shokakibyo Gakkai Zasshi, 1997, 94(7): 464-468.

[633] Lam AK, Carmichael R, Gertrau D, et al. Clinicopathological significance of synchronous carcinoma in colorectal cancer[J]. Am J Surg, 2011, 202(1): 39-44.

[634] Asakawa H, Koido S, Torii A, et al. Alterations of p53 gene, microsatellite instability and proliferation associated antigen Ki-67 in the synchronous multiple colorectal cancers[J]. Nihon Shokakibyo Gakkai Zasshi, 2001, 98(11): 1263-1271.

第二章

预防与筛查

第一节 预　防

多原发肿瘤预防的对象主要指第一原发肿瘤长期生存者，第一原发肿瘤的预防措施亦通常适用于多原发肿瘤的预防。

目前，无论是对第一原发肿瘤还是多原发肿瘤的预防，首先是对全民进行科普知识宣传与教育，增强自我防范意识，并付诸行动，筑牢肿瘤发生的第一道防线。

无论是第一原发肿瘤还是多原发肿瘤预防，培养良好的生活习惯、生活方式尤为重要。吸烟、饮酒、肥胖等是肿瘤发生的高危因素已得到全球医学界的广泛认同，因此，对吸烟的第一原发肿瘤幸存者需进行戒烟教育，力劝戒烟，并减少酒精摄入[1]。

对于超重和肥胖明显的第一原发肿瘤女性患者，尤其是乳腺癌患者，应控制饮食量与种类，加强运动，控制体重，密切监测双侧乳腺或对侧乳腺第二原发肿瘤发生的可能性[2-8]。Friedenreich 等[9]报道，若体力活动增加到每周 5 天中度或剧烈强度活动 30~60min，可预防 9%~19% 的肿瘤发生。一项针对乳腺癌长期生存者的随机试验显示[2]，低脂饮食干预在 60 个月的随访后显著降低了复发事件的风险，包括新的对侧乳腺癌的发生。

环境因素，如辐射、过度的日光照射、病毒感染等亦是肿瘤发生的重要因素之一，故应尽可能避免接触环境中的致癌物，远离核辐射场所，避免长时间、强烈的阳光照射。

肠道多发性息肉，尤其是锯齿状息肉是多原发肠道内肿瘤发生的潜在危险因素，无论是第一原发肿瘤患者还是第二原发肿瘤患者，结肠镜检查并摘除已有的息肉是一种积极的预防性策略。

一般而言，对伴有 Lynch 综合征的第一原发肿瘤患者，为减少或避免异时性结肠癌的发生,应行广泛性结肠切除,如结肠全切除或次全切除[10]。

为预防子宫内膜癌或结直肠癌的发生,对有 MMR 基因缺失的第一原发肿瘤患者,应从 30～35 岁开始每年行子宫内膜活检或妇科超声检查,如无生育要求可考虑行预防性子宫/双附件切除;从 20～25 岁起,每 1～2 年进行 1 次肠镜检查[11]。

对于存在 BRCA 基因突变的第一原发肿瘤乳腺癌患者,建议行预防性输卵管-卵巢切除术(RRSO)[12],该手术可有效降低乳腺癌患者发生第二原发肿瘤卵巢癌、输卵管癌的风险。Curtin 等[13]的研究发现,25% 的 BRCA 基因突变的乳腺癌患者,在进行 RRSO 术后,术后病理显示存在卵巢肿瘤。

对于第一原发肿瘤(如头颈部鳞癌、乳腺癌、肺癌、食管癌、纵隔淋巴瘤、宫颈癌等)局部治疗的选择,应严格遵守治疗规范与指南,如需放射治疗,尽量使用精准放射治疗,如三维适形放射治疗、适形调强放射治疗、立体定向放射治疗、螺旋断层放射治疗、图像引导放射治疗、质子放射治疗等[14],以降低射线对周围正常组织的放射性损伤,防止第二原发肿瘤的发生。

对于第一原发肿瘤系统治疗的选择,如新辅助治疗、辅助治疗及晚期舒缓治疗,亦应遵守治疗规范与指南,包括方案药物组成、剂量、用药时间、用药周期等。对于乳腺癌、急性白血病、淋巴瘤、软组织肉瘤等第一原发肿瘤患者,需慎用拓扑异构酶抑制剂Ⅱ、烷化剂类、抗代谢类等细胞毒性药物,尤其需避免长期、大剂量使用细胞毒性药物,防止因治疗而发生第二原发肿瘤[15-16]。

对于激素受体阳性的第一原发性乳腺癌患者,其辅助治疗中推荐使用选择性雌激素受体调节剂或芳香化酶抑制剂,因其可降低对侧乳腺癌发生的风险。据报道[17-21],他莫昔芬可使对侧乳腺癌发病率降低约 1/3、阿那曲唑与来曲唑可使对侧乳腺癌发病风险降低 45%～53%。早期乳腺癌试验者协作组(Early Breast Cancer Trialists' Collaborative Group,EBCTCG)的研究表明[17],他莫昔芬治疗可使对侧乳腺癌风险显著降低,从每年 0.6% 降至每年 0.4%。ATAC 试验组报道[22],在绝经后妇女中,将阿那曲唑与他莫昔芬比较,显示阿那曲唑可使绝经后妇女的对侧乳腺癌风险大大降低。亦有学者推荐他莫昔芬用于绝经前和绝经后乳腺癌一级预防,推荐雷洛昔芬用于绝经后乳腺癌一级预防[23-24]。郑丽等[25]的研究发现,对于 ER、PR 阳性的乳腺癌患者,进行内分泌治疗,可显著降低第二原发肿瘤卵巢癌的发生率。

但在长期使用他莫昔芬的女性乳腺癌患者中,需特别注意子宫内膜的变化,以便及时发现子宫内膜癌的发生。

有研究报道[26-27],在头颈部鳞状细胞癌患者中,异维甲酸(13-顺式维甲酸)可降低第二原发肿瘤发生的风险。

肠溶阿司匹林可用于结肠癌幸存者和其他结肠癌风险增加的肿瘤幸存者的化学预防[28],有研究者报道[29],使用肠溶阿司匹林可使遗传性非息肉性结肠癌患者的结肠癌发病率降低50%以上,晚期发病率降低28%。

对于长期口服避孕药是否可增加第一、第二原发肿瘤发生风险存在争议[30]。Phd 等[31]认为,长期使用避孕药可使乳腺癌的风险增加,不建议第一原发肿瘤幸存者长期口服避孕药。但 Hannaford 等[32]的研究发现,曾经使用口服避孕药相比于从未使用口服避孕药的第一原发肿瘤患者,患子宫内膜癌的风险更低。

表 2-1 预防要点与方法

预防要点	预防方法
科普宣传教育	采用不同方式(现场、网络等)、不同地点(医院、社区、乡村)广泛讲解多原发肿瘤科普知识,印发科普知识手册
培养良好生活习惯	对吸烟的第一原发肿瘤幸存者需进行戒烟教育,力劝戒烟,并减少酒精摄入
	对于超重和肥胖明显的第一原发肿瘤女性患者,尤其是乳腺癌患者,应控制饮食量与种类(如低脂、低糖等),加强运动,控制体重
	尽可能避免接触环境中的致癌物
	避免长时间、强烈的阳光照射,以防止第二原发肿瘤,如皮肤癌、皮肤黑色素瘤的发生
医学干预	对伴有肠道息肉的第一原发肿瘤患者,建议内镜下治疗
	对伴有 Lynch 综合征的第一原发肿瘤患者,建议广泛性结肠切除,如结肠全切除或次全切除
	对伴有 MMR 基因突变的第一原发肿瘤患者,应从30~35岁开始每年行子宫内膜活检或妇科超声检查,如无生育要求可考虑行预防性子宫/双附件切除
	对存在 BRCA 基因突变的第一原发肿瘤乳腺癌患者,建议行预防性输卵管-卵巢切除术(RRSO)

续表

预防要点	预防方法
医学干预	对于第一原发肿瘤局部治疗的选择，应严格遵守治疗规范与指南，如需放射治疗，尽量使用精准放射治疗，如三维适形放射治疗、适形调强放射治疗、立体定向放射治疗、螺旋断层放射治疗、图像引导放射治疗、质子放射治疗等，降低射线对周围正常组织的放射性损伤
	对于第一原发肿瘤系统治疗的选择，如新辅助治疗、辅助治疗及晚期舒缓治疗，应严格遵守治疗规范与指南，包括方案药物组成、剂量、用药时间、用药周期等；应慎用拓扑异构酶抑制剂Ⅱ、烷化剂类、抗代谢类等细胞毒性药物，尤其需避免长期、大剂量使用细胞毒性药物
	对于激素受体阳性的第一原发乳腺癌患者，需使用选择性雌激素受体调节剂或芳香化酶抑制剂
	对于第一原发肿瘤结肠癌长期幸存者，建议使用肠溶阿司匹林
	对于第一原发肿瘤头颈部鳞状细胞癌长期幸存者，可考虑使用异维甲酸（13-顺式维甲酸）
	长期口服避孕药可能增加第二原发肿瘤发生风险，一般不建议第一原发肿瘤幸存者长期口服避孕药

第二节 筛 查

在第一原发肿瘤诊治后可能长期生存的患者，应对其中发生第二原发肿瘤的高危人群进行密切监测，以及时发现第二原发肿瘤。

一、多原发肿瘤发生风险评估要求

（1）要求肿瘤科所有医务人员，包括外科、内科、放射治疗科医师及相关护理人员对多原发肿瘤专业知识有较充分的了解，增强专业医务人员对多原发肿瘤风险评估和高风险人群筛查重要性的认识，使多原发肿瘤患者得到早期诊断、早期治疗[33-34]。

（2）对于任何第一原发肿瘤长期生存者，必须对其家族遗传史、工作环境、生活习惯、体重或体重指数，以及放射治疗、化学治疗、内分泌治疗等情况进行全面了解，充分评估其第二原发肿瘤发生的风险[35-37]。

二、多原发肿瘤筛查对象与筛查方法

目前指南建议,对于曾有 30 年烟龄的第一原发肿瘤患者继续吸烟或最近才戒烟(戒烟后不足 15 年),此类人群为低剂量螺旋 CT 筛查肺癌的对象。

Shankar 等[38]对 532 例乳腺癌患者进行了年龄分组研究,发现 20~40 岁年龄组患者对侧罹患第二原发乳腺癌的发病率为 83.3%。因此,对于绝经前第一原发肿瘤乳腺癌的患者,需要每 0.5~1 年进行 1 次对侧乳腺的 B 超检查[39]。

有学者建议[40],下咽癌及喉癌为第一原发肿瘤的患者,电子内镜检查应列为常规检查。

对于有结肠癌家族史和(或)Lynch 综合征的第一原发肿瘤幸存者,第二原发性结肠癌的风险最大[41],应考虑早期开始结肠镜检查,并根据结肠镜检查结果确定后续筛查的间隔时间。

Lynch 综合征患者应每 1~2 年进行 1 次筛查,而那些有家族肿瘤史和确定息肉的患者应每 5 年进行 1 次结肠镜检查。

美国妇科肿瘤协会建议,对至少有 1 位一级或二级亲属合并子宫内膜癌和其他 Lynch 综合征相关性肿瘤,或已知一级或二级亲属中有 MMR 基因突变的人群,推荐行基因检测。

第一原发消化道肿瘤手术切除后,产生多原发肿瘤的致病因素仍可能存在,有发生异时性消化道多原发肿瘤的倾向[42-43]。大量研究表明,消化道内镜检查是发现、诊断第二原发肿瘤的重要手段。因此,对消化道单原发肿瘤进行根治术后的患者,应坚持术后长期内镜随访,定期复查[44-45]。

合理的内镜随访方案是异时性多原发肿瘤早期发现的最佳方法,严格的内镜随访可使 96.6% 的第二原发肿瘤早期发现。日本学者[46]随访了 175 例多原发胃癌患者,发现第一原发肿瘤术后 6 个月内随访胃镜,可帮助检出 19% 漏诊的第二原发肿瘤。邓兰树等[47]指出,对于第一原发肿瘤结直肠内癌的高危患者,术后每半年行 CEA 检测、钡剂灌肠及纤维结肠镜检查 1 次,两年后每年 1 次,直至 5 年;同时可在 3 年内每 3~6 个月行 B 超、CT 检查 1 次。

对于有一级或二级亲属患卵巢癌家族史的第一原发肿瘤女性患者,可

上篇 多原发肿瘤
第二章 预防与筛查

考虑进行筛查,筛查方法包括每 2~6 个月测定血清 CA125 和(或)经阴道超声检查[29,48]。

有早期前列腺癌家族史(65 岁以前确诊)的肿瘤患者或 BRAC1 或 BRCA2 基因突变的男性患前列腺癌的风险增加[49-50],对于这些高危人群,肿瘤筛查应从 45 岁开始,检查方法包括前列腺 B 超检查及测定血清前列腺特异性抗原。

Miyoshi 等[51]对单发胃癌与多原发胃癌患者 MSI-L 出现的频率进行了比较,发现两者之间具有统计学意义,认为 MSI-L 可能是预测多原发胃癌的有效分子标记物。

HPV 的检测可能有助于预测第二原发肿瘤的发生风险[52]。

有早期黑色素瘤家族史(50 岁以前确诊)的第一原发肿瘤幸存者,应每年进行 1 次皮肤检查,且每月进行 1 次自我皮肤检查。

表 2-2 筛查对象与筛查方法

分类	内容
筛查对象	对于易感人群,如儿童肿瘤幸存者、免疫缺陷的第一原发肿瘤患者、有肿瘤家族遗传史的第一原发肿瘤患者通常视为第二原发肿瘤发生的高危人群,是监测与筛查的重点对象
	对于携带 BRAC1 或 BRCA2 基因突变、确诊 Lynch 综合征、或有卵巢癌家族史的第一原发肿瘤女性幸存者,应进行妇科肿瘤常规筛查
	有肿瘤家族史,伴有 BRAC1 或 BRCA2 基因突变者或在 10~30 岁期间接受过胸部放射治疗的第一原发肿瘤女性患者,应每年对乳房进行筛查
	对于一级或二级亲属有卵巢癌家族史的第一原发肿瘤女性患者,可考虑进行卵巢癌的常规筛查
	接受头颈部、胸部、盆腔放射治疗的第一原发肿瘤患者随访时间至少在 10 年以上,主要监测、筛查照射野及周围组织、器官(如甲状腺、乳腺、肺、子宫等)
	对于罹患乳腺癌或妇科恶性肿瘤的女性患者,术后随访至少 5 年以上[5]

续表

分类	内容
筛查方法	常规影像学筛查，主要包括 B 超、CT、MRI。甲状腺、乳腺通常可选择 B 超检查，必要时乳腺可选择 MRI；肺部筛查推荐 CT（包括平扫、增强、薄层）
	PET/CT 不作为首选推荐
	内镜检查，包括鼻咽镜、支气管镜、胃镜、肠镜、膀胱镜、宫腔镜等，若发现异常，需行组织活检
	肿瘤血清标志物检测，如 CEA、AFP、CA199、CA724、CA153、CA125、PSA 等
	遗传学检测，如 Lynch 综合征基因检测

参考文献

[1] Parsons A, Daley A, Begh R, et al. Influence of smoking cessation after diagnosis of early stage lung cancer on prognosis: systematic review of observational studies with meta-analysis [J]. BMJ, 2010, 340(211): b5569.

[2] Chlebowski RT, Blackburn GL, Thomson CA, et al. Dietary Fat Reduction and Breast Cancer Outcome: Interim Efficacy Results From The Women'S Intervention Nutrition Study [J]. J Natl Cancer Inst, 2006, 98(24): 1767-1776.

[3] Prentice RL, Thomson CA, Caan B, et al. Low-Fat Dietary Pattern and Cancer Incidence in the Women'S Health Initiative Dietary Modification Randomized Controlled Trial[J]. J Natl Cancer Inst, 2007, 99(20): 1534-1543.

[4] 陈学燕，李利亚，万冬桂，等. 双侧原发性乳腺癌两侧肿瘤病灶的差异性分析[J]. 浙江医学，2020，42(1)：39-43.

[5] McTiernan A, Irwin M, Von Gruenigen V. Weight, Physical activity, diet, and Prognosis in breast and gynecologic cancers[J]. J Clin Oncol, 2010, 28(26): 4074-4081.

[6] Ibrahim EM, Al-Homaidh A. Physical activity and survival after breast cancer diagnosis: meta-analysis of published studies[J]. Med Oncol, 2011, 28(3): 753-765.

[7] Sternfeld B, Weltzien E, Quesenberry CP, et al. Physical activity and risk of recurrence and mortality in breast cancer survivors: findings from the LACE study[J]. Cancer Epidemiol Biomarkers Prev, 2009, 18(1): 87-95.

[8] Sternfeld B, Weltzien E, Quesenberry CP, et al. Physical activity and risk of recurrence and mortality in breast cancer survivors: findings from the LACE study[J]. Cancer Epidemiol Biomarkers Prev, 2009, 18(1): 87-95.

[9] Friedenreich CM, Neilson HK, Lynch BM. State of the epidemiological evidence on physical activity and cancer prevention[J]. Eur J Cancer, 2010, 46(14)：2593-2604.

[10] 徐立斌, 邵永孚, 赵东兵, 等. 同时性多原发大肠癌的外科治疗及预后因素分析[J]. 中华肿瘤杂志, 2005, 27(7)：435-437.

[11] Stoffel EM, Mangu PB, Gruber SB, et al. Hereditary colorectal cancer syndromes：American Society of Clinical Oncology Clinical Practice Guideline endorsement of the familial risk - colorectal cancer：European Society for Medical Oncology Clinical Practice Guidelines [J]. J Clin Oncol, 2015, 33(2)：209-217.

[12] 宋楠, 燕鑫. 乳腺和卵巢相关的多发性原发癌的研究进展[J]. 现代妇产科进展, 2013, 22(4)：325-327.

[13] Curtin JE, Barakat RR, Hoskins WJ. Ovarian disease in women with breast cancer[J]. Obstet Gynecol, 1994, 84(3), 449-452.

[14] 刘玉连, 赵徵鑫, 张文艺, 等. 质子放射治疗的现状与展望[J]. 中国医学装备, 2017, 14(7)：139-143.

[15] Travis LB, Holowaty EJ, Bergfeldt K, et al. Risk of leukemia after platinum - based chemotherapy for ovarian cancer[J]. N Engl J Med, 1999, 340(5)：351-357.

[16] Travis LB, Andersson M, Gospodarowicz M, et al. Treatment - associated leukemia following testicular cancer[J]. J Natl Cancer Inst, 2000, 92(14)：1165-1171.

[17] Ebct CG. Effects of chemotherapy and hormonal therapy for early breast cancer on recurrence and 15 - year survival：an overview of the randomised trials[J]. Lancet, 2005, 365(9472)：1687-1717.

[18] Group AT. Results of the ATAC(Arimidex, Tamoxifen, Alone or in Combination)trial after completion of 5 years adjuvant treatment for breast cancer[J]. Lancet, 2005, 365(9453)：60-62.

[19] Vogel VG, Costantino JP, Wicke MDL, et al. Update of the National Surgical Adjuvant Breast and Bowel Project Study of Tamoxifen and Raloxifene(STAR)P - 2 Trial：Preventing Breast Cancer[J]. Cancer Prev Res (Phila), 2010, 3(6)：696-706.

[20] Group TBC. Letrozole Therapy Alone or in Sequence with Tamoxifen in Women with Breast Cancer[J]. Lancet, 2009, 361：766-776.

[21] Coates AS, Keshaviah A, Thurlimann B, et al. Five Years of Letrozole Compared With Tamoxifen As Initial Adjuvant Therapy for Postmenopausal Women With Endocrine - Responsive Early Breast Cancer：Update of Study BIG 1 - 98[J]. J Clin Oncol, 2007, 25(5)：486-492.

[22] Phbp JC, Phd IS, Mdp MB, et al. Effect of anastrozole and tamoxifen as adjuvant treatment for early - stage breast cancer：10 - year analysis of the ATAC trial[J]. Lancet Oncol, 2010, 11(12)：11341-11351.

[23] Vogel VG, Cosnjtino JP, Wickeam DL. Effects of Tamoxifen VS Raloxifene on the Risk of Developing Invasive Breast Cancer and Other Disease Outcomes[J]. JAMA, 2006, 295: 2727-2741.

[24] Fisher B, Costanto JP, Wickerham DL, et al. Tamoxifen for the Prevention of Breast Cancer: Current Status of the National Surgical Adjuvant Breast and Bowel Project P-l Study [J]. J Natl Cancer Inst, 2005, 97(22): 1652-1662.

[25] 郑丽, 张丽娜, 顾林, 等. 44例乳腺卵巢双原发癌的临床特点与预后分析[J]. 中华普通外科杂志, 2016, 31(6): 482-485.

[26] Fadlor-Khur I, Xim ES. The Impact of Smoking Status, Disease Stage, and Index Tumor Site on Second Primary Tumor Incidence and Tumor Recurrence in the Head and Neck Retinoid Chemoprevention Trial[J]. Cancer Epidemiol Biomarkers Prev, 2001, 10: 823-829.

[27] Mayne ST, Cartmel B. Chemoprevention of Second Cancers[J]. Cancer Epidemiol Biomarkers Prev, 2006, 15(11): 2033-2037.

[28] Chan AT, Arber N, Burn J, et al. Aspirin in the Chemoprevention of Colorectal Neoplasia: An Overview[J]. Cancer Prev Res (Phila), 2012, 5(2): 164-178.

[29] Mdps JB, Mdpa MG, Mdpf M, et al. Long-term effect of aspirin on cancer risk in carriers of hereditary colorectal cancer: an analysis from the CAPP2 randomised controlled trial[J]. Lancet, 2011, 378(9809): 2081-2087.

[30] Collaborative Group On Epidemiological Studies Of Ovarian Cancer. Ovarian cancer and oral contraceptives: collaborative reanalysis of data from 45 epidemiological studies including 23257 women With ovarian cancer and 87 303 controls[J]. Lancet, 2008, 371(9609): 303-314.

[31] Phd GFGM, Phd BCTM. The use of hormonal contraception and its protective role against endometrial and ovarian cancer[J]. Best Pract Res Clin Obstet Gynaecol, 2010, 24(1): 29-38.

[32] Hannaford PC, Selvaraj S, Elliott AM, et al. Cancer risk among users of oral contraceptives: cohort data from the Royal College of General Practitioner'S oral contraception study[J]. BMJ, 2007, 335(7621): 651-658.

[33] Corkum M, Hayden JA, Kephart G, et al. Screening for new primary cancers in cancer survivors compared to non-cancer controls: a systematic review and meta-analysis[J]. J Cancer Surviv, 2013, 7(3): 455-463.

[34] Shin DW, Baik YJ, Kim YW, et al. Knowledge, attitudes, and practice on second primary cancer screening among cancer survivors: a qualitative study[J]. Patient Education & Counseling, 2011, 85(1): 74-78.

[35] Shin DW, Kim Y, Baek YJ, et al. Oncologists experience with second primary cancer

screening: current practices and barriers and potential solutions[J]. Asian Pac J Cancer Prev, 2012, 13(2): 671-678.

[36] Cybulski C, Nazarali S, Narod SA. Multiple primary cancers as a guide to heritability[J]. Int J Cancer, 2014, 135(8): 1756-1763.

[37] 叶岚, 艾毅钦, 吴星娆, 等. 宫颈癌合并乳腺癌 7 例临床分析[J]. 实用妇产科杂志, 2016, 32(3): 229-232.

[38] Shankar A, Roy S, Malik A, et al. Contralateral breast cancer: a clinico-pathological study of second primaries in opposite breasts after treatment of breast malignancy[J]. Asian Pac J Cancer Prev, 2015, 16(3): 1207-1211.

[39] Anwar SL, Prabowo D, Avanti WS, et al. Characteristics and the associated risk factors of the development of bilateral breast cancers: a case-control study[J]. Ann Med Surg, 2020, 60(11): 285-296.

[40] Liu WS, Chang YJ, Lin CL, et al. Secondary primary cancer in patients with head and neck carcinoma: the differences among hypopharyngeal, laryngeal, and other sites of head and neck cancer[J]. Eur J Cancer Care, 2014, 23(1): 36-42.

[41] Hampel H. Referral for cancer genetics consultation: a review and compilation of risk assessment criteria[J]. J Med Genet, 2004, 41(2): 81-91.

[42] Rosso S, Terracini I, Riccefi F, et al. Multiple prinmry tumours: incidence estimation in the presence of competing risks[J]. Popul Health Metr, 2009, 7(5): 1-10.

[43] VazLuis I, Macedo R, Teixeira E, et al. Clinical characteristics of patients with lung cancer and metaehronousor synchronous tumours with other locations[J]. Rev Port Pneumol, 2010, 16(3): 391-405.

[44] Hosokawa O, Kaizaki Y, Watanabe K, et al. Endoscopic surveilianee for gastric remnant cancer. Dfterearlv cancer surgery[J]. Endoscopy, 2002, 34(6): 469-473.

[45] 夏金荣, 缪才良. 上消化道多原发癌临床分析[J]. 中华消化内镜杂志, 2000, 17(2): 80-90.

[46] Kato M, Nishida T, Yamamoto K, et al. Scheduled endoscopic surveillance controls secondary cancer after curative endoscopic resection for early gastric cancer: a multicentre retrospective cohort study by Osaka University ESD studygroup[J]. Gut, 2013, 62(10): 1425-1432.

[47] 邓兰树, 吴祝东, 杨少华. 大肠多原发癌 8 例临床分析[J]. 中国实用外科杂志, 1994, 14(1): 47-48.

[48] Rosenthal A, Jacobs I. Familial ovarian cancer screening[J]. Best Pract Res Clin Obstet Gynaecol, 2006, 20(2): 321-338.

[49] Liede A, Karlan BY, Narod SA. Cancer Risks for Male Carriers of Germline Mutations in BRCA1 or BRCA2: A Review of the Literature[J]. J Clin Oncol, 2004, 22(4): 735-

742.

[50] Wolf AMD, Wender RC, Etzioni RB, et al. American Cancer Society Guideline for the Early Detection of Prostate Cancer: Update 2010[J]. CA Cancer J Clin, 2010, 60(2): 70-98.

[51] Miyoshi E, Haruma K, Hiyama T, et al. Microsatellite in stability is a genetic marker for the development of multiple gastric cancers[J]. Int J Cancer, 2001, 95(6): 350-353.

[52] Saito Y, Ebihara Y, Ushiku T, et al. Negative human papillomavirus status and excessive alcohol consumption are significant risk factors for second primary malignancies in Japanese patients with oropharyngeal carcinoma[J]. Jpn J Clin Oncol, 2014, 44(6): 564-569.

第三章

检查、诊断与治疗

第一节 检 查

多原发肿瘤检查与第一原发肿瘤初始基线检查基本相同,主要包括全身影像学检查、内镜检查(如鼻咽镜、支气管镜、胃镜、肠镜、膀胱镜、宫腔镜等)及新发病灶组织(内镜活检、穿刺活检、腔镜活检等)病理学检查(包括常规病理、免疫组化、分子基因检测等)、遗传学检查及肿瘤标志物检测等。

一、影像学检查

常规影像学检查包括 B 超、消化道造影、CT(平扫与增强)、MRI(头颅、骨骼、软组织、脊髓、盆腔等)、全身骨扫描,必要时可选择全身 PET/CT 检查。

目前,内镜检查技术及成像清晰度、放大倍数皆有明显提高,可清晰显示多种腔道黏膜上皮早期、微小及表浅病变[1],对于发现的可疑病灶内镜下可直接进行组织活检,早期、微小及表浅病变可行内镜下切除,以及单发、多发性息肉可行内镜下治疗。

近年来,随着碘染色技术、窄带成像内镜(narrow band imaging,NBI)、卢戈氏碘染色等新型技术的发展,更加有效地减少了单纯白光内镜可能引起的漏诊或误诊,使得内镜下消化系统多原发肿瘤的确诊率明显提高。

卢戈氏碘染色可发现食管多处黏膜病变[2-3],有学者指出[4],卢氏碘染色联合 NBI 进行观察较单独应用白光及 NBI 更易检测出多发食管病变,尤其是食管早期癌。

日本 Ribeiro 等[5]的研究显示,在 553 例胃癌患者中,内镜检查发现了

19例同时性多原发肿瘤,第二原发肿瘤多为早期肿瘤,为及时手术治疗提供了重要信息。2018年,王沧海等[6]报道了10年来胃镜下诊断胃肿瘤患者358例,食管癌患者201例,单发胃食管早期癌患者68例;胃食管多原发肿瘤12例,其中同时多原发肿瘤9例,异时多原发肿瘤3例。作者指出,多原发胃食管肿瘤,尤其是第二原发病灶多为早期肿瘤,内镜易漏诊,应用放大内镜、NBI及化学染色方法可避免漏诊。朱一苗等[7]报道了1例8年间先后胃、食管发现5处腺癌、鳞癌及不典型增生的患者。

有研究报道[8-9],同时性结直肠内多原发癌可发生于结直肠任一部位,可为同一肠段、邻近肠段或不同肠段,大多发生在直肠、乙状结肠、升结肠。有学者报道[10-11],同时性结直肠内多原发癌以发生在同一肠段或相邻肠段者居多,也有学者报道以相隔较远肠段者较多[12]。

目前,结肠镜检查被用作整个结直肠肿瘤术前监测的标准方法,不仅可发现单一原发肿瘤部位,也可发现多原发肿瘤位置,以及评估肿瘤大小、组织活检。因此,对结直肠癌患者而言,术前全结肠镜检查应尽可能常规进行。

临床上,借助X射线气钡双重造影、CT、MRI等检查及术中探查、术中肠镜等检查可提高同时性结直肠内多原发癌的诊断率,降低漏诊率[13]。CT仿真结肠镜检查(computed demographic colonography,CTC)是一种对充气扩张和清洁肠道提供分层和腔内成像的新技术。Neri等[14]认为,CTC对大肠癌的敏感性和特异性分别是86%和100%,可发现异时性和同时性肿瘤,缺点是无法识别细微的黏膜病变或肠壁表面变化,同时不能取活检,假阳性率较高。

PET/CT目前在多发肿瘤部位的诊断与鉴别诊断中具有很高价值,且多原发肿瘤在PET/CT中的表现有其独特的特点,与常规影像学检查相比,更易发现多原发肿瘤,尤其是针对第一原发肿瘤远处转移与第二原发肿瘤的鉴别[15-16]。

Xu等[17]的研究报道,PET/CT诊断第二原发肿瘤的敏感性可达到95.24%。Pang等[18]利用PET/CT筛查了19例多原发肿瘤患者,发现了38个各器官不同类型的病灶,多为胃肠道、肺部恶性肿瘤。Malik等[19]对591例食管癌患者行PET/CT检查,发现多原发肿瘤55例。

二、组织病理学检查

组织病理学检查是最基本的检查,亦是多原发肿瘤诊断的关键条件。

Froio 等[20]对 40 篇文献中 10 例单原发肺癌、189 例多原发肺癌组织学类型进行了比较分析,结果发现,10 例单原发性支气管肺癌为多形性癌,由 2~3 种类型肿瘤细胞组成。多原发肺癌中,82 例异时性和 107 例同时性有着相同的组织学类型,58 例组织学类型不同的肺多原发癌中 51 例为双原发癌,7 例为三原发癌。

郭春梅等[21]报道,同时性多原发结直肠癌病理仍以腺癌为主,且以高、中分化腺癌更为多见。但也有研究显示[22],黏液腺癌在同时性多原发结直肠癌患者中的发生率较单原发结直肠癌患者更高(13.0% vs 3.7%)。

三、免疫组化检查

免疫组化标记对原发肿瘤的诊断,以及在不同原发肿瘤之间、原发肿瘤与转移肿瘤之间的鉴别诊断起着举足轻重的作用,且对某些单原发或多原发肿瘤治疗原则的确定具有重要指导意义,如结直肠癌的微卫星(MS)状态(4 个免疫标记:MLH1、MSH2、MSH6、PMS2)[23],乳腺癌、胃癌等 HER-2(++时,需行 FISH 检测),乳腺癌 ER、PR、AR 状态,等等。

Kadara 等[24]通过免疫组化分析 CK19、p53、CEA、Hup-1、PE-10 和 Ki-67 蛋白表达,对临床诊断为肺多原发癌患者及转移癌患者进行二次诊断,结果显示,7 例临床标准诊断为多原发肿瘤中的 6 例及 8 例临床诊断为转移癌中的 5 例被重新诊断为多原发性肺癌。

四、分子基因检测

分子基因检测结果是不能进行局部治疗(如手术、放射治疗等)而进行靶向治疗(针对特定的致癌驱动基因)药物选择的唯一依据,亦是某些家族遗传性肿瘤诊断的重要指标。

目前,分子基因检测(包括杂合性缺失和基因突变)已广泛应用于多原发肿瘤的诊断与鉴别诊断中,包括 DNA 分子标记技术、致癌驱动基因突变检测技术、二代测序(next-generation sequencing, NGS)技术[25-29],NGS 具有通量大、可同时检测多种未知基因突变的优势[30]。

Froio 等[31]对一个同时性肺内多原发癌患者的 3 个肿瘤灶(左肺上叶周围型腺癌及支气管内鳞癌,左肺下叶小细胞神经内分泌癌)进行了 40 个染色体位点的杂合性缺失(loss of heterozygosity, LOH)分析,结果显示,各个肿瘤灶的 LOH 存在差异,这种差异表现为不同肿瘤病灶有不同的染色体位点突变,不同肿瘤病灶存在相同的染色体突变位点,但突变方式不同。该结果表明这3个肿瘤病灶相互独立,属于多克隆起源,为肺多原发癌;亦提示基因分析在肺部多灶肿瘤中区分肺多原发及肺癌肺内转移具有重要意义。

Dacic等[32]通过分析p53蛋白表达、染色体3p缺失、k-ras基因突变,证明了5例同时性肺多原发肿瘤患者的11个肿瘤病灶有各自独立起源,而确诊为同时性多原发肺内癌。

有研究者认为[33],检测外周血有核细胞DNA损伤程度,有利于肺多原发肿瘤与转移癌的鉴别。

五、肿瘤标志物检测

肿瘤标志物检测指标主要有CEA、AFP、CA199、CA153、CA125、PSA(前列腺特异性抗原)等,AFP、PSA对原发性肝细胞癌、前列腺癌的诊断有一定的特异性,而Cyclin D1、p53和Ki-67的高表达与多原发肿瘤恶性生物学行为相关,其高表达通常提示肿瘤分化程度差、侵袭性高和早期转移[34]。

表3-1 多原发肿瘤检查方法

项目	内容	证据等级
影像学检查	B超,消化道造影、CT(平扫与增强),MRI(头颅、骨骼、软组织、脊髓、盆腔等),全身骨扫描	1类
	PET/CT(必要时)	3类
组织病理学检查	所有获得的肿瘤组织需进行常规病理学检查	1类
免疫组化检查	所有获得的肿瘤组织需进行常规免疫标记或特定免疫标记检测	1类
分子基因检测	DNA分子标记,或致癌驱动基因突变检测,或二代测序(NGS)	2A类
肿瘤标志物检测	CEA、AFP、CA199、CA153、CA125、PSA等	2A类

第三章 检查、诊断与治疗

第二节 诊 断

一、漏诊分析

因多原发肿瘤发生部位的广泛性,以及其本身的复杂性与多样性,加之临床医生对多原发肿瘤认识不足,往往只满足于一处病灶的诊断,而忽视了其他病灶,且在第一原发肿瘤诊治后若干时间,发现远处新病灶,多认为是肿瘤转移,而未考虑是第二、第三原发肿瘤;另外,活检病理取材不当,导致假阴性。因此,多原发肿瘤临床上极易漏诊[35-38]。王沧海等[6]对12例食管早期多原发肿瘤的胃镜活检组织病理分析发现,12例第二原发肿瘤中,10例为早期癌及高级别瘤变,与单原发早期癌的形态大小无差异,易于漏诊。

2005年,日本学者报道[39],上消化道内多原发肿瘤在确诊的恶性肿瘤中的检出率为1.6%~3.8%。20世纪60年代,中国报道上消化道内多原发癌检出率为1.12%~1.15%,1985—1990年间有报道其检出率仅为1.67%[40]。1998年,中国学者报道[41],上消化道多原发肿瘤漏诊率极高,可高达83.3%~100%。

近年来,随着临床医生对多原发肿瘤的重视及检测技术的进步,中国上消化道内多原发癌的检出率呈现逐步增高的趋势,上消化道内多原发癌检出率达到1.99%~2.42%[42-44]。肖杨等[40]报道的13例上消化道多原发癌,1988年以前发现的5例术前全部漏诊,1989年以后发现的8例多原发癌术前全部确诊。徐丽芳等[45]统计了1995—2000年检出的上消化道内多原发癌35例中,1998—2000年检出病例为1995—1997年的4倍。

值得注意的是,在多原发肿瘤诊断中,排除第一原发肿瘤转移尤为重要,否则将误诊、误治。Mamounas等[46]在1382例曾患乳腺癌患者的尸检报告中指出,多原发癌的发生率为11.4%,其中有10.6%多原发癌患者在生前被误诊为转移癌。

目前,临床上对组织学类型不同和(或)位于不同器官的多灶肿瘤,诊断多原发癌较为容易;然而,对于多灶肿瘤具有相同组织学类型时,仅通过影像学表现及组织学形态准确区分多原发肿瘤和转移癌仍十分困难[47-48]。

二、总体诊断标准

目前,多原发肿瘤的诊断主要依赖于影像学和组织病理学(包括免疫组化、分子病理等)。结合多项研究报道[49-58],其总体诊断标准为每个肿瘤必须独立存在于不同器官或同一器官不同部位、每个肿瘤具有各自不同的病理学特征,同一单一器官及对称性同侧器官肿瘤间须间隔一定距离的正常组织(2cm以上),通过影像学及组织病理学检查排除了第一原发肿瘤转移。

三、双侧原发乳腺癌诊断

若双侧病理类型相同,当满足以下条件之一者,可被认为是双侧原发乳腺癌[59]。

(1)双侧乳腺癌均为原位或早期癌,区域淋巴结无转移。
(2)双侧乳腺癌分化程度不同。
(3)次发侧病灶位于外上象限,首发侧无区域淋巴结转移。
(4)双侧乳腺癌间隔5年以上,无区域复发或远处转移。

以6个月为界限,可分为同时性双侧原发性乳腺癌(synchronous bilateral primary breast cancer,SB-PBC)与异时性双侧原发性乳腺癌(metachronous bilateral primary breast cancer,MB-PBC)。

在乳腺多原发肿瘤描述中,乳腺外多原发肿瘤定义为肿瘤病灶位于非乳腺部位,即不包括对侧乳腺癌。

四、肺内多原发癌诊断

1975年,Martini和Melamed对50例肺内多原发癌(multiple primary lung cancers,M-PLC)患者的临床病例数据进行归纳总结,提出了M-PLC的诊断标准,即Martini-Melamed标准[60]。

肺内多原发癌是指有2个或2个以上肺部恶性病变,不包括第一原发肺癌的肺内转移(同侧肺或对侧肺)。

同时性肺内多原发癌是一种特殊类型的肺癌,至少发现2个原发肿瘤,组织学相同或不同,但发生在不同的节段、肺叶或肺,可在同侧或对侧肺,可起源于原位癌,且无淋巴结转移。

异时性肺内多原发癌是具有不同组织学类型的肺癌,或起源于原位癌，无淋巴结转移，且在诊断时没有肺外转移[61-63]。

肺内多原发癌病理学特征以腺癌为主，鳞癌次之[64]。临床上，当出现同侧或对侧肺内同时性或异时性组织病理学相同的肿瘤时，如肺腺癌、肺鳞癌，要鉴别是多原发癌还是转移癌难度相当大[65]。

有学者认为[66-69]，对主要驱动基因的体细胞突变进行检测、数十个基因靶向测序，以及杂合性缺失、染色体重排等多种分子检测，可识别同一患者体内受外在环境改变及内在基因变异影响的多个病灶的克隆性，从而将原发肿瘤与转移肿瘤区分开来。

Warth 等[70]指出，在分子谱上具有高度相似性的病灶往往是转移性病灶而非多原发肿瘤。Rens 等[71]通过 p53 突变分析对 31 例同时性和异时性肺内多原发癌患者的 64 个病灶进行了研究，其中 21 例患者的肿瘤表现出不同的 p53 突变，明确了多原发肿瘤的诊断，其中 1 例患者的肿瘤不符合 Martini-Melamed 的诊断标准；此外，2 例患者的肿瘤带有相同的基因突变，提示为转移性病灶；另有 8 例患者仅通过 p53 突变分析不能得出明确诊断。Shimizu 等[72]认为，增加基因组测序 panel 的基因数目可有效提高鉴别诊断的敏感性。

目前，二代测序(NGS)技术可作为肺内多原发癌与肺转移癌鉴别的一个准确可靠的检测工具。全外显子(whole-exome sequencing，WES)组以及全基因组(whole-gene sequencing，WGS)测序可提供更全面的基因组信息来准确区分肺内多原发癌与肺转移癌[73]。Ezer 等[74]使用 NGS 对 61 例多原发肺腺癌患的 131 个病灶进行了分析，发现 50% 以上的基因突变类型为 KRAS 突变，且明确指出大多数患者的不同部位肿瘤分子学结果存在差异。Roepman 等[75]通过常规组织学特征、免疫组化、p53 蛋白表达、TP53 突变分析以及 50 基因 panel 测序系统分析了 50 例肺内多原发癌患者的 111 个病灶，TP53 突变分析在大多数情况下无法得出明确诊断，而使用 50 基因 panel 测序时，仅 2 例无法明确判断。Mansuet-Lupo 等[76]基于 NGS 技术联合组织分子算法区分肺部多个肿物性质，发现 EGFR L858R 是肺内多原发腺癌最频繁的突变。

然而孙芩玲等[77]指出，多基因 panel 测序成本费用高昂以及对样本质量要求极高，对每位患者的单个肿瘤进行基因分析至少目前临床上难以广泛开展。

一般而言，肺内多原发癌的诊断需结合临床表现、影像学特征及组织病理学等进行[25],Belardinilli 等[78]利用影像学、组织病理学和 NGS 技术,对 10 例多原发肺腺癌患者中的 24 个病灶进行了回顾性分析,结果表明,这些方法具有高度一致性。

影像学检查在肺内多原发癌诊断中具有普遍价值,肺内多原发癌与单发肺癌的影像学特点相似,主要表现为类圆形或圆形的孤立结节状阴影,密度不均,边缘毛糙,呈分叶状及毛刺征[79]。

Liu 等[80]报道,PET/CT 的 SUVmax 值在多原发肺癌与肺转移癌之间有显著性差异。目前,已将不同的影像学表现和生物标志物(如核素)代谢摄取的差异,作为区分第二原发肺癌和单一原发肺癌转移或复发的诊断标准之一[81]。

五、多原发肿瘤临床或病理分期

目前,尚无多原发肿瘤统一分期,但通常根据影像学检查、术后组织病理检查进行各自原发肿瘤临床分期及病理分期。

然而,对于同时性多原发肿瘤存在多处转移灶时,则难以进行准确的临床分期,因通常难以根据常规病理,甚至免疫组化判断是哪一个原发肿瘤发生的转移,如 2 个或 2 个以上的原发肿瘤病灶病理均为腺癌或鳞癌时。

肝、肺、骨骼是恶性实体肿瘤最常见转移的部位,当这些部位转移灶病理为腺癌或鳞癌,若同时存在原发乳腺癌、肺腺癌或肺鳞癌、食管鳞癌、胰腺腺癌、结直肠腺癌、宫颈鳞癌等,则很难确定是哪一个原发肿瘤或多个原发肿瘤发生的转移。

在同一食管或胃内,多原发肿瘤起源通常是多中心和(或)多时相的,不同肿瘤进展阶段不尽相同,多原发肿瘤中的不同肿瘤可能存在早期癌与早期癌共存、早期癌与中晚期癌共存、中晚期癌与中晚期癌共存等现象。有研究报道[82-83],上消化道多原发癌中食管早期癌,相较于胃、十二指肠早期癌更为常见。

第三章 检查、诊断与治疗

表 3-2 多原发肿瘤相关诊断标准

分类	诊断指标
总体诊断标准	每个肿瘤必须独立存在于不同器官或同一器官不同部位； 每个肿瘤具有各自不同的病理学特征； 同一单一器官（如甲状腺、食管、胃、结直肠等）及对称性同侧器官（如乳腺、肺、肾脏、卵巢等）肿瘤间须间隔一定距离的正常组织（2cm 以上）； 通过影像学及组织病理学检查（包括免疫组化、基因检测），排除第一原发肿瘤转移
双侧原发乳腺癌诊断标准	双侧乳腺组织中分别找到原位癌成分，如导管癌、小叶癌等； 双侧乳腺癌病理组织类型不同； 双侧乳腺癌病理组织类型相同者，而先发侧无局部复发、无淋巴转移及其他远处转移者； 原发癌好发部位多在外上象限，生长在乳腺实质中，边界不清，常有浸润；转移癌多见于对侧乳腺内侧或尾部脂肪组织中，呈扩张性生长，常为多发； 第一原发乳腺癌治疗后 5 年以上对侧发生的乳腺癌
肺内多原发癌诊断标准	同时性 MPLC 的诊断标准： 不同病灶之间相互独立； 不同病灶的组织学类型不同； 若组织学的类型相同，则进一步辨别多个病灶的解剖区域，多个病灶共同引流区域应无肿瘤累及，且诊断过程中无肺外转移，不同病灶解剖区域不同
	异时性 MPLC 的诊断标准： 不同病灶组织学类型不同； 原位癌引起的新病变、另一个肺叶或另一个肺出现第二原发肿瘤； 排除了在这两种肿瘤中常见的肺外转移和淋巴结转移
食管内多原发癌诊断标准	每个肿瘤灶必须经组织病理证实，并排除食管壁内浸润转移与术后局部复发； 每个肿瘤灶必须独立存在； 每个肿瘤灶之间有一定距离的正常食管组织； 以浸润程度最深、长度最大者为第一原发癌，其他为第二、第三等原发癌

续表

分类	诊断指标
胃内多原发癌诊断标准	每个肿瘤灶必须经组织病理证实，并排除胃内浸润转移与术后局部复发； 每个肿瘤灶必须独立存在； 每个肿瘤灶之间有一定距离的正常胃壁组织； 以浸润程度最深、侵犯范围最大者为第一原发癌，其他为第二、第三等原发癌
结直肠内多原发癌诊断标准	每个肿瘤灶必须经组织病理证实； 每一肿瘤为独立起源，具有相同或不相同的病理学形态； 肿瘤发生在结直肠内不同部位，两处病变一般间隔正常肠壁 5cm 以上； 排除家族性腺瘤样息肉病
Lynch 综合征诊断标准	其中 1 例为另 2 例的一级亲属； Lynch 综合征相关性肿瘤累及连续 2 代或 2 代以上家族成员； 其中至少 1 例发病年龄 <50 岁； 结直肠癌患者要排除家族性腺瘤样息肉； Lynch 综合征相关性肿瘤经病理证实
放射治疗相关多原发癌诊断标准	有接受第一原发肿瘤放射治疗的病史； 第二原发肿瘤发生于第一原发肿瘤照射野内； 第二多原发肿瘤与第一原发肿瘤的病理类型不同； 具有第二原发肿瘤的潜伏期（第一原发肿瘤放射治疗结束至第二原发肿瘤发生的时间，通常为 10~15 年）
多原发肿瘤与转移瘤的鉴别诊断要点	转移瘤多发生在肝、肺和骨骼等，而多原发肿瘤有相对应的位置； 在影像学表现上，转移瘤常为多发、密度均匀、轮廓清晰的圆形灶，而多原发肿瘤为孤立病灶； 当第一原发肿瘤无复发且无周围淋巴结转移时，发现其他部位的肿瘤，应考虑为多原发肿瘤

表 3-3 多原发肿瘤 Warran-Gates、IARC/IACR 与 SEER 诊断标准

Warran-Gates 标准	IARC/IACR 标准（世界范围）	SEER 标准（北美地区）
各个肿瘤须经组织细胞学证实为恶性肿瘤； 各个肿瘤的病理类型不同； 排除肿瘤转移； 肿瘤发生在不同部位，两者无关联	Warran-Gates 标准： 同一器官的不同部位发生的、病理类型相同的多个癌灶，不论肿瘤发生时间间隔的长短，均被视为同一个原发恶性肿瘤，即多灶癌，而非多原发肿瘤。 同时性多原发肿瘤：间隔时间 <6 个月 异时性多原发肿瘤：间隔时间 >6 个月	Warran-Gates 标准： 同一器官上不同部位发生的多个原发癌，即使病理类型相同，只要肿瘤发生间隔时间超过 2 个月，也被视作多原发肿瘤

第三节 治 疗

一、治疗原则

目前尚无统一、公认的多原发肿瘤标准治疗方案，但大多数学者认为[84-91]，一旦确诊为多原发肿瘤，必须组织多学科团队(multidisciplinary team，MDT)讨论，通常需遵照个体化治疗原则，通过对各原发肿瘤的病理类型、临床分期、患者身体耐受情况等进行全面评估，制定各原发肿瘤最佳治疗方案，在治疗方法上达成一致意见或共识。

一般而言，可手术切除者，应尽量采取根治性手术治疗，不能行根治性手术的患者可进行放射治疗、化学治疗、分子靶向治疗、免疫治疗等综合治疗以延长患者生存期。张立玮等[92]报道了一例历时25年，胃、十二指肠及结肠等脏器发生五原发肿瘤、6个肿瘤病灶，异时性癌兼同时性癌，经过4次手术、1次内镜下治疗，获得了长期生存。

在多原发肿瘤整合治疗过程中，外科手术占有极其重要的地位。对于可手术患者，应首选手术，除非有手术禁忌证或患者拒绝手术。Adebonojo等[93]指出，对于大部分多原发肿瘤患者而言，积极采取外科手术治疗更为合适。董莉莉等[94]报道，对于第二原发肿瘤为肺癌的患者，肺癌手术切除患者的2年生存率为85.5%，而未行手术患者的2年生存率仅为53.3%，二者有显著性差异。孙晓卫等[95]研究发现，对于不能根治性手术切除的多原发肿瘤患者，即使是接受姑息性手术，中位生存时间亦是未手术患者的3倍。张真等[96]报道141例多原发肿瘤，对手术与非手术进行比较研究，结果表明，双原发肿瘤手术切除患者较双原发肿瘤非手术切除患者的中位OS延长41个月。叶天仪等[97]对34例中33例双原发肿瘤患者行手术治疗，19例子宫内膜癌、17例结直肠癌术后放化学治疗，2年生存率为84.3%，5年生存率为63.1%。伍国号等[98]的研究结果显示，对于放射治疗诱发的多原发鼻咽癌患者，手术治疗3年、5年无瘤生存率均明显高于单纯放射治疗组。

异时性多原发肿瘤治疗的最大挑战之一是评估能否行外科手术切除，在考虑手术治疗时，必须仔细评估两种肿瘤的可治愈性，如果这2种肿瘤均有治愈的潜力，则每个肿瘤皆应单独治疗。

一般而言，若2个原发肿瘤位置距离较远，第一原发肿瘤行手术治疗或放射治疗和化学治疗后，不影响第二原发肿瘤的治疗；若2个原发肿瘤位置距离较近，对于异时性多原发肿瘤，由于第一原发肿瘤治疗后粘连、解剖结构改变等原因，难以进行第二次手术，或经过放射治射治疗，影响组织结构和血供，对第二原发肿瘤可采用放化学治疗等治疗方法[99]。

对于同时性食管、胃、结直肠内多原发肿瘤，若肿瘤表浅（黏膜内）、体积小，可经内镜切除；若肿瘤侵犯较深、范围较大则需同期或分期手术治疗（腹腔镜手术或开腹手术）[100]。

对于乳腺癌发生异时性第二原发妇科肿瘤的治疗策略，多数学者认为[101-103]，一旦确诊是多原发肿瘤而并非转移癌，应积极采取根治性手术措施。

对于不能耐受手术或广泛转移无法手术的多原发肿瘤患者，给予规范的系统治疗，可延长患者生存期[104-105]。

表3-4 多原发肿瘤基本治疗原则

分类	治疗原则
总体原则	多学科讨论
	通过对各原发肿瘤的病理类型、临床分期、患者身体耐受情况等进行全面评估，制定各原发肿瘤最佳治疗方案
	无论是同时性多原发肿瘤，还是异时性多原发肿瘤，其分子靶向治疗药物（包括针对驱动基因阳性、抗肿瘤新生血管生成）、免疫检查点抑制剂均可参考各自相应肿瘤NCCN指南或ESMO指南推荐
同时性多原发肿瘤	对于同时性多原发肿瘤，治疗前需完成准确的各自临床分期
	对于同时性多原发肿瘤临床分期均为早期的患者，首选同期或分期手术切除；如果患者只能耐受分期手术，则对生物学行为差（如分化差）的肿瘤首先进行手术切除
	对于同时性多原发肿瘤临床分期均为中期（局部进展期）的患者，可考虑同期或分期手术切除，或新辅助治疗后再同期或分期手术切除，或同步或序贯放射治疗联合内科系统治疗（包括化学治疗、分子靶向治疗、免疫检查点抑制剂治疗）
	对于同时性多原发肿瘤临床分期均为晚期的患者，以全身系统治疗为主，或联合舒缓性局部治疗（如恶性心包腔积液、胸腔积液、腹腔积液的腔内药物灌注治疗，脑、骨等转移灶的放射治疗，肝转移灶肝动脉化学治疗灌注与栓塞等）

续表

分类	治疗原则
同时性多原发肿瘤	对于同时性多原发肿瘤临床分期，一种原发肿瘤为早期、另一种原发肿瘤为晚期，一般先针对晚期原发肿瘤进行内科系统治疗，待晚期原发肿瘤缩小（近期疗效评价达到 PR）且病情稳定在 6 月以上者，可考虑早期原发肿瘤手术切除
	对于同时性多原发肿瘤细胞毒药物的选择，应首先选择对 2 种或 2 种以上原发肿瘤均有效、且指南推荐的药物，如同时性肺癌与食管癌、胃癌、卵巢癌、宫颈癌、三阴性乳腺癌等可选择铂类（如顺铂、奈达铂）、紫杉醇类药物（如多西紫杉醇、白蛋白结合型紫杉醇），同时性晚期胃癌与结直肠癌可选择铂类（如奥沙利铂）、氟尿嘧啶类药物（如氟尿嘧啶、卡培他滨等）、伊立替康，同时性胰腺癌与晚期结直肠癌可选择伊立替康、氟尿嘧啶类药物（如氟尿嘧啶、卡培他滨等），等等
异时性多原发肿瘤	对于异时性多原发肿瘤，除第一原发乳腺癌术后分子靶向治疗在 6 个月内未完成辅助治疗外，绝大多数第一原发实体肿瘤均在术后 6 个月完成了辅助治疗。因此，对于异时性第二原发肿瘤的治疗原则与第一原发瘤相同，可参考相应肿瘤 NCCN 指南或 ESMO 指南等推荐
	对于异时性多原发肿瘤细胞毒药物的选择，无论早期、晚期、新辅助、辅助、舒缓治疗，第二、第三等原发肿瘤均以指南推荐药物为准，可参考相应肿瘤 NCCN 指南或 ESMO 指南等推荐
	第一原发肿瘤为早期肿瘤的患者，经过手术治疗和（或）辅助治疗后，无复发、转移： 若第二原发肿瘤临床分期为早期时，首选手术切除第二原发肿瘤； 若临床分期为局部晚期时，可选择新辅助治疗或同步或序贯放射治疗联合内科系统治疗；若临床分期为晚期时，除肿瘤急症（如大出血、胃肠道梗阻与穿孔等）外，一般选择内科系统治疗和（或）联合舒缓性放射治疗（如脑、骨转移等局部放射治疗）
	第一原发肿瘤为局部进展期的患者，未进行根治性手术切除，但通过同步或序贯放射治疗联合内科系统治疗后，肿瘤得到充分控制，且疾病稳定≥1 年： 若第二原发肿瘤临床分期为早期时，可对第二原发肿瘤进行手术切除； 若临床分期为局部晚期时，可选择新辅助治疗或同步或序贯放射治疗联合内科系统治疗；若临床分期为晚期时，除肿瘤急症（如大出血、胃肠道梗阻与穿孔等）外，一般选择内科系统治疗和（或）联合舒缓性放射治疗（如脑、骨转移等局部放射治疗）
	第一原发肿瘤为晚期的患者，第二原发肿瘤无论何种临床分期，除肿瘤急症（如大出血、胃肠道梗阻与穿孔等）外，一般选择内科系统治疗和（或）联合舒缓性放射治疗（如脑、骨转移等局部放射治疗）

二、肺内多原发癌的治疗

对于肺内多原发癌的治疗,目前没有统一的权威性治疗指南指导,关键在于早发现、早诊断、早治疗。首先考虑手术,且治疗后的随访亦极其重要[106]。IASLC指出,多原发肺癌是各不相关的肿瘤,应根据每一个肺部肿瘤的情况单独进行TNM分期[107]。

肺内多原发癌患者预后取决于多种因素[108],但Kim等[109]的研究发现,仅接受支持治疗而不进行抗肿瘤治疗是肺内多原发癌患者预后差的独立危险因素。Dai等[110]指出,多次手术与单次手术治疗疗效相当。

肺内多原发癌的治疗方案应结合患者的临床特征、肿瘤发生部位、肿瘤临床分期、第一原发癌的既往治疗方案等进行综合评估,以确定合理的、可行的治疗方案。对于TNM分期为Ⅰ~Ⅱ期的肺内多原发癌患者,在充分评估患者身体情况的基础上,且无手术禁忌证的情况下,首选的治疗方式仍是手术切除。对于TNM分期较晚或无法耐受手术的患者,应积极进行化学治疗、放射治疗、免疫治疗、靶向治疗。

(一)同时性肺内多原发癌

对于确诊为同时性肺内多原发癌后,应评估两个肺癌病灶是否均可行手术切除。多数学者认为[70,111],多个独立原发肺癌的治疗方法与单一原发肺癌的治疗方法相同,在没有明显禁忌证的情况下建议手术切除,并应尽量选择两个肿瘤均可完全解剖性切除的手术方式。若患者身体可耐受,且多个肿瘤病灶同时具备手术条件,可行同期手术治疗;若不适于同期手术,可根据肿瘤恶性程度、进展速度、预后影响等情况进行综合评估,选择分期手术。如果肺功能储备有限,则患者可能需接受1个或2个病灶的局限性切除,或接受非手术的局部治疗。有研究报道[111-112],同时性肺内2个原发肿瘤病灶均切除的患者,很大一部分患者长期生存超过5年。

对于同时性肺内多原发癌的患者,非手术治疗(放射治疗、化学治疗、靶向治疗、免疫治疗等)可能有一定作用,既可以2个病灶均治疗,也可在2个原发病灶皆需手术切除但认为患者不能耐受时与分期手术切除联合。Zhang等[113]报道了1例同时性肺内多原发癌患者,对其进行了3个周期的新辅助帕博利珠单抗治疗,观察到实性癌灶显著缩小,混合性及纯磨玻璃癌灶不缩小。

有研究表明[114-116]，立体定向放射治疗是同时性肺内多原发癌有效治疗方法，且毒性可耐受，是不能耐受手术或拒绝手术患者的首选治疗手段。

对同时性肺内多原发癌患者而言，如果患者已接受Ⅱ期或Ⅲ期肿瘤切除，则推荐辅助化学治疗、靶向治疗（针对EGFR敏感性突变患者）[117]。

（二）异时性肺内多原发癌

异时性肺内多原发癌患者，通常在第一原发肺癌治疗过程中已接受过常规治疗，如手术、新辅助治疗或辅助治疗。对于这类患者，只要具备手术条件，应行第二原发肺癌的手术治疗。Shen等[118]报道，约2/3的异时性肺内多原发癌患者可行手术切除，接受切除术的患者中约1/3为局限性切除术。

三、上消化道内多原发肿瘤治疗

上消化道内多原发肿瘤的治疗，一般遵循各肿瘤相应的处理原则，即根据各病灶的部位、临床分期，选择不同的治疗方法[119]。

有研究报道[120-123]，对于上消化道内多原发早期癌，除手术切除外，可选择单独内镜微创治疗，如对多原发癌灶中的食管重度异型增生/原位癌和黏膜内癌、胃腺上皮高级别上皮内瘤变，采用内镜黏膜切除术（EMR）、内镜黏膜剥离术（ESD）、多环套扎黏膜切除术（MBM）；对于早期癌与进展期癌共存的多原发癌患者，可采用内镜治疗早期病灶、手术治疗进展期病灶。

Kimir等[124]认为，早期胃内多原发癌淋巴结浸润和血行转移与单发癌相当或很少，术后生存率与单发相似。因此，早期胃内多原发癌无须扩大手术范围，若每一处病变符合治疗标准，可行内镜下治疗。Seto等[125]指出，内窥镜黏膜切除术对早期胃内多原发癌是可行的，只要没有黏膜下浸润，病灶不超过2cm，亦没有淋巴结转移。

四、同时性结直肠内多原发癌治疗

目前，尚无针对同时性结直肠内多原发癌标准治疗方案，但通常与单原发结直肠癌相似。一般需根据患者年龄、身体状况、肿瘤数量和位置、分化程度、结直肠切除范围，以及可能的吻合口，制订个体化的治疗方案。

同时性结直肠内多原发癌的手术治疗需针对肿瘤不同的位置选择不同的手术方案。李晨等[126]建议，肿瘤灶位于相隔肠段时可行相应肠段根治性切除术，当位于同一肠段或相邻肠段时，应行连续性肠段切除术。切除相应肠段后，需观察剩余肠段血供情况。Lee 等[127]研究显示，对于相隔较远的癌灶实行分段切除较广泛切除在并发症发生率及异时性癌发生率方面并无差异，且保留了功能肠段，预后更好。

腹腔镜手术创伤小，患者恢复快，相对于传统开腹手术，术后感染及术后肠粘连的概率大大降低。有研究报道[128-131]，腹腔镜辅助同步肠吻合术、腹腔镜同时性结直肠内多原发癌根治术是一种安全、可行的手术方法。

参考文献

[1] 王贵齐，魏文强，吕宁，等. 应用内镜普查研究食管癌高发区贲门癌的发病情况[J]. 中国肿瘤临床，2003，30(3)：156-158.

[2] Hori K, Okada H, Kawahara Y, et al. Lugol – voiding lesions are an important risk factor for a second primary squamous cell carcinoma in patients with csosphageal cancer or head and neck cancer[J]. Am J Gastroenterol, 2011, 106(5)：858-866.

[3] Sun D, Shi Q, Li R, et al. Experience in Simultaneous Endoscopic Submucosal Dissection Treating Synchronous Multiple Primary Early Esophageal Cancers[J]. J Laparoendosc Adv Surg Tech A, 2019, 29(7)：921-925.

[4] 赵丽，张晓梅，孙刚，等. 色素内镜-食管多原发癌早期诊断的有效手段[J]. 胃肠病学和肝病学杂志，2017，26(5)：534-535.

[5] Ribeiro UJr, Jorge UM, Safatle – Ribeiro AV, et al. Clinicopathologic and immunohistochemistry characterization of synchronous multiple primary gastric adenocarcinoma[J]. J Gastrointest Surg, 2007, 11(3)：233-239.

[6] 王沧海，吴静，刘红，等. 胃食管早期多原发肿瘤12例分析[J]. 首都医科大学学报，2018，39(5)：680-684.

[7] 朱一苗，潘文胜. 异时性多原发上消化道肿瘤[J]. 实用肿瘤杂志，2014，29(5)：457-460.

[8] 刘刚，史良会. 19例同时性多原发性结直肠癌临床诊疗分析[J]. 齐齐哈尔医学院学报，2017，38(23)：2782-2783.

[9] 牛丽云，张峻岭，刘天野，等. 结直肠同时性多原发癌的临床病理特征和预后分析

[J]. 中华胃肠外科杂, 2018, 21(1): 41-45.

[10] Eu KW, Seow-Choen F. Synchronous colorectal cancer in an Oriental population[J]. Int J Colorectal Dis, 1993, 8(4): 193-196.

[11] Latournerie M, Jooste V, Cottet V, et al. Epidemiology and prognosis of synchronous colorectal cancers[J]. Br J Surg, 2008, 95(12): 1528-1533.

[12] 申占龙, 叶颖江, 王杉. 多原发结直肠癌的临床病理特点[J]. 中华消化外科杂志, 2011, 10(1): 53-56.

[13] Kim MS. Detection and treatment of synchronous lesions in colorectal cancer: the clinical implication of perioperative colonoscopy[J]. World J Gastroenterol, 2007, 13(30): 4108-4111.

[14] Neri E, Giusti P, Battolla L, et al. Colorectal cancer: role of CT colonography in preoperative evaluation after incomplete colonoscopy[J]. Radiology, 2002, 223: 615-619.

[15] Xu GZ, Guan DJ, He ZY. ^{18}F-FDG PET/CT for detecting distant metastases and second primary cancers in patients with head and neck cancer. A meta-analysis[J]. Oral Oncol, 2011, 47(7): 560-565.

[16] Ishimori T, Patel PV, Wahl RL. Detection of unexpected additional primary malignancies with PET/CT[J]. J Nucl Med, 2005, 46(5): 752-757.

[17] Xu H, Zhang M, Zhai G, et al. The clinical significance of ^{18}F-FDG PET/CT in early detection of second primary malignancy in cancer patients[J]. J Cancer Res Clin Oncol, 2010, 136(8): 1125-1134.

[18] Pang L, Liu G, Shi H, et al. Nineteen cases with synchronous multiple primary cancers studied by ^{18}F-FDG PET/CT[J]. Hell J Nucl Med, 2017, 20(1): 36-40.

[19] Malik V, Johnston C, Donohoe C, et al. F-18-FDG PET-detected synchronous primary neoplasms in the staging of esophageal cancer incidence, cost, and impact on management [J]. Clin Nucl Med, 2012, 37(12): 1152-1158.

[20] Froio E, DAdda T, Fellegara G, et al. Uterinestatic to the lung as large-cell neuroendocrine carcinoma with synchronous sarcoid granulomatosis[J]. Lung Cancer, 2009, 64(3): 371-377.

[21] 郭春梅, 吴静, 刘红, 等. 多原发大肠癌临床病理特点及诊治分析[J]. 中华消化内镜杂志, 2019, 36(10): 731-736.

[22] Arakawa K, Hata K, Nozawa H, et al. Prognostic significance and clinicopathological features of synchronous colorectal cancer[J]. Anticancer Res, 2018, 38(10): 5889-5895.

[23] Yokozaki H, samba H, Fujimoto JY. Microsatellite instabilities in gastric cancer patients with multiple primary cancers[J]. Int J Oncol, 1999, 14(1): 151-155.

[24] Kadara H, Wistuba H. Field cancerization in non-small cell lung cancer: implications in

disease pathogenesis[J]. Proc Am Thorac Soc, 2012, 9(2): 38-42.

[25] Asmar R, Sonett JR, Singh G, et al. Use of oncogenic driver mutations in staging of multiple primary lung carcinomas: a single-center experience[J]. J Thorac Oncol, 2017, 12(10): 1524-1535.

[26] Weinberg BA, Gowen K, Lee TK, et al. Comprehensive genomic profiling aids in distinguishing metastatic recurrence from second primary cancers[J]. Oncologist, 2017, 22(2): 152-157.

[27] Murphy SJ, Harris FR, Kosari F, et al. Using genomics to differentiate multiple primaries from metastatic lung cancer[J]. J Thorac Oncol, 2019, 14(9): 1567-1582.

[28] Huang J, Behrens C, Wistuba I, et al. Molecular analysis of synchronous and metachronous tumors of the lung: impact on management and prognosis[J]. Ann Diagn Pathol, 2001, 5(6): 321-329.

[29] van Rens MT, Eijken EJ, Elhers JR, et al. p53 mutation analysis for definite diagnosis of multiple primary lung carcinoma[J]. Cancer, 2002, 94(1): l88-196.

[30] Metzker ML. Sequencing technologies - the next generation[J]. Nat Rev Genet, 2010, 11(1): 31-46.

[31] Froio E, D'Adda T, Fellegara G, et al. Three different synchronous primary lung tumours: a case report with extensive genetic analysis and reviwc of the literature[J]. Lung cancer, 2008, 59(3): 395-402.

[32] Dacic S. Dilemmas in lung cancer staging[J]. Arch Pathol Lab Med, 2012, 136(10): 1194-1197.

[33] 周渝斌, 沈诚, 杜恒, 等. 外周血有核细胞DNA损伤检测在肺多原发癌患者诊断中的临床价值[J]. 肿瘤防治研究, 2015, 42(04): 373-377.

[34] Dong M, Wei H, Hou JM, et al. Possible prognostic significance of p53, cyclin D1 and Ki-67 in the second primary malignancyof patients with double primary malignancies[J]. Int J Clin Exp Pathol, 2014, 7(7): 3975-3983.

[35] 李海亮, 张勇, 李晓磊, 等. 食管鳞状细胞癌壁内浸润的临床病理研究[J]. 宁夏医学杂志, 2010, 32(12): 1166-1168.

[36] 吴道宏, 吴洲红, 吴本俨, 等. 多原发早期胃癌临床病理特征及预后分析[J]. 中国肿瘤临床与康复, 2009, 16(1): 19-21.

[37] 汪栋, 金岚, 姚宏伟, 等. 35例同时性多原发结直肠癌患者临床诊疗分析[J]. 首都医科大学学报, 2018, 39(3): 413-417.

[38] 付金金, 黄载伟, 林英豪, 等. 39例多原发结直肠癌的临床研究[J]. 南方医科大学学报, 2013, 33(4): 578-581.

[39] Natsugoe S, Matsumoto M, Okumura H, et al. Multiple primary carcinomas with esophageal squamous cell cancer: clinical pathologic outcome[J]. World J Surg, 2005, 29

(1)：46-49.

[40] 肖杨，王发恒，朱德祥，等．食管多原癌及食管癌伴消化道恶性肿瘤[J]．肿瘤防治研究，1993，20(4)：280-281．

[41] 解建，王连生，孟凡利，等．上消化道同时性多原发性肿瘤漏诊原因及其防治——附28例分析[J]．中国肿瘤临床与康复，1998，5(2)：43-44．

[42] 陈建华，张成阳，王世芳，等．食管胃双原发癌临床病理分析[J]．肿瘤研究与临床，2004，16(1)：52-53．

[43] 林汉利，郑昌京．食管癌538例内镜病理分析——附多源癌13例[J]．实用医学杂志，2009，25(19)：3291-3293．

[44] 李小毅，钟定荣，陈思，等．胃癌合并其他器官原发癌103例分析[J]．中国普外基础与临床杂志，2012，19(1)：43-47．

[45] 徐丽芳，朱丽．上消化道多发癌53例临床分析[J]．实用肿瘤学杂志，2002，16(3)：222-223．

[46] Mamounas EP, Perez-Mesa C, Penetrante RB, et al. Patterns of occurrence of second primary non-mammary malignancies in breast cancer patients: results from 1382 consecutive autopsies[J]. Surg Oncol, 1993, 2(3): 175-185.

[47] Yuan L, Liu LX, Che GW. The advancement of predictive diagnosis and molecular mechanism in multiple primary lung cancer[J]. Chin J Cancer, 2010, 29(5): 575-578.

[48] Tanvetyanon T, Finley DJ, Fabian T, et al. Prognostic factors for survival after complete resections of synchronous lung cancers in multiple lobes: pooled analysis based on in dividual patient data[J]. Ann Oncol, 2013, 24(4): 889-894.

[49] Warren S, Gates O. Multiple primary malignant tumors: a survey of the literature and a statistical study[J]. Am Cancer, 1932, 16(8): 1358-1414.

[50] 朱莉菲，薛鹏，王理伟．65例多原发癌的临床回顾性研究[J]．复旦学报(医学版)，2010，37(5)：591-593．

[51] 钟海鸣，陈景胜，吴昱冶，等．多原发癌86例临床分析[J]．广东医学院学报，2009，27(4)：433-434．

[52] 王帆，郭瑞嵩，韩海鱼，等．多原发癌384例临床分析[J]．实用医技杂志，2009，16(12)：960-961．

[53] Rovatti M, Gerosa E, Turi V, et al. Multiple primary malignant neoplasms[J]. Minerva Chir, 1995, 50(11): 909-958.

[54] Detterbeck FC, Jones DR, Kernstine KH, et al. Lung cancer. Special treatment issues[J]. Chest, 2003, 123(1 Sup-pl): 244S-258S.

[55] Registries IAOC. International rules for multiple primary cancers[J]. Asian Pac J Cancer Prev, 2005, 6(1): 104-106.

[56] Working Group Report. International rules for multiple primary cancers (ICD-0 third

edition)[J]. Eur J Cancer Prev, 2005, 14(4): 307-308.

[57] Ferlay J, Soerjomataram I, Ervik M, et al. GLOBOCAN 2012 v1.1, Cancer incidence and mortality worldwide: IARC cancer base No. 11[J]. Int J Cancer, 2014, 136(5): e359-e386.

[58] Moertel CG, Dockerty MB, Baggenstoss AH. Multiple primary malignant neoplasms[J]. Cancer, 1961, 14(1): 221-237.

[59] Chaudary MA, Millis RR, Hoskins EO, et al. Bilateral primary breast cancer: a prospective study of disease incidence[J]. Br J Surg, 1984, 71(9): 711-714.

[60] Martini N, Melamed MR. Multiple primary lung cancers[J]. J Thorac Cardiovasc Surg, 1975, 70(4): 606-612.

[61] Chen TF, Xie CY, Rao BY, et al. Surgical treatment to multiple primary lung cancerpatients: a systematic review and meta-analysis[J]. BMC Surg, 2019, 19(1): 185.

[62] Li X, Hu B, Li H, et al. Application of artificial intelligence in the diagnosis of multiple primary lung cancer[J]. Thorac Cancer, 2019, 10(11): 2168-2174.

[63] 彭岳, 王晖, 谢厚耐, 等. 同时性多原发肺腺癌的外科治疗及预后[J]. 中国肺癌杂志, 2017, 20(2): 107-113.

[64] Jiang L, He J, Shi X, et al. Prognosis of synchronous and metachronous multiple primary lung cancers: Systematic review and meta-analysis[J]. Lung Cancer, 2015, 87(3): 303-310.

[65] Fonseca A, Detterbeck FC. How many names for a rose: Inconsistent classification of multiple foci of lung cancer due to ambiguous rules[J]. Lung Cancer, 2014, 85(1): 7-11.

[66] Takamochi K, Oh S, Matsuoka J, et al. Clonality status of multifocal lung adenocarcinomas based on the mutation patterns of EGFR and K-ras[J]. Lung Cancer, 2012, 75(3): 313-320.

[67] Patel SB, Kadi W, Walts AE, et al. Next Generation Sequencing A Novel Approach to Distinguish Multifocal Primary Lung Adenocarcinomas from Intrapulmonary Metastases[J]. J Mol Diagn, 2017, 19(6): 870-882.

[68] Chiang CL, Tsai PC, Yeh YC, et al. Recent advances in the diagnosis and management of multiple primary lung cancer[J]. Cancers (Basel), 2022, 14(1): 242.

[69] Chang JC, Alex D, Bott M, et al. Comprehensive next-generation sequencing unambiguously distinguishes separate primary lung carcinomas from intrapulmonary metastases: comparison with standard histopathologic approach[J]. Clin Cancer Res, 2019, 25(23): 7113-7125.

[70] Warth A, Macher-Goeppinger S, Muley T, et al. Clonality of multifocal non-small cell lung cancer: implications for staging and therapy[J]. Eur Respir J, 2012, 39(6): 1437-

1442.

[71] Rens M, Eijken E, Elbers J, et al. p53 mutation analysis for definite diagnosis of multiple primary lung carcinoma[J]. Cancer, 2002, 94(1): 188-196.

[72] Shimizu S, Yatabe Y, Koshikawa T, et al. High frequency of clonally related tumors in cases of multiple synchronous lung cancers as revealed by molecular diagnosis[J]. Clin Cancer Res, 2000, 6(10): 3994-4013.

[73] Allen EMV, Wagle N, Stojanov P, et al. Whole-exome sequencing and clinical interpretation of formalin-fixed, paraffin-embedded tumor samples to guide precision cancer medicine[J]. Nat Med, 2014, 20(6): 682-688.

[74] Ezer N, Wang H, Corredor AG, et al. Integrating NGS-derived mutational profiling in the diagnosis of multiple lung adenocarcinomas[J]. Cancer Treat Res Commun, 2021, 29(4): 100484-100494.

[75] Roepman P, Heuvel AT, Scheidel KC, et al. Added Value of 50-Gene Panel Sequencing to Distinguish Multiple Primary Lung Cancers from Pulmonary Metastases: A Systematic Investigation-ScienceDirect[J]. J Mol Diagn, 2018, 20(4): 436-445.

[76] Mansuet-Lupo A, Barritault M, Alifano M, et al. Proposal for a combined histomolecular algorithm to distinguish multiple primary adenocarcinomas from intrapulmonary metastasis in patients with multiple lung tumors[J]. J Thorac Oncol, 2019, 14(5): 844-856.

[77] 孙芩玲, 叶联华, 黄云超, 等. 多原发肺癌的临床特征及预后因素分析[J]. 癌症, 2022, 41(4): 191-199.

[78] Belardinilli F, Pernazza A, Mahdavian Y, et al. A multidisciplinary approach for the differential diagnosis between multiple primary lung adenocarcinomas and intrapul-monary metastases[J]. Pathol Res Pract, 2021, 220(4): 153387-153396.

[79] Zhou LN, Wu N, Li M. Diagnostic value of multi-slice spiral CT in synchronous multiple primary lung cancer[J]. Ai Zheng Jin Zhan, 2012, 10(1): 64-68.

[80] Liu Y, Tang Y, Xue Z, et al. SUVmax Ratio on PET/CT May Differentiate Between Lung Metastases and Synchronous Multiple Primary Lung Cancer[J]. Acad Radiol, 2020, 27(5): 618-623.

[81] Detterbeck FC, Nicholson AG, Franklin WA, et al. The IASLC lung cancer staging project: summary of proposals for revisions of the classification of lung cancers with multiple pulmonary sites of involvement in the forth-coming eighth edition of the TNM classification[J]. J Thorac Oncol, 2016, 11(5): 639-650.

[82] 苏若瑟, 王其山. 食管与胃相对同时性双原发癌32例临床分析[J]. 中国内镜杂志, 2004, 10(3): 67-68.

[83] 宋丽杰, 吴华星, 付丽娜, 等. 同时性食管多原发癌99例内镜检查分析[J]. 实用肿瘤学杂志, 2008, 22(3): 244-245.

[84] Hyjata K, Sipita J, Grenman R, et al. Panendoscopy and synchronous second primary cancer patients[J]. Eur Arch otorhinolarynol, 2005, 262(1): 17-20.

[85] Kim SH, Kim HJ, Lee JI, et al. Multiple primary cancers including colorectal cancer[J]. J Korean Soc Coloproctol, 2008, 24(7): 467-472.

[86] Giardiello C, Angelone G, Iodice G, et al. Diagnosis, therapy, and follow up in synchronous colorectal cancer of the colon[J]. G Chir, 2001, 22(4): 122-124.

[87] 孙海燕, 潘战宇, 张新伟, 等. 40例多原发癌姑息治疗多学科会诊临床分析[J]. 中国肿瘤临床, 2016, 43(15): 674-678.

[88] 孙海涛, 王南, 刘艺, 等. 184例多原发恶性肿瘤临床特征及其预后分析[J]. 现代肿瘤医学, 2023, 31(8): 1530-1535.

[89] Xue X, Xue Q, Wang N, et al. Early clinical diagnosis of synchronous multiple primary lung cancer[J]. Oncol Lett, 2012, 3(1): 234-237.

[90] Tsunezuka Y, Matsumoto I, Tamura M, et al. The results of therapy for bilateral multiple primary lung cancers: 30 years experience in a single centre[J]. Eur J Surg Oncol, 2004, 30(7): 781-785.

[91] Gu HL, Zeng SX, Chang YB, et al. Multidisciplinary treatment based on surgery leading to long-term survival of a patient with multiple a synchronous rare primary malignant neoplasms: A case report and literature review[J]. Oncol Lett, 2015, 9(3): 1135-1141.

[92] 张立玮, 丛庆文, 王十杰, 等. 多原发癌五次手术及内镜治疗长期生存一例[J]. 中华医学杂志, 1998, (12): 946.

[93] Adebonojo SA, Moritz DM, Danby CA. The results of modem surgical therapy formultiple primary lung cancers[J]. Chest, 1997, 112(3): 693-701.

[94] 董莉莉, 牛艳洁, 潘峰, 等. 第二原发癌为肺癌的多原发癌患者临床分析[J]. 临床与病理杂志, 2017, 37(4): 724-728.

[95] 孙晓卫, 詹友庆, 李威, 等. 58例多原发性胃癌分析[J]. 中国肿瘤临床, 2007, 34(5): 261-265.

[96] 张真, 蔡昌豪, 吴本俨. 141例多原发恶性肿瘤的临床分析[J]. 中华老年多器官疾病杂志, 2008, 7(2): 128-131, 144.

[97] 叶天仪, 姚洪文, 吴令英, 等. 34例子宫内膜癌合并结直肠癌双原发癌的临床特征及其与Lynch综合征关系分析[J]. 中国肿瘤临床, 2015, 42(8): 432-436.

[98] 伍国号, 陈福进, 曾宗渊, 等. 放射诱发的第二原发性恶性肿瘤的临床治疗[J]. 中华肿瘤杂志, 2003, 25(3): 275-277.

[99] Morita M, Kimura Y, Yamashita N, et al. Surgical strategies for esophageal cancer associated with head and neck cancer[J]. Surg Today, 2014, 44(9): 1603-1610.

[100] Morita M, Kimura Y, Saeki H, et al. Surgical resection for esophageal cancer synchronously

or metachronously associated with head and neck cancer[J]. Ann Surg Oncol, 2013, 20(7): 2434-2439.

[101] 李小平, 魏丽惠, 王悦, 等. 13例子宫内膜癌合并多原发恶性肿瘤临床分析[J]. 中国妇科临床杂志, 2001, 2(1): 11-13.

[102] 帖晓静. 首发为乳腺癌的相关多原发癌23例临床分析[J]. 中国医药科学, 2011, 1(16): 164-164.

[103] 李倩, 王纯雁. 乳腺癌术后再发卵巢癌的预防与诊治[J]. 中国实用妇科与产科杂志, 2017, 33(4): 371-376.

[104] Ishibashi-Kanno N, Yamagata K, Uchida F, et al. Usefulness of esophagogastro-duodenoscopy and ^{18}F-fluorodeoxyglucose positronemission tomography in detecting synchronous multiple primary cancers with oral cancer[J]. J Oral Maxillofac Surg, 2017, 21(4): 391-396.

[105] Li QW, Zhu YJ, Zhang WW, et al. Chemoradiotherapy for synchronous multiple primary cancers with esophageal squamous cell carcinoma: a case-control study[J]. J Cancer, 2017, 8(4): 563-569.

[106] Gregoire J. Guiding principles in the management of synchronous and metachronous primary non-small cell lung cancer[J]. Thorac Surg Clin, 2021, 31(3): 237-254.

[107] Detterbeck FC, Boffa DJ, Kim AW, et al. The eighth edition lung cancer stage classification[J]. Chest, 2017, 151(1): 193-203.

[108] Waller DA. Surgical management of lung cancer with multiple lesions: implication of the new recommendations of the 8th edition of the TNM classification for lung cancer[J]. J Thorac Dis, 2018, 10(S22): S2686-S2691.

[109] Kim SW, Kong KA, Kim DY, et al. Multiple primary cancers involving lung cancer at a single tertiary hospital: Clinical features and prognosis[J]. Thorac Cancer, 2015, 6(2): 159-165.

[110] Dai L, Yang HL, Yan WP, et al. The equivalent efficacy of multiple operations for multiple primary lung cancer and a single operation for single primary lung cancer[J]. J Thorac Dis, 2016, 8(5): 855-861.

[111] Finley DJ, Yoshizawa A, Travis W, et al. Predictors of Outcomes after Surgical Treatment of Synchronous Primary Lung Cancers[J]. J Thorac Oncol, 2010, 5(2): 197-205.

[112] Stella F, Luciano G, Dell'Amore A, et al. Pulmonary Metastases from NSCLC and MPLC (Multiple Primary Lung Cancers): Management and Outcome in a Single Centre Experience[J]. Heart Lung Circ, 2016, 25(2): 191-195.

[113] Zhang C, Yin K, Liu SY, et al. Multiomics analysis reveals a distinct response mechanism in multiple primary lung adenocarcinoma after neoadjuvant immunotherapy[J]. J Immunother Cancer, 2021, 9(4): e002312.

[114] Owen D, Olivier KR, Mayo CS, et al. Outcomes of stereotactic body radiotherapy(SBRT) treatment of multiple synchronous and recurrent lung nodules[J]. Radiat Oncol, 2015, 10(43): 1-8.

[115] Chang JY, Liu YH, Zhu Z, et al. Stereotactic ablative radiotherapy: A potentially curable approach to early stage multiple primary lung cancer[J]. Cancer, 2013, 119(18): 3402-3410.

[116] Griffioen GH, Lagerwaard FJ, Haasbeek CJA, et al. Treatment of multiple primary lung cancers using stereotactic radiotherapy, either with or without surgery[J]. Radiother Oncol, 2013, 107(3): 403-408.

[117] Marcel T, Van Rens A, Hans R, et al. Prognostic Assessment of 2, 361 Patients Who Underwent Pulmonary Resection for Non-small Cell Lung Cancer, Stage Ⅰ, Ⅱ, and ⅢA[J]. Chest, 2000, 117(2): 374-379.

[118] Shen KR, Meyers BF, Larner JM, et al. Special Treatment Issues in Lung Cancer[J]. Chest, 2007, 132(3): 290S-305S.

[119] 马少华, 杨合利, 梁震, 等. 综合治疗食管多原发癌22例[J]. 中华胃肠外科杂志, 2011, 14(9): 702-704.

[120] Shimada H, Makuuchi H, Chino O, et al. Recent advances of endoscopic treatment for esophageal cancer[J]. Nihon Geka Gakkai Zasshi, 2008, 109(1): 10-14.

[121] 张立玮, 土士杰, 于卫芳, 等. 早期贲门癌及癌前病变的内镜微创治疗研究[J]. 中国肿瘤临床. 2008, 35(22): 1261-1264.

[122] Wang SJ, Wu ML, Zhang LW, et al. The value of endoscopic mucosal resection for dysplasia and early-stage cancer of the esophagus and gastric cardia[J]. Zhonghua Zhong Liu Za Zhi, 2008, 30(11): 853-857.

[123] Becker V, Mhouj M, Schmid RM, et al. Multimodal endoscopic therapy for multifocal intraepithelial neoplasia and superficial esophageal squamous cell carcinoma a case series[J]. Endoscopy, 2011, 43(4): 360-364.

[124] Kimir Takeshita, Masao Tani, Tooru Honda. Treatment of Primary Multiple Early Gastric Cancer: From the view point of clinicopathologic Features[J]. World J Surg, 1997, 21(8): 832-836.

[125] Seto Y, Nagawa H, Muto T. Treatment of multiple early gastric cancer[J]. Jpn J Clin Oncol, 1996, 26(3): 134-138.

[126] 李晨, 郭玉霖, 陈贵进, 等. 同时性多原发结直肠癌临床诊治分析[J]. 解放军医学院学报, 2016, 37(7): 735-738.

[127] Lee BC, Yu CS, Kim J, et al. Clinicopathological features and surgical options for synchronous colorectal cancer[J]. Medicine, 2017, 96(9): e6224-e6231.

[128] Li ZT, Wang DW, Wei YW, et al. Clinical outcomes of laparoscopic-assisted

synchronous bowel anastomoses for synchronous colorectal cancer: initial clinical experience [J]. Oncotarget, 2017, 8(6): 10741-10747.

[129] Inada R, Yamamoto S, Takawa M, et al. aparoscopic resection of synchronous colorectal cancers in separate specimens[J]. Asian J Endosc Surg, 2014, 7(3): 227-231.

[130] 李慧诚, 刘习红, 王希, 等. 腹腔镜同时性多原发结直肠癌根治术[J]. 中华消化外科杂志, 2013, 12(6): 443-446.

[131] Takatsu Y, Akiyoshi T, Nagata J, et al. Surgery for synchronous colorectal cancers with double colonic anastomoses: a comparison of laparoscopic and open approaches[J]. Asian J Endosc Surg, 2015, 8(4): 429-433.

第四章

预后、随访与康复

第一节 预后情况

一、生存率的计算

目前,对于多原发肿瘤患者生存时间的计算方法没有统一标准,且存在一定分歧,尤其是异时性多原发肿瘤患者的生存计算。

有学者认为[1],对于异时性多原发肿瘤患者的生存时间应从第一原发肿瘤确诊时间算起,因从第二原发肿瘤计算生存时间会减少有用信息;而另一些学者认为[2-4],应从第二原发肿瘤的发生时间计算较为合理,因第二原发肿瘤的发生后才能定义为该患者为多原发肿瘤患者,若从第一原发肿瘤开始计算,则往往出现多原发肿瘤患者的1年、3年、5年预后与单发肿瘤者无差异甚至较单发肿瘤好的结果,这似乎与事实不相符。因此,有较多的学者支持第二种观点。但是,多原发肿瘤预后受多种因素影响,且部分多原发肿瘤患者预后不一定劣于单原发肿瘤患者。

二、总体预后

由于计算方法上的不同,文献报道的多原发肿瘤年生存率存在较大差异。有学者报道[5],多原发肿瘤的10年生存率为69.3%;而张稚淳等[6]报道的120例多原发肿瘤患者,3年、5年生存率分别为48.3%和37.5%。易胜中等[7]报道了281例肺癌和肺外器官肿瘤组成的多原发肿瘤,115例第一原发肿瘤为肺癌、第二原发肿瘤为肺或肺外器官(A组),166例第一原发肿瘤为肺外器官、第二原发肿瘤为肺(B组)。从第一原发癌确诊算起,A、B两组中位生存时间分别为69.0个月和87.5个月,5年生存率分别为59.0%和70.0%,B组优于A组。从第二原发癌确诊算起,A、B两组中位 OS 时间分别为 25.0 个月和 28.0 个月，5 年生存率分别为 10.5% 和 13.5%，两者无显著性差异。

亦有生存期极长的中国个案报道，如许刚等[8]报道了 1 例四原发癌，分别为结肠腺癌、膀胱低级别尿路上皮癌、肾脏透明细胞癌、食管腺鳞癌，截止报道时（2019 年），距离首次发病的结肠癌 33 年、膀胱癌 8 年、肾癌 2 年，膀胱癌复发 4 次，但无远处转移，至报道时患者仍生存。吴建国等[9]报道了 1 例消化道异时性多原发肿瘤患者，经多次手术后，生存期达到 35 年。

另外，第一、第二等原发肿瘤部位不同，其远期生存亦有明显不同。不同的作者报道的手术根治性切除术后的病理分期为 Ⅱ 期的肺内多原发癌患者 5 年生存率有很大差异，区间为 0%～79%[10-13]。张琦等[14]报道了 118 例同时性多原发肺内癌，3 年、5 年生存率分别为 92.37%、82.20%；作者认为，是否吸烟、术后有无辅助治疗、病理类型、淋巴结是否转移、分化程度，以及是否位于同一肺叶是该类患者生存的独立预后因素。Takamochi 等[15]报道，多原发肺内腺癌患者的 3 年、5 年生存率分别为 82.1% 和 77.3%；Yang 等[16]的研究结果显示，双侧多原发肺内腺癌患者的 3 年、5 年生存率分别为 84.5% 和 75.0%；二者报道的结果相似。

Rose 等[17]的研究显示，第二原发散发型子宫内膜癌的 5 年生存率约为 80%，多原发结直肠内癌的 5 年生存率约为 60%。一项长达 26 年的流行病学调查数据显示[18]，乳腺癌作为第一原发肿瘤的多原发肿瘤患者的 5 年生存率仅有 25%。

三、预后相关因素

多数学者认为[19-25]，多原发肿瘤患者的预后与肿瘤临床或病理分期、肿瘤分化程度、肿瘤部位分布、两种肿瘤发生的间隔时间、治疗方式以及患者年龄等多种因素相关。

孙海涛等[26]报道了 184 例多原发肿瘤，单因素分析表明，性别、年龄、第一原发肿瘤分期、吸烟史、同时性或异时性是影响多原发肿瘤生存的预后因素；多因素分析显示，第一原发肿瘤临床分期是影响多原发肿瘤预后的独立危险因素。李小毅等[27]认为，胃内多原发癌的预后与肿瘤的病理类型、临床分期、病灶的位置及根治程度等因素有关。Tae Kyung 等[28]对 90 例第一原发肿瘤胃癌患者再发第二原发肿瘤的观察发现，相较于第一原发肿瘤胃癌分期,第二原发肿瘤分期对于患者预后影响更大。Eom 等[29]指出,胃癌合并其他器官多原发肿瘤患者的主要死因是其他器官的原发肿瘤,而非胃癌。但董锐增[30]认为,第一原发肿瘤胃癌是该类患者最主要的死因,这可能是因为国外多原发肿瘤患者中早期胃癌的比例较高[31]。

有学者认为[32-33],多原发肿瘤患者的生存期很大程度上取决于恶性程度最高的原发肿瘤。肖飞等[34]指出,多原发肺鳞癌患者预后较早期发现的肺周边型原位腺癌及微浸润腺癌相差很多,且不同病理类型患者转移程度及治疗敏感度不同,从而导致患者预后及生存状况的不同。

何萍等[35]的研究表明,淋巴结是否转移、病灶是否位于同一肺叶均是影响同时性多原发肺内癌患者预后及生存状况的独立危险因素。孙芩玲等[36]报道了120例多原发肺内癌,均经手术病理确诊,患者手术后3年、5年生存率分别为87.5%(105/120)、79.2%(95/120);Cox多因素分析结果显示,年龄>65岁、既往有吸烟史、Ki-67>50%、最大肿瘤直径>2cm及淋巴结转移可能为多原发肺内癌预后不良因素。郭海法等[37]认为,较小的肿瘤直径与多原发肺内癌预后良好相关。Wang等[38]对肺内多原发癌的研究显示,第一原发肿瘤诊断年龄(≥60岁)、同时性多原发肿瘤、第一原发肿瘤为肺癌且其分期≥Ⅱ期为其预后欠佳的独立危险因素。有学者报道[39-40],吸烟对多原发肺内癌预后可产生严重的负面影响。

有研究报道[41],乳腺多原发癌的类型、有无淋巴结转移是乳腺多原发肿瘤患者预后的独立影响因素。同时性双侧乳腺癌ER、PR一致阳性、Ki-67一致性低表达患者预后最佳,ER、PR一致阴性、Ki-67一致性高表达患者预后最差[42-44]。

牛丽云等[45]的研究表明,同时性多原发结直肠内癌患者年龄≤65岁、肿瘤分期Ⅲ和Ⅳ期以及肿瘤的病理类型为未分化癌或黏液腺癌是结直肠癌术后5年复发的危险因素;且有研究报道[46],同时性多原发结直肠癌的存在、原发肿瘤大小≥6.5cm是异时性多原发结直肠癌的独立危险因素。

Aydiner等[47]认为,性别对多原发肿瘤患者的预后无明显影响,但也有文献报道,女性患者预后优于男性患者[48]。

(一)多原发肿瘤、单原发肿瘤与预后

对于多原发肿瘤与单原发肿瘤预后是否存在差异,目前存在争议,主要有3种观点,①二者无差异;②单原发肿瘤优于多原发肿瘤;③多原发

第四章　预后、随访与康复

肿瘤优于单原发肿瘤。

(1) 有学者认为[49-51]，多原发肿瘤患者与单发肿瘤患者的预后无明显差异，且多原发肿瘤患者预后与原发肿瘤的个数无关。

Bhattacharyya 等[52]通过对头颈部第二原发癌与第一原发癌进行配对研究，结果显示，头颈部第二原发癌患者的生存率可能较第一原发癌差，但无统计学意义。Wang 等[53]对第二原发性小细胞肺癌与第一原发小细胞肺癌的比较发现，在疗效、中位生存期方面二者无显著性差异。

(2) 有学者认为单原发肿瘤患者预后优于多原发肿瘤患者，Boute 等[54]指出，单原发头颈部肿瘤患者预后较头颈部多原发肿瘤患者预后好。魏先锋等[55]认为，头颈部多原发肿瘤预后不良的原因是多原发肿瘤多发生于老年患者，身体素质差，伴随疾病多；多原发癌发病隐匿，临床上对原发癌评估不足或随访不严密而易漏诊、误诊，延误诊治；第一原发癌的治疗(如放射治疗)影响了第二原发肿瘤的治疗。

有研究报道[56-57]，单原发乳腺癌患者的总体生存率明显优于多原发乳腺癌患者。在乳腺多原发肿瘤患者中，多原发肿瘤发生数量越多，预后越差，发生间隔时间较长，预后较好[58]。MD 安德森癌症中心的一项基于4198 例乳腺癌保乳治疗的随访数据发现[59]，单原发乳腺癌患者的预后明显优于多原发乳腺癌患者。韩国学者报道的数据显示[60]，单原发乳腺癌与多原发乳腺肿瘤的 5 年生存率、10 年生存率有显著差异，单一乳腺癌患者的预后显著优于多原发乳腺癌。有研究者指出[61-62]，多原发乳腺肿瘤患者的预后还取决于第二原发肿瘤的类型、恶性程度及其对治疗的反应。Lee 等[20]随访了 8204 例乳腺癌患者，所有患者均行根治性乳腺癌切除手术，其中 858 例患者患有多原发肿瘤。伴有多原发肿瘤的 0～Ⅰ期乳腺癌患者较不伴多原发肿瘤患者的生存率明显降低，而对于Ⅱ～Ⅲ期乳腺癌伴和不伴多原发肿瘤患者的生存率差异无统计学意义。

一项研究显示[63]，同时性多原发结直肠癌患者的 5 年无复发生存率低于单发结直肠癌患者(65.3% vs 75.1%)。

(3) 有学者认为[64-65]，多原发肿瘤患者预后不差于单原发肿瘤患者，尤其是异时性多原发肿瘤患者的预后要优于单原发肿瘤术后复发或转移的患者。Jiao 等[66]统计分析了 6545 例肿瘤患者资料，72 例为多原发肿瘤，其中位生存时间为 15.7 年，5 年生存率为 56%；而单发肿瘤转移的患者中位生存期仅为 6 月。Kim 等[25]指出，多原发肺内癌患者多数在肿瘤早期即被诊断，其预后优于单原发肺癌术后复发和远处转移的患者，且随着肿瘤发生间隔时间的延长，预后越好。

一项基于 SEER 数据的研究显示[67]，多原发食管癌患者相对于单原发食管癌而言，预后更好、生存期更长，食管特异性死亡率更低。Ha 等[68]的观察发现，与第一原发性胃癌相比，患者的生存受第二原发肿瘤的影响更大。张培趁等[69]报道了 48 例胃肠道多原发性肿瘤，同时性多原发肿瘤经手术治疗预后与单一原发肿瘤相似，异时性多原发肿瘤预后优于单一原发肿瘤。van Leersum 等[70]的研究显示，单发性结直肠癌预后差于多原发结直肠癌。

还有研究报道，多原发肿瘤、单原发肿瘤的预后与随访时间长短有关。韩国开展了一项关于肾脏多原发肿瘤的大型回顾性研究[71]，分析结果显示，多原发肿瘤组和单原发肿瘤组患者的 10 年生存率分别为 60.9%、63.1%，差异无统计学意义（$P > 0.05$）；但在随访的前 8 年，多原发肿瘤组患者的总生存率高于单发肿瘤组，可能由于单发肿瘤组患者多处于晚期，生存期较短；而 8 年后单原发肿瘤组患者的总生存率高于多原发肿瘤组，可能由于多原发肿瘤组患者受第二原发肿瘤的影响，生存期缩短。

（二）两个原发肿瘤间隔时间长短与预后

相关研究报道[72-73]，第一原发肿瘤与第二原发肿瘤中位时间间隔为 5~8 年。一般而言[74]，多原发肿瘤中，2 个原发肿瘤发生的间隔时间长短与患者预后呈正相关。有学者发现[75-76]，第一原发肿瘤与第二原发肿瘤之间间隔时间越短，其预后相对越差，且间隔时间 <12 个月预后最差，而 >60 个月的患者预后较好。有学者分析其原因，可能是两次肿瘤发生的时间间隔过短，当发生第二原发肿瘤时，被第一原发肿瘤破环的免疫系统尚未完全修复，不能被再次触发而发挥其免疫防御等功能[66]。

（三）同时性、异时性多原发肿瘤与预后

一般而言，多原发肿瘤中异时性多原发肿瘤较多见，第一原发肿瘤在第二原发肿瘤诊断时已经过治疗，部分患者经治疗后甚至可达无瘤生存状态，故相对于第一原发肿瘤，第二原发肿瘤对多原发肿瘤患者预后影响更大。

恶性程度最高的肿瘤病灶对异时性多原发肿瘤患者生存期往往起决定性作用，而异时性多原发肿瘤的数量与异时性多原发肿瘤患者生存期

第四章 预后、随访与康复

无关[77]。

同时性与异时性多原发肿瘤患者生存存在差异,但二者谁优谁劣目前存在一定分歧。

(1)多数学者认为[78-80],异时性多原发肿瘤患者预后优于同时性多原发肿瘤患者。Ikeda 等[5]报道,多原发肿瘤 10 年总生存率为 69.3%,其中同时性多原发肿瘤为 40.1%,异时性多原发肿瘤为 75.2%,二者差异显著。朱莉非等[81]回顾性分析了 65 例多原发肿瘤,结果发现,同时性与异时性多原发患者中位生存期分别为 1.9 年和 4.3 年,两者的生存期差异有统计学意义。范黎等[82]在对多原发肿瘤患者预后因素分析中指出,两肿瘤的发病时间间隔越短,预后越差,尤以同时性、恶性程度高的多原发肿瘤预后最差。

张欣欣等[83]报道,头颈部多原发肿瘤的 3 年、5 年总生存率(OS)分别为 84.6%、75.7%,其中同时性多原发肿瘤的 3 年、5 年 OS 分别为 56.4%、37.6%,异时性多原发肿瘤的 3 年、5 年 OS 分别为 92.2%、84.2%,两组间比较异时性多原发肿瘤的 OS 明显高于同时性多原发肿瘤。Kyun 等[21]报道,乳腺多原发肿瘤患者 10 年生存率同时性多原发为 40.1%、异时性多原发为 75.2%,异时性乳腺多原发肿瘤患者其各个原发肿瘤间隔时间越长,预后越好,其中间隔 1 年内的多原发肿瘤预后最差,而间隔 5 年以上,其预后最好。郑希希等[41]报道了 226 例乳腺癌多原发肿瘤患者,中位随访时间平均为 84.75(4.1~384.5)个月,226 例患者的 3 年、5 年 OS 率分别为 91.7%、82.9%,无淋巴结转移、异时性多原发乳腺肿瘤患者预后更好。Carmichael 等[84]的研究发现,同时性双侧乳腺原发癌(S-BPBC)的生存率较异时性双侧乳腺原发癌(M-BPBC)及单侧乳腺癌(unilateral breast cancer,UBC)低,SBPBC 比 MBPBC 和 UBC 远处转移的风险性高。

Pairolero 等[85]报道,单原发肺癌原位复发后手术治疗的肺癌患者 2 年生存率仅有 23%,而异时性多原发肺癌手术治疗后 2 年生存率可达 52%。Kang 等[86]回顾性分析了多次肺切除术治疗的多原发肺内癌患者,发现异时性多原发肺内癌患者组的 5 年无病生存率、总生存率高于同时性多原发肺内癌,5 年累积复发率更低。奥婷等[87]报道了 94 例肺癌合并其他原发肿瘤,第一原发肿瘤为肺癌者 30 例,第一原发为其他肿瘤者 64 例,肺癌为第一原发癌者的生存率低于其他肿瘤为第一原发癌者(中位生存时间 39

个月 vs 97 个月，$P<0.001$），同时性多原发肿瘤 22 例，异时性多原发肿瘤 72 例，中位生存时间分别为 23 个月和 96 个月，异时性多原发肿瘤者生存率较高，1 年、3 年、5 年生存率分别为 91.5%、72.4% 和 56.5%。

Panosetti 等[88]报道，上消化道相关多原发肿瘤中，异时性多原发肿瘤 5 年生存率为 55%，而同时性多原发肿瘤仅为 18%。有研究者发现[89-90]，上消化道多原发肿瘤与单原发肿瘤患者的预后无明显差异；在多原发肿瘤中，异时性多原发肿瘤预后明显较同时性多原发肿瘤好，异时性多原发癌发病的间隔时间对其预后影响较大，即间隔时间越短，预后越差，而性别、年龄、发病部位等均不是影响多原发癌预后的主要因素。Baba 等[91]回顾性研究分析了 538 例食管癌患者，其中 163 例为多原发肿瘤，158 例为双原发癌，5 例为三原发癌，结果显示，同时性多原发癌的患者总生存期更短，是其独立预后因素。Ikeda 等[5]对第一原发肿瘤胃癌后发生第二原发肿瘤患者的预后进行了研究，发现同时性多原发肿瘤以及异时性多原发肿瘤患者的 10 年累积生存率具有显著差异，其生存率分别为 40.1% 和 75.2%。

Watanabe 等[92]对 96 例结直肠癌合并胃癌双原发癌的研究发现，异时性多原发肿瘤的 5 年生存率为 84.3%，高于同时性多原发肿瘤（47.1%），2 个原发癌的间隔时间越长，预后越好。何建军[93]对 2025 例中国多原发结直肠癌患者的生存进行了荟萃分析，结果显示，同时性多原发结直肠癌 3 年、5 年、10 年、15 年生存率分别为 64.3%、44.6%、26.3%、9.4%，异时性多原发结直肠癌为 69.6%、59.2%、45.0%、36.7%，10 年、15 年二者生存有显著性差异，异时性者明显优于同时性者。

（2）亦有研究报道[94-97]，同时性多原发结直肠癌的预后较单原发结直肠癌要好或相当。

（四）治疗方式与预后

多原发肿瘤患者的预后与能否早期诊断并及时进行规范化治疗包括根治性手术、辅助化学治疗、放射治疗等综合治疗方法的应用密切相关，因此早期发现、早期诊断、早期治疗对多原发肿瘤患者预后具有重要意义[98]。Kim 等[26]指出，只接受最佳支持治疗的多原发肺癌患者若无抗肿瘤治疗，其预后极差。

手术被认为是多原发肿瘤可治愈的唯一方式，其治疗疗效优于合并转移的单原发肿瘤[99]。多数学者认为[100-102]，接受以手术治疗为主的综合治疗的多原发肿瘤患者其生存预后明显优于单纯接受手术治疗的患者。有研究报道[103-104]，确诊为早期的肺内多原发癌患者（尤其是同时性）通过手术切除，可获得治愈性结果。Nie 等[105]对包含1788名患者的26项研究进行了荟萃分析，发现手术治疗对同时性多原发肺内癌的生存预后是有益的。

已有研究证实[106-107]，目前发现的消化系统多原发肿瘤中以早期相对多见，因此对于该类患者，给予根治性手术治疗，大多可获得较好的临床获益，进而明显改善患者预后及生存质量。

有研究显示[108-109]，对于不能耐受手术的多原发食管内癌患者，给予合理的放射治疗和化学治疗，可有效延长患者生存率及改善患者生存质量，5年生存率可达26%~45%。彭岳等[110]指出，同时性多原发肺腺癌术后是否接受化学治疗亦是影响患者预后的因素之一。

第二节　医生随访与患者康复

表4-1　医生对多原发肿瘤患者的随访要求及患者自身康复要领

分类	内容
随访要求	对于第二、第三等原发肿瘤患者完成治疗后，主管医生要进行全程管理，密切监测与随访
	主管医生需根据第二、第三等原发肿瘤的组织学类型、分化程度、临床或病理分期，以及患者年龄、性别、职业、生活方式、家族遗传史等制订个体化的随访方案与实施计划，建立随访档案
	随访档案主要内容包括：患者姓名、性别、年龄、职业、生活习惯、家族史，第一、第二、第三等原发肿瘤组织病理学（免疫组化、基因检测情况），临床或病理分期，具体治疗方法，疗效评价，不良事件发生及处理情况，等等
	随访检查主要内容包括：患者一般状态（ECOG-PS评分）、影像学检查（包括B超、CT、MRI、全身骨扫描，PET/CT不做特别推荐）、内镜检查、常规肿瘤标志物检测等
	随访截止时间，对于多原发肿瘤患者通常需要终生随访

续表

分类	内容
患者自身康复要领	需客观、正确认识及对待所患疾病，保持良好的心态，树立战胜癌症的坚强信念
	需严格遵守主管医生制订的随访方案与计划，坚持正确的、科学的、规范的康复方法
	经常观看由专业协会、学会主办的肿瘤相关科普知识及健康教育讲座
	绝不能信奉迷信、传奇广告（包括各种网络、电视广告，广告传单，各种宣传标语等）、祖传秘方，以及江湖神医、游医
	纠正不良生活习惯，如戒烟、戒酒，尽量低脂饮食，多食蔬菜、豆制品
	合理、适当运动（包括健身、旅游等），保证足够的休息或睡眠
	主动、积极参加社会交谊活动或社会公益活动
	保持或寻找、培养至少1种有利于自己身心健康的爱好，如音乐、书法、绘画、钓鱼、养鸟、种花、旅游、手工等，以缓解各种心理压力
	减少家庭各种矛盾，建立良好的家庭氛围；充分获得家庭成员的理解和支持
	在身体状况、心理状态允许的情况下，可重返较轻松的工作岗位

参考文献

[1] Heron DE, Komarnicky LT, Hyslop T, et al. Bilateral breast carcinoma: risk factors and outcomes for patients with synchronous and metachronous disease[J]. Cancer, 2000, 88(12): 2739-2750.

[2] Liang X, Li D, Geng WJ, et al. The prognosis of synchronous and metachronous bilateral breast cancer in Chinese patients[J]. Tumour Biol, 2013, 34(2): 995-1004.

[3] Kumagai Y, Kawano T, Nakajima Y, et al. Multiple primary cancers associated with esophageal carcinoma[J]. Surg Today, 2001, 31(10): 872-876.

[4] Koide N, Yazawa K, Koike S, et al. Oesophageal cancer associated with other primary cancers: A study of 31 patients[J]. J Gastroenterol Hepatol, 1997, 12(9-10): 690-694.

[5] Ikeda Y, Saku M, Kawanaka H, et al. Features of second primary cancer in patients with gastric cancer[J]. Oncology, 2003, 65(2): 113-117.

[6] 张稚淳，贾梦冉，丁皓，等.120例多原发肿瘤临床分析[J].肿瘤防治研究, 2019, 46

(2): 153-158.

[7] 易胜中, 张德超, 王永岗, 等. 肺癌和肺外器官恶性肿瘤组成的多原发癌281例临床分析. 癌症, 2006, 25(6): 731-735.

[8] 许刚, 卜珊珊, 王修身. 原发性四重癌1例报道[J]. 肿瘤防治研究, 2019, 46(12): 1141-1142.

[9] 吴建国, 卢正茂, 罗天航, 等. 消化系多原发癌多次手术存活35年1例报告[J]. 中国实用外科杂志, 2011, 31(6): 544-547.

[10] Vodicka J, Spidlen V, Simdnek V, et al. Surgical therapy of pulmonary metastases of colorectal cancer-ten-year results[J]. Rozhl Chit, 2012, 91(2): 81-86.

[11] Obuchi T, Saito T, 1wasaki A. Frequency of multiple primary cancers in the lung and other organs in hemodialysis patients[J]. Gen Thorac Cardiovasc Surg, 2012, 60(8): 489-493.

[12] Arai J, Tsuchiya T, Oikawa M, et al. Clinical and molecular analysis of synchronous double lung cancer[J]. Lung Cancer, 2012, 77(82): 281-287.

[13] 陈颖, 赵明芳, 曲秀娟, 等. 30例多原发癌回顾性分析[J]. 中国医科大学学报, 2012, 41(4): 340-342.

[14] 张琦, 谢国明, 陈科, 等. 同时性多原发肺癌患者生存状况及其影响因素分析. 浙江医学, 2019, 41(15): 1655-1656, 1659.

[15] Takamochi K, Oh S, Matsuoka J. Clonality status of multifocal lung adenocarcinomas based on the mutation patterns of EGFR and K-ras[J]. Lung Cancer, 2012, 75(3): 13-20.

[16] Yang H, Sun Y, Yao F, et al. Surgical therapy for bilateral multiple primary lung cancer[J]. Ann Thorac Surg, 2016, 101(3): 1145-1152.

[17] Rose PG, Herterick EE, Boutselis JG, et al. Multiple primary gynecologic neoplasms[J]. Am J Obstet Gynecol, 1987, 157(2): 261-267.

[18] Mariotto AB, Rowland JH, Ries LA, et al. Multiple cancer prevalence: a growing challenge in long-term survivorship[J]. Cancer Epidemiol Biomarkers Prev, 2007, 16(3): 566-571.

[19] Jiang Y, Miao Z, Wang J, et al. Clinical characteristics and prognosis associated with multiple primary malignant tumors in non-Hodgkin lymphoma patients[J]. Tumori, 2019, 105(6): 474-482.

[20] Lee J, Park S, Kim S, et al. Characteristics and Survival of Breast Cancer Patients with Multiple Synchronous or Metachronous Primary Cancers[J]. Yonsei Med J, 2015, 56(5): 1213-1220.

[21] Kyun KB, Jeong OS, Song JY, et al. Clinical Characteristics and Prognosis Associated with Multiple Primary Cancers in Breast Cancer Patients[J]. J Breast Cancer, 2018, 21(1): 62-69.

[22] Niu L, Zhang J, Liu T, et al. Clinicopathological characteristics and prognosis analysis of

colorectal synchronous multiple primary cancer[J]. Chinese Journal of Gastrointestinal Surgery, 2018, 21(1): 41-45.

[23] Chen MC, Huang WC, Chan CH, et al. Impact of second primary esophageal or lung cancer on survival of patients with head and neck cancer[J]. Oral Oncology, 2010, 46(4): 249-254.

[24] 王鑫洪, 林考兴. 多原发恶性肿瘤病因及发病特点[J]. 中国老年学杂志, 2013, 33(20): 5216-5217.

[25] Kim SW, Kong KA, Kim DY, et al. Multiple primary cancers involving lung cancer at a single tertiary hospital: Clinical features and prognosis[J]. Thorac Cancer, 2015, 6(2): 159-165.

[26] 孙海涛, 王南, 刘艺, 等. 184例多原发恶性肿瘤临床特征及其预后分析[J]. 现代肿瘤医学, 2023, 31(8): 1530-1535.

[27] 李小毅, 钟定荣, 陈思, 等. 胃癌合并其他器官原发癌103例分析[J]. 中国普外基础与临床杂志, 2012, 19(1): 43-47.

[28] Tae Kyung HA, An JY, Youn HG, et al. Surgical Outcome of Synchronous Second Primary Cancer in Patients with Gastric Cancer[J]. Yonsei Med J, 2007, 48(6): 981-7.

[29] Eom BW, Lee HJ, Yoo MW, et al. Synchronous and metachronous cancers in patients with gastric Cancer[J]. J Surg Oncol, 2008, 98(2): 106-110.

[30] 董锐增, 师英强, 叶廷伟, 等. 胃癌合并其他器官原发癌74例临床分析[J]. 中华胃肠外科杂志, 2010, 13(2): 125-128.

[31] Lim SB, Jeong SY, Choi HS, et al. Synchronous gastric CanCer in primary sporadic colorectal cancer patients in Koma[J]. Int J Colorectal Dis, 2008, 23(1): 61-65.

[32] Powell S, Tarchand G, Rector T, et al. Synchronous and metachronous malignancies: analysis of the Minneapolis Veterans Affairs(VA) tumor registry[J]. Cancer Causes Control, 2013, 24(8): 1565-1573.

[33] Lopez-Oliva CLL, Yun JY, Kim HS, et al. Extremity soft tissue sarcoma with multiple primary malignancies-Characteristics and outcome[J]. European Journal of Surgical Oncology the Journal of the European Society of Surgical Oncology & the British Association of Surgical Oncology, 2016, 42(4): 567-573.

[34] 肖飞, 梁朝阳. 多原发肺癌的诊断治疗及预后判断[J]. 中华胸心血管外科杂志, 2014, 30(8): 499-501, 509.

[35] 何萍, 顾霞, 关玉宝, 等. 同时性多中心原发性肺癌37例临床病理分析[J]. 中华肿瘤防治杂志, 2013, 20(5): 357-360.

[36] 孙芩玲, 叶联华, 黄云超, 等. 多原发肺癌的临床特征及预后因素分析[J]. 癌症, 2022, 41(4): 191-199.

[37] 郭海法, 毛锋, 张辉, 等. 同时性多原发肺癌的预后及生存相关因素研究[J]. 中国

肺癌杂志, 2017, 20(01): 21-27.

[38] Wang H, Hou J, Zhang G, et al. Clinical characteristics and prognostic analysis of multiple primary malignant neoplasms in patients with lung cancer[J]. Cancer Gene Ther, 2019, 26(11-12): 419-426.

[39] Teng J, Xu J, Jiao J, et al. Radiofrequency ablation of synchronous multiple primary lung cancer assisted by a magnetic navigation system: a case report[J]. Ann Palliat Med, 2020, 9(2): 478-482.

[40] Goto T, Hirotsu Y, Mochizuki H, et al. Mutational analysis of multiple lung cancers: Discrimination between primary and metastatic lung cancers by genomic profile[J]. Oncotarget, 2017, 8(19): 31133-31143.

[41] 郑希希, 贾勇圣, 史业辉, 等. 乳腺癌多原发癌的临床病理特征及预后分析[J]. 中国肿瘤临床, 2017, 44(05): 219-223.

[42] 牛一茹, 吴焕文, 梁智勇. 同时性双侧乳腺癌的临床病理学特征及预后分析[J]. 中华病理学杂志, 2020, 49(5): 435-440.

[43] Dhadlie S, Whitfield J, Hendahewa R. Synchronous bilateral breast cancer: a case report of heterogeneous estrogen receptor status[J]. Int J Surg Case Rep, 2018, 53: 102-106.

[44] Baretta Z, Olopade OI, Huo D. Heterogeneity in hormone-receptor status and survival outcomes among women with synchronous and metachronous bilateral breast cancers[J]. Breast, 2015, 24(2): 131-136.

[45] 牛丽云, 张峻岭, 刘天野, 等. 结直肠同时性多原发癌的临床病理特征和预后分析[J]. 中华胃肠外科杂志, 2018, 21(1): 41-45.

[46] Kato T, Alonso S, Muto Y, et al. Tumor size is an independent risk predictor for metachronous colorectal cancer[J]. Oncotarget, 2016, 7(14): 17896-17904.

[47] Aydiner A, Karadeniz A, Uygun K, et al. Multiple primary neoplasms at a single institution: differences between synchronous and metachronous neoplasms[J]. Am J Clin Oncol, 2000, 23(4): 364-370.

[48] Li F, Zhong WZ, Niu FY, et al. Multiple primary malignancies involving lung cancer[J]. BMC Cancer, 2015, 15: 696-701.

[49] Izmajłowicz B, Kornafel J, Blaszczyk J. Multiple Neoplasms Among Cervical Cancer Patients in the Material of the Lower Silesian Cancer Registry[J]. Adv Clin Exp Med, 2014, 23(3): 433-440.

[50] Fumihiro S, Koji Y, Naoko M, et al. Postoperative Management of Multiple Primary Cancers Associated with Non-small Cell Lung Cancer[J]. Anticancer Res, 2018, 38(6): 3773-3778.

[51] Shoji F, Yamazaki K, Miura N, et al. Postoperative management of multiple primary cancers associated with nonsmall cell lung cancer[J]. Anticancer Res, 2018, 38(6): 3773-3778.

[52] Bhattacharyya N, Nayak VK. Survival outcomes for second primary head and neck cancer: a matched analysis[J]. Otolaryngol Head Neck Surg, 2005, 132(1): 63-68.

[53] Wang XW, Liu L, Wang YW, et al. Clinical course of patients with small cell lung cancer as second primary malignancy[J]. The Chinese-German Journal of Clinical Oncology, 2005, 4(5): 297-300.

[54] Boute P, Page C, Biet A, et al. Epidemiology, prognosis and treatment of simultaneous squamous cell carcinomas of the oral cavity and hypopharynx[J]. Eur Ann Otorhinolary, 2014, 131(5): 283-287.

[55] 魏先锋, 李丽. 头颈部多原发癌[J]. 临床耳鼻咽喉头颈外科杂志, 2010, 24(12): 573-576.

[56] Wei JL, Jiang YZ, Shao ZM. Survival and chemotherapy-related risk of second primary malignancy in breast cancer Patients: a SEER-based study[J]. Int J Clin Oncol, 2019, 24(8): 934-940.

[57] 侯丁丁, 凌煜玮, 康骅. 乳腺癌患者并发第二原发甲状腺癌的诊治现状[J]. 新医学, 2017, 48(8): 515-518.

[58] Kim BK, Oh SJ, Song JY, et al. Clinical Characteristics and Prognosis Associated with Multiple Primary Cancers in Breast Cancer Patiems[J]. J Breast Cancer, 2018, 21(1): 62-69.

[59] Min YM, Ph D, Cormier JN, et al. Other Primary Malignancies in Breast Cancer Patients Treated with Breast Conserving Surgery and Radiation Therapy[J]. Ann Surg Oncol, 2013, 20(5): 1514-1521.

[60] Raymond JS, Hogue CJR. Multiple primary tumours in women following breast cancer, 1973-2000[J]. Br J Cancer, 2006, 94(11): 1745-1750.

[61] 杨韵, 王宁霞. 合并第二原发癌的乳腺癌患者的病理特征及预后[J]. 暨南大学学报(自然科学与医学版), 2018, 39(2): 127-130, 148.

[62] Arakawa K, Hata K, Nozawa H, et al. Prognostic significance and clinicopathological features of synchronous colorectal cancer[J]. Anticancer Res, 2018, 38(10): 5889-5895.

[63] Kozawa E, Sugiura H, Tsukushi S, et al. Multiple primary malignancies in elderly patients with high-grade soft tissue sarcoma[J]. Int J Clin Oncol, 2014, 19(2): 384-390.

[64] Yang L, Parkin DM, Ferlay J, et al. Estimates of cancer incidence in China for 2000 and projections for 2005[J]. Cancer Epidemiol Biomarkers Prev, 2005, 14(1): 243-250.

[65] 孙俊杰, 李双庆. 多原发癌病因及发病机制的探索[J]. 中国全科医学, 2017, 20(9): 1136-1141.

[66] Jiao F, Yao LJ, Zhou J, et al. Clinical features of multiple primary malignancies: a retrospective analysis of 72 Chinese patients[J]. Asian Pac J Cancer Prev, 2014, 15(1):

331-334.

[67] Hu Z, Zhang M, Wang Z, et al. An observational study on the clinical features of esophageal cancer followed by multiple primary cancers[J]. Future Oncol, 2019, 15(6): 601-610.

[68] Ha TK, An JY, Youn HG, et al. Surgical outcome of synchronous secondprimary cancer in patients with gastric cancer[J]. Yonsei Med J, 2007, 48(6): 981-987.

[69] 张培趁, 程骏, 余作黔, 等. 48例胃肠道多原发性肿瘤的临床分析[J]. 浙江临床医学, 2005, 7(1): 15-16.

[70] van Leersum NJ, Aalbers AG, Snijders HS, et al. Synchronous colorectal carcinoma: a risk factor in colorectal cancer surgery[J]. Dis Colon Rectum, 2014, 57(4): 460-466.

[71] Joung JY, Kwon WA, Lim J, et al. Second primary cancer risk among kidney cancer patients in korea: a population-based cohort study[J]. Cancer Res Treat, 2018, 50(1): 293-301.

[72] Kim JY, Song HS. Metachronous double primary cancer after treatment of breast cancer[J]. Cancer Res Treat, 2015, 47(1): 64-71.

[73] Shoji F, Yamazaki K, Kouso H, et al. Clinicopathological Features and Outcome of Lung Cancer Patients with Hematological Malignancy[J]. Ann Surg Oncol, 2016, 23(2): 633-637.

[74] 孙红梅, 鲍云华, 郑丽平, 等. 多原发癌46例临床分析[J]. 中华老年多器官疾病杂志, 2016, 15(8): 609-612.

[75] Corso G, Veronesi P, Santomauro GI, et al. Multiple primary non-breast tumors in breast cancer survivors[J]. J Cancer Res Clin Oncol, 2018, 144(5): 979-986.

[76] Lv M, Zhang X, Shen Y, et al. Clinical analysis and prognosis of synchronous and metachronous multiple primary malignant tumors[J]. Medicine, 2017, 96(17): 1-8.

[77] 赵明芳, 刘云鹏. 四重原发性恶性肿瘤1例及文献复习[J]. 中国医科大学学报, 2006, (3): 325.

[78] Kim JH, Rha SY, Kim C, et al. Clinicopathologic features of metachronous or synchronous gastric cancer patients with three or more primary sites[J]. Cancer Res Treat, 2010, 42(4): 217-224.

[79] Liu YY, Chen YM, Yen SH, et al. Multiple primary malignancies involving lung cancer-clinical characteristics and prognosis[J]. Lung Cancer, 2002, 35(2): 189-194.

[80] Oeffinger KC, Baxi SS, Novetsky Friedman D, et al. Solid tumor second primary neoplasms: who is at risk, what can we do? [J]. Semin Oncol, 2013, 40(6): 676-689.

[81] 朱莉菲, 薛鹏, 王理伟. 65例多原发癌临床回顾性研究[J]. 复旦学报, 2010, 37(5): 591-593.

[82] 范黎, 于钊, 任军, 等. 61例多原发癌的病种分布和预后分析[J]. 第四军医大学学

报，2002，23(1)：95-96.

[83] 张欣欣，颜芳，刘明波，等.伴多原发癌的头颈部恶性肿瘤的临床特征分析[J]. 中华耳鼻咽喉头颈外科杂志，2016，51(7)：491-496.

[84] Carmichael AR, Bendall S, Lockerbie L, et al. The long-term outcome of synchronous bilateral breast cancer is worse than metachronous or unilateral tumours[J]. Eur J Surg Oncol, 2002, 28：388-391.

[85] Pairolero PC, Williams DE, Bergstralh EJ, et al. Postsurgical Stage I Bronchogenic Carcinoma：Morbid Implications of Recurrent Disease[J]. Ann Thorac Surg, 1984, 38(4)：331-338.

[86] Kang X, Zhang C, Zhou H, et al. Multiple pulmonary resections for synchronous and metachronous lung cancer at two Chinese centers[J]. Ann Thorac Surg, 2020, 109(3)：856-863.

[87] 奥婷，孙军平，肖永久，等.94例肺癌合并其他原发恶性肿瘤生存分析[J]. 解放军医学院学报，2016，37(5)：432-436.

[88] Panosetti E, Luboinski B, Mamelle G, et al. Multiple synchronous and metachronous cancers of the upper aerodigestive tract：a nine-year study[J]. Laryngoscope, 1989, 99(12)：1267-1273.

[89] 黄进丰，赫捷.同期食管癌和胃癌的临床特征和预后分析[J]. 中华外科杂志，2008，46(9)：674-676.

[90] Bmie F, Plaisant N, Millat B, et al. Treatment and prognosis of early multiple gastric cancer[J]. Eur J Surg Oneol, 2003, 29(5)：511-514.

[91] Baba Y, Yoshida N, Kinoshita K, et al. Clinical and Prognostic Features of Patients With Esophageal Cancer and Multiple Primary Cancers：A Retrospective Single-institution Study[J]. Ann Surg, 2018, 267(3)：478-483.

[92] Watanabe M, Kochi M, Fujii M, et al. Dual primary gastric and colorectal cancer：is the prognosis better for synchronous or metachronous?[J]. Am J Clin Oncol, 2012, 35(5)：407-410.

[93] 何建军.中国人2025例多原发结直肠癌荟萃分析[J]. 中华胃肠外科杂志，2006，9(3)：225-229.

[94] Lam AK, Chan SS. Synchronous colorectal cancer：clinical, pathological and molecular implications[J]. World J Gastroenterol, 2014, 20(22)：6815-6820.

[95] Chen HS. Synchronous and early metachronous colorectal adenocarcinoma：analysis of prognosis and current trends[J]. Dis Colon Rectum, 2000, 43(8)：1093-1099.

[96] Oya M, Takahashi S, Okuyama T, et al. Synchronous colorectal carcinoma：clinico-pathological features and prognosis[J]. Jpn J Clin Oncol, 2003, 33(1)：38-43.

[97] Kaibara N, Koga S. Synchronous and metachronous malignancies of the colon and rectum in

Japan with special reference to a coexisting early cancer[J]. Cancer, 1984, 54(9): 1870-1874.

[98] 杨建光, 李晓霞, 孔凡民. 多原发癌临床特征分析[J]. 现代肿瘤医学, 2011, 19(12): 2551-2553.

[99] Hu B, Castillo E, Harewood L, et al. Multifocal epithelial tumors and field cancerization from loss of mesenchymal CSL signaling[J]. Cell, 2012, 149(6): 1207-1220.

[100] 孙百顺, 张耀, 贾振庚. 多原发癌26例临床资料回顾性分析[J]. 中国煤炭工业医学杂志, 2013, 16(8): 1346-1349.

[101] 王亚兵, 王家和. 必须重视多原发癌的临床研究[J]. 肿瘤学杂志, 2002, 8(5): 294-296.

[102] 王晓斌, 白松, 吕国利. 重复癌的病因及诊疗方案的探讨和展望[J]. 中国老年保健医学, 2011, 9(6): 61-63.

[103] Reinmuth N, Stumpf A, Stumpf P, et al. Characteristics and outcome of patients with second primary lung cancer[J]. Eur Respir J, 2013, 42(6): 1668-1676.

[104] Xue X, Xue Q, Wang N, et al. Early clinical diagnosis of synchronous multiple primary lung cancer[J]. Oncol Lett, 2012, 3(1): 234-237.

[105] Nie Y, Wang X, Yang F, et al. Surgical prognosis of synchronous multiple primary lung cancer: systematic review and meta-analysis[J]. Clin Lung Cancer, 2021, 22(4): 341-350.

[106] Otowa Y, Nakamura T, Takiguchi G, et al. Safety and benefit of curative surgical resection for esophageal squamous cell cancer associated with multiple primary cancers[J]. Eur J Surg Oncol, 2016, 42(3): 407-411.

[107] Shirai K, Tamaki Y, Kitamoto Y, et al. Prognosis was not deteriorated by multiple primary cancers in esophageal cancer patients treated by radiotherapy[J]. J Radiat Res, 2013, 54(4): 706-711.

[108] 陈意标, 张汉雄, 蒋振东, 等. 三维适形放疗联合同期化疗治疗食管多发癌的临床观察[J]. 肿瘤研究与临床, 2013, 25(1): 22-24.

[109] Li QW, Zhu YJ, Zhang WW, et al. Chemoradiotherapy for synchronous multiple primary cancers with esophageal squamous cell carcinoma: a case-control study[J]. J Cancer, 2017, 8(4): 563-569.

[110] 彭岳, 王晖, 谢厚耐, 等. 同时性多原发肺腺癌的外科治疗及预后[J]. 中国肺癌杂志, 2017, 20(2): 107-113.

下 篇
不明原发肿瘤

第五章

总　论

第一节　基本概念

在既往文献中[1-7]，不明原发肿瘤（carcinomas of unknown primary，CUP）有多种名称，如"原发灶不明转移癌"、"隐匿性原发肿瘤"（occult primary tumor）、"原发灶未知或隐匿性肿瘤（unknown or occult primary tumour）"、"来源未知的癌或腺癌（carcinoma or adenocarcinoma of unknown primary）"、"来源不明的转移癌（metastases of unknown origin）"、"原发肿瘤未知的转移癌（metastases from unknown primary tumours）"、"来源未确定的肿瘤（tumour of unknown or unidentified origin）"，本书使用"不明原发肿瘤"之名。

关于不明原发肿瘤的定义，一直存在分歧。1997年，希腊学者Biasoulis等[8]，指出，CUP是指首先发现转移灶而缺乏原发肿瘤表现，经详细询问病史、体格检查及辅助检查均无法明确原发灶的一组特异类型的肿瘤。2010年，英国国家卫生与临床优化研究所（National Institute for Health and Clinical Excellence，NICE）在其公布的《原发灶不明转移癌诊治指南》中，将CUP定义为经组织学确认的转移性上皮来源癌或神经内分泌肿瘤，且经全面检查，包括详细的病史询问、体格检查、血液学检查、尿粪检查、肿瘤标志物检测、免疫组化、内镜，以及多种影像学，如X线、CT、MRI、PET/CT、乳腺钼靶等，并由专家进一步判定，最终仍未确定组织起源的恶性肿瘤，不包括非上皮来源的黑色素瘤、肉瘤、淋巴瘤、生殖细胞瘤等。

2022年，欧洲肿瘤内科学会（European Society for Medical Oncology，ESMO）在其发布的关于《原发性不明肿瘤：ESMO诊断、治疗和随访临床实践指南》中指出[9]，CUP是指经标准化检查后仍无法确定导致转移的原发肿瘤的肿瘤。美国国家综合癌症网络(National Comprehensive Cancer Network，NCCN)对隐匿性原发肿瘤使用的定义是指经组织学证实的转移性肿瘤，其原发部位在标准的预处理评估中无法确定，病理类型包括腺癌、鳞癌、未分化癌、神经内分泌癌、生殖细胞瘤等，不包括淋巴瘤、软组织肉瘤等。目前，多采用NCCN指南的定义[10-14]。

第二节 流行病学

一、发病情况

不同的国家、地区及不同的作者、不同的报道时间，CUP发病率略有差异，一般为(6~16)/10万，占所有恶性肿瘤的2.3%~7.8%，为第八大常见肿瘤，死亡率位列第四[15-26]；仅有20%~27%的患者死亡前才明确原发肿瘤[27-28]；有学者报道[29-30]，在20%~50%的CUP患者中，即使在尸检后亦无法明确原发肿瘤。

2000年，Greenlee等[31]报道的比例较高，CUP占全部恶性肿瘤的5%~10%。2011年，Massard等[29]报道，CUP占所有恶性肿瘤的3%~5%。丹麦2009—2013年男性为2.5%、女性为3.2%，英国2014年为3.0%，美国2017年为2.0%[33]。

对1973—2008年SEER数据库的分析发现[34]，随着时间的推移、诊断方法的改进，不明原发肿瘤发生比例一直呈下降趋势。据估计[35]，2022年美国诊断出30620例CUP，仅占美国所有癌症的2%。

CUP发病率随年龄增长而增加，平均诊断年龄为60岁，高发年龄段为60~75岁，男性高于女性[36-38]。

二、转移部位

CUP的自然病程与原发灶明确的肿瘤不同，具有侵袭性强、早期易发生转移、短期内即表现出与转移部位相关的症状和体征，以及转移方式的不可预知性。Pavlidis等[14]报道，约33%的CUP患者被诊断时在3个或更多器官中已发生转移。据报道[39]，CUP转移部位十分广泛，在CUP发现的转移部位中，常见的转移部位有淋巴结、肝、肺、骨骼和脑实质，少见的有卵巢、骨髓、脑膜、胸膜、腹膜等。根据尸检病例研究结果[40]，CUP

患者最常见的原发肿瘤部位是肺(27%)和胰腺(24%),其次是肝/胆管(8%)、肾或肾上腺(8%)、结肠(7%),以及生殖器官(前列腺2%、睾丸0.3%、卵巢/子宫4%、子宫颈0.7%)等。

Grau等[28]报道,CUP中淋巴结为最常见的转移部位,约占15%;脏器转移约占85%,其中腹腔内转移占35%~50%,骨转移占5%~25%。Gallagher等[41]的研究发现,CUP最常见的转移部位是淋巴结(占30%),其次是骨(占15%~28%),其他部位较少(占15%)。王成锋等[37]统计分析了1273例CUP,除淋巴结转移外,其他部位有肝脏8.6%;骨骼7.6%,包括椎骨、胸骨、颅骨、锁骨、肩胛骨、骨盆、肱骨、肋骨、髋骨、腓骨等;肺5.1%、卵巢3.6%、脑2.6%、腹腔1.6%。少见部位有腹膜、盆腔、胸壁、阴道、皮肤;更少见的部位有腹壁、大网膜、肾、乳腺、甲状腺、胰腺、胸膜、肾上腺、胸腺、腮腺、肠系膜、眼眶内、睾丸、精索、外阴。黑砚等[42]报道了22例眼眶转移性肿瘤,其中有3例原发肿瘤不明,其他原发肿瘤为乳腺癌、肺癌、甲状腺癌、宫颈癌、直肠类癌、下肢黑色素瘤、腹膜后恶性副神经节瘤及神经母细胞瘤。

(一)淋巴结转移

相关文献报道,CUP常见的淋巴结转移部位为颈部淋巴结、腋窝淋巴结和腹股沟淋巴结。

颈部淋巴结十分丰富,约300枚,且颈部淋巴是全身淋巴的一个重要交汇区,全身淋巴液均可引流至此。因此,理论上讲,全身恶性实体肿瘤细胞均可经淋巴系统到达颈部淋巴结[43]。

鼻咽部肿瘤可经咽后壁外侧淋巴结汇入颈内静脉上区淋巴结,即Ⅱ区;口底及舌部肿瘤侵犯淋巴管可进入Ⅰ区淋巴结,包括颏下淋巴结和颌下淋巴结,少数可进入颈深淋巴结;喉癌及喉咽癌较易转移至Ⅱ区及Ⅲ区。亦有胸部、腹部及乳腺等处的原发肿瘤转移至颈部淋巴结,但主要转移至左锁骨上区淋巴结,转移至颌下、上颈部甚或颈后三角区极少见。

据报道[44],淋巴结转移部位以颈部淋巴结高发,而颈部淋巴结转移癌约70%来源于头颈部原发肿瘤,锁骨上区CUP的原发肿瘤绝大部分发生在胸部器官。康炜东等[45]报道,在43例颈部淋巴结转移癌中,原发于鼻咽的转移癌为27.9%,原发于喉的为25.6%,原发于喉咽和甲状腺的均为11.6%;原发灶为肺癌3例,口底癌2例,舌癌1例,胃癌及乳腺癌各1

例,有 2 例原发肿瘤不明。王成锋等[37]统计分析了 1273 例 CUP 患者,淋巴结转移最多见,占 67.0%,其中颈部淋巴结占 69.1%(包括锁骨上淋巴结 149 例)、未注明部位占 17.6%、多处淋巴结占 4.0%、腹股沟淋巴结占 3.6%、腋淋巴结占 3.2%,其他少见部位有纵隔淋巴结、颌下淋巴结、肺门淋巴结与耳后淋巴结等。

(二)骨转移

恶性实体肿瘤骨转移的发生率较高,60%~80% 恶性实体肿瘤患者伴有骨转移。不明原发肿瘤骨转移(bone metastases from cancer of unknown primary,BM-CUP)是一类经病理证实为骨转移癌但经详细询问病史、体格检查和影像学检查后仍不能明确其原发解剖部位的肿瘤。

骨是恶性实体肿瘤仅次于肺、肝的第三大转移好发部位[11],张新涛等[46]统计分析了 897 例骨转移瘤,原发肿瘤以肺癌最常见(26.0%),其次为不明原发肿瘤(24.0%)、前列腺癌(7.8%)、肝癌(6.3%)、胃肠道恶性肿瘤(5.7%)、乳腺癌(3.8%)、鼻咽癌(3.2%)、甲状腺癌(2.3%)。BM-CUP 占 CUP 的比例,Rougraff 等[47]报道为 3%~4%,Conroy 等[48]报道为 0.9%。中国学者报道的比例一般较高,曹来宾等[49]报道的比例最高,为 27.03%。在徐栋梁等[50]报道的 390 例骨转移肿瘤中,原发肿瘤依次为肺癌、前列腺癌、乳腺癌、原发性肝癌、胃肠道癌;脊柱转移占 47.7%,其次为骨盆 18.2%、股骨 15.4%、肋骨 12.6%,全身多处转移占 20.5%。首先被发现的原发肿瘤仅 29.7%,不明原发肿瘤为 24%。但叶癘飞等[51]报道的 408 例转移骨肿瘤中,不明原发肿瘤仅 18 例,占 4.41%。

一般而言,肿瘤骨转移有一定的规律性[52-55],好发于 41 岁以上的患者;肺癌、前列腺癌、乳腺癌、肝癌为最常见的原发肿瘤,且以脊柱转移最为常见,其次为骨盆、股骨、肋骨,影像学表现以溶骨性破坏为主。

原发肿瘤来源不明的脊柱转移瘤,国内既往报道约占骨转移瘤的 25% 左右,国外报道为 3%~4%[44]。中国学者报道的比例明显高于国外,在王丰等[56]报道的 481 例脊柱转移瘤中,不明原发肿瘤 93 例,占所有脊柱转移瘤的 19.3%。

相关文献报道[57-58],易发生骨转移的常见原发肿瘤为乳腺癌、前列腺癌、鼻咽癌、肺癌和甲状腺癌,其中男性患者前列腺癌骨转移最为常见,女性患者乳腺癌骨转移最为多见[58],约 70% 的乳腺癌患者在自然病程中可发生骨转移[59]。张新涛等[46]对897例转移骨肿瘤的原发肿瘤进行了分析，在男性中由多到少依次为肺癌、不明原发肿瘤、前列腺癌、肝癌，女性为肺癌、不明原发肿瘤、乳腺癌、胃肠道癌，无论男性、女性，不明原发肿瘤均居第2位。在张小军等[60]报道的640例脊柱转移肿瘤中，原发肿瘤由多到少依次为肺癌、肝癌和胃癌、不明原发肿瘤、前列腺癌、女性乳腺癌，不明原发肿瘤居第3位；王丰等[56]对481例脊柱转移瘤进行了流行病学分析，结果发现，原发肿瘤由多到少依次为肺癌、不明原发肿瘤、肾癌、女性乳腺癌、肝癌，男性依次为肺癌、不明原发肿瘤、肾癌、肝癌、前列腺癌；女性依次为肺癌、不明原发肿瘤、乳腺癌、甲状腺癌、胃肠道癌；无论男女，不明原发肿瘤均居第2位。在叶骉飞等[51]报道的408例转移性骨肿瘤中，发病年龄最早的是乳腺癌（57.68岁），最晚是前列腺癌（72.33岁），脊柱转移为74.02%、肋骨为61.27%、骨盆为38.24%、股骨为23.53%、胸骨为15.44%。

从20世纪80年代开始，一系列研究显示[61-66]，肺癌是不明原发肿瘤骨转移最常见的原发肿瘤。Vandecandelaere等[65]报道，在过去的40年中，不明原发肿瘤骨转移患者中已查明的原发肿瘤主要来自肺癌，其次是肾透明细胞癌、前列腺癌和甲状腺癌。Nottebaert等[64]研究分析了51例不明原发肿瘤骨转移患者，发现肺癌占已查明原发肿瘤的52%。Rougraff等[62]对40例当时诊断不明原发肿瘤骨转移的患者进行了回顾性诊断分析，发现肺癌占已查明原发肿瘤的63%。

（三）脑转移

脑转移瘤发生率为原发脑肿瘤的4~10倍，成人脑转移瘤前5位原发肿瘤为肺癌（40%~60%）、乳腺癌（10%）、黑色素瘤（3.5%）、结肠癌（2.8%）和肾癌（1.2%），占脑转移瘤的80%。

原发灶来源不明的脑转移瘤（brain metastasis of unknown primary cancer, BM-CUP）指有脑转移瘤的临床表现、影像学特征，或活检证实为脑转移恶性肿瘤，但病史、体格检查及相关实验室检查未能找出原发部位的转移瘤[67]。Taillibert等[68]报道，临床上约15%的脑转移瘤患者未能发现其原发肿瘤，占实体肿瘤脑转移的3%~5%，占所有肿瘤脑转移患者的15%~40%，年发病率为12/10万，平均年龄为51~55岁，男性多见。但中国学者报道的比例较高，张继良等[69]报道了640例脑转移癌，不明原发肿瘤 123 例，占 20.7%；其他明确的原发肿瘤为肺癌 338 例、乳腺癌与消化道肿瘤 43 例、卵巢癌 18 例、鼻咽癌 14 例。石易鑫等[70]对 159 例脑转移癌进行了回顾性分析，结果表明，有明确原发肿瘤部位或颅内转移灶病理结果的患者占 67.9%，不明原发肿瘤患者为 32.1%，近 1/3 的患者无法明确原发肿瘤。

不明的脑转移瘤约 85% 的病灶位于大脑半球，通常在大脑中动脉和大脑后动脉的分水岭区；多发生在顶叶，其次是额叶、枕叶和小脑，基底节和丘脑等部位少见。穆林森等[71]报道了 26 例不明的脑转移瘤病灶位于额叶 8 例、顶叶 13 例、枕叶 1 例、小脑 3 例、基底节区 1 例。

另外，临床上脑膜转移瘤（leptomeningeal metastasis，LM）并不少见，是指转移肿瘤细胞在脑和脊髓的软膜内弥漫播散或呈多个局灶性浸润，表现为脑、颅神经和脊髓受损的中枢神经系统转移癌的一种特殊类型。然而，脑膜转移灶的病理学诊断通常比较困难，且亦存在原发肿瘤不易发现[72-73]。Posner 等[74]对 1970—1976 年 2375 例晚期肿瘤患者进行尸检发现，9% 的患者合并硬脑膜转移瘤（intracranial dural matastasis，IDM），与软脑膜癌发生率相近，其中仅累及硬脑膜者占 4%，原发肿瘤多为乳腺癌、前列腺癌、神经母细胞瘤等。Laigle - Donadey 等[75]对 1904—2003 年报道的 198 例 IDM 进行分析表明，原发肿瘤依次为前列腺癌（19.7%）、乳腺癌（16.7%）、肺癌（11.1%）、胃癌（7.6%）、血液系统恶性肿瘤（6.1%），而 9.6% IDM 患者难以明确原发肿瘤。

（四）卵巢转移

卵巢转移癌，有研究报道[76]，有 5% ~ 30% 的卵巢癌是转移性肿瘤。卵巢转移癌的原发肿瘤可来源于全身各部位，非生殖系统包括胃、结肠、直肠、乳腺、胰腺、小肠、阑尾、腹膜、肾、膀胱、输尿管、黑色素瘤等；生殖系统包括子宫体、子宫颈、输卵管，其中胃肠道是最常见的肿瘤原发部位（39%）；其次是乳腺（28%）、子宫内膜（20%）；其他部位少见（13%）[77-78]。

卵巢转移癌多发生于绝经前女性，发病年龄在 40 ~ 48 岁之间[79-80]。Lee 等[76]报道，42.9% 的转移卵巢癌患者有原发恶性肿瘤病史，54.5% 的患者同时发现原发肿瘤和转移卵巢癌，有极少数患者不能明确原发肿瘤。

（五）胸膜、腹膜转移

恶性实体肿瘤胸膜、腹膜转移导致的主要结果即胸腹腔积液，恶性胸腹腔积液为晚期恶性肿瘤患者常见合并症之一,约占所有积液的45%。

恶性胸膜腔积液占各种原因胸膜腔积液的25%~53%,引起恶性胸膜腔积液的常见原发肿瘤有胸膜间皮瘤、淋巴瘤、肺癌、乳腺癌、食管癌、胃癌、胰腺癌、骨与软组织肿瘤、卵巢癌、宫颈癌等。

恶性腹膜腔积液常见原发肿瘤为卵巢癌、胃肠道肿瘤、肝胆胰腺肿瘤、子宫内膜癌等。

恶性浆膜腔积液的诊断首先是排除良性疾病,通常情况下,1~2次的脱落细胞学检查阳性率很低,而腔镜下浆膜组织活检有较大的创伤,晚期肿瘤患者依从性较低。因此,获得病理学诊断有一定难度;且即使有明确的病理学诊断,而少数患者很难明确原发肿瘤。Saif等[81]报道,有高达20%的恶性腹膜腔积液原发肿瘤不明。

(六)骨髓转移

骨髓转移癌是指原发于骨髓外的组织或器官的恶性肿瘤细胞转移至骨髓而引起的临床及血液学改变的疾病。

实体肿瘤骨髓转移率极低,在已明确的实体肿瘤患者中,行骨髓活检的患者有17.7%~25%发生骨髓转移[82]。Tyagi等[83]检测了2860例实体肿瘤患者骨髓标本,有22例发生骨髓转移,发生率仅为0.8%。Kucukzeybek等[84]评估了3345例骨髓活检标本,有58例被诊断为肿瘤骨髓转移(发生率为1.7%)。

在儿童中,侵犯骨髓的最常见实体肿瘤为尤文氏肉瘤、横纹肌肉瘤和神经母细胞瘤[85],成人中骨髓转移癌原发肿瘤以乳腺癌、前列腺癌、胃癌、肺癌多见[86];一些少见的骨髓转移实体肿瘤有肉瘤、原发性肝癌、结肠癌、黑色素瘤、鼻咽癌、肾细胞癌等[87]。

Kucukzeybek等[84]报道,骨髓转移癌中原发肿瘤乳腺癌占59%、胃癌占15.3%、前列腺占10.2%和肺癌占7.7%。Huang等[88]报道了83例实体肿瘤骨髓转移,胃癌为39%,前列腺癌为19%,肺癌为15%。但Chandra等[89]研究发现,骨髓转移发生率最高的原发肿瘤是前列腺癌,其次为肺癌和胃肠道肿瘤。Mohanty等[90]亦指出,实体肿瘤骨髓转移前列腺癌最常见,其次是乳腺癌、肺癌、结肠癌。

虽然实体肿瘤骨髓转移率很低,但在实体肿瘤骨髓转移中,不明原发肿瘤所占比例则较高。有研究报道[91-92],不明原发肿瘤占所有肿瘤骨髓转移的 32.8%～72%。Kucukzeybek 等[84]报道，在 58 例实体肿瘤骨髓转移的患者中，有 32.8%的患者原发肿瘤不明。Xiao 等[93]回顾性分析了 10112 例非血液学肿瘤骨髓样本，有 50%的患者原发肿瘤不明。陈朴等[91]对 106 例实体肿瘤骨髓转移癌患者进行了分析，结果显示，原发肿瘤不明的患者占 46%。弓长丽等[94]对 72 例老年骨髓转移癌患者进行了回顾性分析，最后明确原发肿瘤者 44 例，28 例（占 38.9%）原发肿瘤不明。

第三节 发生机制

恶性实体肿瘤转移的主要途径是肿瘤细胞从原发灶脱落，进入血液、淋巴系统，转移到其他组织器官、淋巴结。

目前，CUP 确切的发病因素、发生机制均不十分清楚，有多种理论或观点。

就发生因素而言，吸烟者有罹患 CUP 的风险，这种风险与烟草暴露水平相关，吸烟 1～15 支/天者为不吸烟者 1.8 倍，吸烟 16～25 支/天者为不吸烟者 3.5 倍，吸烟 >25 支/天者为不吸烟者 4.1 倍[95]。CUP 伴有呼吸系统转移患者吸烟的比例（4.9 倍）高于 CUP 伴有肝转移患者（2.0 倍）[96]。

Ⅱ型糖尿病（1.8 倍）和自身免疫性疾病亦与发生 CUP 风险增加有关[97]；多发性肌炎/皮肌炎的相对风险为 3.5 倍，原发性胆汁性肝硬化为 1.8 倍，Addison 病为 1.7 倍[98]。高体重指数、腰围、低社会经济地位可能是 CUP 发生的额外风险因素[99]。

Elrassy 等[100]报道，人乳头状瘤病毒（human papilloma virus，HPV）与头颈部、腹部、骨盆和腹膜后的不明原发鳞状细胞癌有关。

一项基于瑞典家族癌症数据库分析的研究显示[101]，2.8%的不明原发肿瘤病例是家族性的（即父母一方和后代均被诊断为不明原发肿瘤），部分 CUP 患者的发病部位与其一级亲属原发肿瘤部位有显著相关性，许多因 CUP 死亡的患者，其转移灶部位甚至与其亲属中的原发肿瘤部位相同；另外，CUP 与家族中肺癌、肾癌和结直肠癌的发生有关。因此，不明原发肿瘤可能有遗传学基础。

在分子基因层面，有研究表明[102]，CUP 与血管生成激活（50%～89%）、多种癌基因过度表达（10%～30%）、上皮-间质转化标记物或缺氧相关蛋白过表达（16%～25%）、细胞内信号如 AKT 或 MAPK 的激活

（20%~35%）相关，而与肿瘤抑制基因点突变或癌基因激活无关。

就发生机制而言，有学者认为[103]，可能是原发灶过小且生长缓慢或微小原发灶生长受宿主免疫抑制，并发生消退。Komuro 等[104]报道，曾在多种肿瘤中发现肿瘤自发性退化现象。

Lopez-Lzazro[105]指出，一些迁移能力强的肿瘤细胞在早期即扩散到转移部位并改变其微环境，导致在尚未形成可检查发现的原发灶之前已经发生了实质性的转移。Vant Veer 等[36]亦认为，肿瘤发生早期即有转移倾向。但 Rassy 等[106]认为，在 CUP 形成过程中不存在平行进展过程，而是依赖于肿瘤微环境选择性地助力肿瘤细胞在转移部位的生长，同时抑制了具有相同基因型的肿瘤细胞在原发部位的生长。

有学者将肿瘤血液、淋巴转移分为早期转移模式与后期转移模式[107]，在早期转移模式中，肿瘤细胞在经过循环系统到达目的地之后才发生变异，这种模式中转移灶与原发灶的肿瘤细胞基因相似度较低，不易确定原发肿瘤位置。

一些学者还认为[108-111]，CUP 可能因其原发肿瘤太小或位置隐蔽，现有检查方法难以发现。

另外，转移癌的生物学特性可能与原发肿瘤不同，使原发肿瘤尚未发现，患者即死于转移癌。郭伟剑等[112]报道了 24 例原发灶不明的肝转移癌，有 9 例死因明确的患者中有 6 例死于肝转移灶进展所致的肝功能衰竭。

第四节　临床分型与分期

关于不明原发肿瘤的分类，有根据转移组织或器官而分为淋巴结转移癌和脏器转移癌[113]，有根据转移部位而细分为原发灶不明淋巴结转移癌、原发灶不明内脏（包括胸膜、腹膜、硬脊膜）转移癌、原发灶不明骨转移癌、原发灶不明皮肤和软组织转移癌[114]；还有根据病理类型，分为原发灶不明转移性腺癌、原发灶不明转移性鳞癌、原发灶不明转移性低分化癌与未分化癌、原发灶不明转移性神经内分泌癌。

目前，主要根据其对治疗反应及预后进行分类[16]，分为预后良好型（Favourable-subsets）与预后不良型（Unfavourable-subsets），目前多数学者采用此种分类方法。

一般而言,对于可疑 CUP 患者进行系统检查后明确了原发肿瘤,其分期按已知原发肿瘤进行分期,除乳腺癌腋窝淋巴结转移且无脏器转移外,其他 CUP 临床分期均为晚期(Ⅳ期)。

但目前对于不明原发肿瘤尚无任何分期标准,包括 2024 年第 1 版 NCCN 指南亦无明确分期,仅颈部淋巴结 CUP 分期可参考国际抗癌联盟(Union for International Cancer Control,UICC)、AJCC 头颈部恶性肿瘤 TNM 分期标准中的颈部淋巴结转移癌的临床 N 分期。

表 5-1 CUP 临床分型

分型	肿瘤
预后良好型	位于正中线的低分化癌(性腺外的胚胎肿瘤); 女性腹膜腔乳头状腺癌; 女性局限于腋窝淋巴结转移性腺癌; 颈部淋巴结转移性鳞癌; 孤立性腹股沟腺癌或鳞癌; 低分化神经内分泌癌; 伴有前列腺特异性抗原(PSA)升高的男性骨转移癌; 单发的、体积较小的、潜在可切除的转移性肿瘤
预后不良型	肝或其他脏器的转移性腺癌、鳞癌; 恶性腹水(腺癌、鳞癌); 多发脑转移癌(腺、鳞癌); 多发肺/胸膜转移性(恶性胸水)腺癌、鳞癌; 多发骨转移性腺癌(可疑前列腺癌除外)、鳞癌; 骨髓转移癌

参考文献

[1] Catanla VC. Treatment of peripheral lymph node metastases of tumors of unknown primary Site [J]. Tumori, 1954, 40(6): 677-685.

[2] Vanden Heule B, Gompel C. Adenocarcinomas of unknown origin. Study of 17 autopsies (author's transl)[J]. Bull Cancer, 1978, 65(4): 389-393.

[3] Sande GM. Metastases of unknown origin in cervical lymph nodes, A case report[J]. East Afr Med J, 1972, 49(3): 240-242.

[4] Barrie JR, Knapper WH, Strong EW. Cervical nodal metastases of unknown origin[J]. CA Cancer J Clin, 1971, 21(2): 112-119.

[5] Röder K. Value of lymphographic examinations for the diagnosis of metastasizing of unknown primary tumors[J]. Radiol Diagn(Berl), 1971, 12(3): 343-349.

[6] Chrzanowska A. Evaluation of the results of treatment of patients with neoplastic metastases from unknown primary focus[J]. Nowotwory, 1969, 19(2): 93-98.

[7] Howet F. Deep malignant epithelial tumors of the neck of unknown origin[J]. Acta Chir Belg, 1951, 50(5): 265-280.

[8] Briasoulis E, Pavlidis N. Cancer of Unknown Primary Origin[J]. Oncologist, 1997, 2(3): 142-152.

[9] Krämer A, Bochtler T, Pauli C, et al. Cancer of unknown primary: ESMO Clinical Practice Guideline for diagnosis, treatment and follow-up[J]. Ann Oncol, 2022, 34(3): 228-247.

[10] Tomuleasa C, Zaharie F, Muresan MS, et al. How to Diagnose and Treat a Cancer of Unknown Primary Site[J]. J Gastrointestin Liver Dis, 2017, 26(1): 69-79.

[11] Pavlidis N, Briasoulis E, Hainsworth J, et al. Diagnostic and therapeutic management of cancer of an unknown primary[J]. Eur J Cancer, 2003, 39(14): 1990-2005.

[12] Pavlidis N, Pentheroudakis G. Cancer of unknown primary site[J]. The Lancet, 2012, 379(9824): 1428-1435.

[13] Bochtler T, Loffler H, Kramer A. Diagnosis and management of metastatic neoplasms with unknown primary[J]. Semin Diagn Pathol, 2017, 26(11): 1-8.

[14] Pavlidis N, Fizazi K. Carcinoma of unknown primary (CUP)[J]. Crit Rev Oncol Hematol, 2009, 69(3): 271-278.

[15] Pavlidis N, Rassy E, Smith-Gagen J. Cancer of unknown primary: Incidence rates, risk factors and survival among adolescents and young adults[J]. Int J Cancer, 2020, 146(6): 1490-1498.

[16] Pavlidis N, Fizazi K. Cancer of unknown primary (CUP)[J]. Crit Rev Oncol Hematol, 2005, 54(3): 243-250.

[17] Varadhachary GR, Raber MN. Cancer of unknown primarysite[J]. N Engl J Med, 2014, 371(8): 757-765.

[18] Dennis JL, Hvidsten TR, Wit EC, et al. Markers of adenocarcinoma characteristic of the site of origin: development of a diagnostic algorithm[J]. Clin Cancer Res, 2005, 11(10): 3766-3772.

[19] Mevio E, Gorini E, Sbrocca M, et al. The role of positron emission tomography (PET) in the management of cervical lymphnodes metastases from an unknown primary tumour[J]. Acta Otorhinolaryngol Ital, 2004, 24(6): 342-347.

[20] 吴志坚, 张永学, 魏昊, 等. ^{18}氟-2-脱氧-D-葡萄 PET/CT 全身显像对不明原发灶肿瘤处理决策的影响[J]. 中华医学杂志, 2007, 87(32): 2253-2256.

[21] Ambrosini V, Nanni C, Rubello D, et al. ^{18}F-FDG PET/CT in the assessment of carcinoma of unknown primary origin[J]. Radiol Med, 2006, 111(8): 1146-1155.

[22] Fencl P, Belohlavek O, Skopalova M, et al. Prognostic and diagnostic accuracy of ^{18}F-FDG-PET/CT in 190 patients with carcinoma of unknown primary[J]. Eur J Nucl Med Mol Imaging, 2007, 34(11): 1783-1792.

[23] Rassy E, Pavlidis N. Progress in refining the clinical management of cancer of unknown primary in the molecular era[J]. Nat Rev Clin Oncol, 2020, 17(9): 541-554.

[24] Jones W, Allardice G, Scott I, et al. Cancers of unknown primary diagnosed during hospitalization: a population-based study[J]. BMC Cancer, 2017, 17(1): 85-96.

[25] Hainsworth JD, Greco FA. Management of patient with cancer of unknown primary site[J]. Oncology(Huntingt), 2000, 14(4): 563-574.

[26] Brewster DH, Lang J, Bhatti LA, et al. Descriptive epidemiology of cancer of unknown primary site in Scotland, 1961-2010[J]. Cancer Epidemiol, 2014, 38(3): 227-234.

[27] Le Chevalier T, Cvitkovic E, Caille P, et al. Early metastatic cancer of unknown primary origin at presentation. Aclinical study of 302 consecutive autopsied patients[J]. Arch Intern Med, 1988, 148(9): 2035-2039.

[28] Grau C, Johansen LV, Jakobsen J, et al. Cervical lymphnode metastases from unknown primary tumors. Results from a national survey by the Danish Society for Head and Neck Oncology[J]. Radiother Oncol, 2000, 55(6): 121-129.

[29] Blaszyk H, Hartmann A, Bjornsson J. Cancer of unknown primary: clinicopathologic correlations[J]. APMIS, 2003, 111(12): 1089-1094.

[30] Hillen HF. Unknown primary tumours[J]. Postgrad Med J, 2000, 76(901): 690-693.

[31] Greenlee RT, Murray T, Bolden S, et al. Cancer statistics, 2000[J]. Cancer J Clin, 2000, 50(1): 7-33.

[32] Massard C, Loriot Y, Fizazi K. Carcinomas of an unknown primary origin-diagnosis and treatment[J]. Nat Rev Clin Oncol, 2011, 8(12): 701-710.

[33] Burglin SA, Hess S, Hilund-Carlsen PF, et al. ^{18}F-FDG PET/CT for detection of the primary tumor in adults with extracervical metastases from cancer of unknown primary: A systematic review and meta-analysis[J]. Medicine(Baltimore), 2017, 96(16): e6713-e6721.

[34] Urban D, Rao A, Bressel M, et al. Cancer of unknown primary: apopulation-based analysis of temporal change and socioeconomic disparities[J]. Br J Cancer, 2013, 109(5): 1318-1324.

[35] Siegel RL, Miller KD, Fuchs HE, et al. Cancer statistics, 2022[J]. CA Cancer J Clin, 2022, 72(1): 7-33.

[36] Van't-Veer LJ, Weigelt B. Road map to metastasis[J]. Nat Med, 2003, 9(8): 999-

1000.

[37] 王成锋，田艳涛，张建伟. 不明原发灶肿瘤1273例报告[J]. 中国微创外科杂志，2007，7(11)：1072-1074.

[38] Levi F, Te VC, Erler G, et al. Epidemiology of unknown primary tumours[J]. Eur J Cancer, 2002, 38(13): 1810-1812.

[39] 赵丽霞，李林，赵祯，等. ^{18}F-FDG PET/CT全身显像在不明原发灶肿瘤中的诊断价值[J]. 四川大学学报(医学版)，2010，41(3)：545-547.

[40] 中国抗癌协会肿瘤标志专业委员会，重庆市医学会精准医疗与分子诊断分会，重庆抗癌协会肿瘤标志物专业委员会. 基于分子指导的原发灶不明肿瘤临床诊治实践的中国专家共识(2023年版)[J]. 中国癌症防治杂志，2023，15(3)：252-262.

[41] Gallagher CJ, Reznek RH. Cancer of unknown primary site[J]. Clin Med, 2008, 8(4): 451-454.

[42] 黑砚，康莉，李月月，等. 22例眼眶转移癌临床病理分析[J]. 眼科，2007，16(6)：403-406.

[43] Huang G, Tian X, Li Y, et al. Clinical characteristics and surgical resection of multifocal papillary thyroid carcinoma: 168 cases[J]. Int J Clin Exp Med, 2014, 7(12): 5802-5807.

[44] 肖光莉，徐国镇，高黎. 原发灶不明的颈部淋巴结转移癌的治疗[J]. 中华放射肿瘤学杂志，2002，11(2)：84-87.

[45] 康炜东，王春贵，壮志，等. 43例老年颈部淋巴结转移癌的来源及分区特征分析[J]. 吉林医学，2016，37(6)：1367-1368.

[46] 张新涛，徐栋梁，谭本前，等. 转移性骨肿瘤897例临床分析[J]. 中国骨肿瘤骨病，2005，4(3)：135-142.

[47] Rougraff BT. Evaluation of the patient with carcinoma of unknown origin metastatic to bone[J]. Clin Orthop Relat Res, 2003, 10(415 Suppl): S105-S109.

[48] Conroy T, Malissard L, Dartois D, et al. Natural history and development of bone metastasis: A propos of 429 cases[J]. Bull Cancer, 1988, 75(9): 845-857.

[49] 曹来宾，王安明，徐爱德，等. 1047例骨转移瘤的影像学诊断[J]. 中华放射学杂志，1997，31(8)：547-551.

[50] 徐栋梁，张新涛，王国海，等. 390例病理确诊转移性骨肿瘤的临床分析[J]. 癌症，2005，24(11)：1404-1407.

[51] 叶骉飞，王斌，代丽，等. 408例恶性肿瘤骨转移临床特征分析[J]. 中国肿瘤临床，2013，40(4)：217-220.

[52] 荆鑫，吴海山，周维京. 转移性骨肿瘤发生机制的研究进展[J]. 中华骨科杂志，2002，22(6)：377-379.

[53] 赵瑞华，樊青霞. 108例恶性肿瘤骨转移的临床分析[J]. 肿瘤基础与临床，2008，21

(4): 316-318.

[54] Ugras N, Yalcinkaya U, Akesen B, et al. Solitary bone etastases of unknown origin[J]. Acta Orthop Belg, 2014, 80(1): 139-143.

[55] Vander Linden YM, Dijkstra SP, Vonk EJ, et al. Prediction of survival in patients with metastases in the spinal column: results based on a randomized trial of radiotherapy[J]. Cancer, 2005, 103(2): 320-328.

[56] 王丰, 伦登兴, 张浩, 等. 脊柱转移瘤481例的流行病学分析[J]. 中国脊柱脊髓杂志, 2017, 27(9): 787-794.

[57] Ferlay J, Shin HR, Bray F, et al. Estimates of world wide burden of cancer in 2008: GLOBOCAN 2008[J]. Int J Cancer, 2010, 127(12): 2893-2917.

[58] Scutellari PN, Antinolfi G, Galeotti R, et al. Metastatic bone disease: strategies for imaging[J]. Minerva Med, 2003, 94(2): 77-90.

[59] Akhtari M, Mansuri J, Newman KA, et al. Biology of breast cancer bone metastasis[J]. Cancer Biol Ther, 2008, 7(1): 3-9.

[60] 张小军, 王臻, 郭征, 等. 640例脊柱肿瘤及瘤样病变的临床流行病学分析[J]. 临床肿瘤学杂志, 2012, 17(6): 543-548.

[61] Katagiri H, Takahashi M, Inagaki J, et al. Determining the site of the primary cancer in patients with skeletal metastasis of unknown origin: a retrospective study[J]. Cancer, 1999, 86(3): 533-537.

[62] Rougraff BT, Kneisl JS, Simon MA. Skeletal metastases of unknown origin: A prospective study of a diagnostic strategy[J]. J Bone Joint Surg Am, 1993, 75(9): 1276-1281.

[63] Shih LY, Chen TH, Lo WH. Skeletal metastasis from occult carcinoma[J]. J Surg Oncol, 1992, 51(2): 109-113.

[64] Nottebaert M, Exner GU, von Hochstetter AR, et al. Metastatic bone disease from occult carcinoma: a profile[J]. Int Orthop, 1989, 13(2): 119-123.

[65] Vandecandelaere M, Flipo RM, Cortet B, et al. Bone metastases revealing primary tumors: Comparison of two series separated by 30 years[J]. Joint Bone Spine, 2004, 71(3): 224-229.

[66] Hemminki K, Riihimaki M, Sundquist K, et al. Site-specific survival rates for cancer of unknown primary according tolocation of metastases[J]. Int J Cancer, 2013, 133(1): 182-189.

[67] Bartelt S, Lutterbach J. Brain metastases in patients with cancer of unknown primary[J]. J Neurooncol, 2003, 64(3): 249-253.

[68] Taillibert S, Le Rhun É. Epidemiology of brain metastases[J]. Cancer Radiother, 2015, 19(1): 3-9.

[69] 张继良, 徐俊玲, 李永丽, 等. 640例脑转移瘤的临床及MRI分析[J]. 中国实用神经

疾病杂志，2008，11(2)：121-123.

[70] 石易鑫，王月坤，邢昊，等. 北京协和医院脑转移瘤多学科协作诊疗经验：159例病例总结[J]. 协和医学杂志，2023，14(2)：306-314.

[71] 穆林森，张红波，陈谦学，等. 原发灶来源不明的脑转移瘤的临床特点及治疗[J]. 中国临床神经外科杂志，2015，20(12)：733-735.

[72] Nayak L，Abrey LE，Lwamoto FM. Intracranial dural metstases[J]. Cancer，2009，115(9)：1947-1953.

[73] Kunii N，Morita A，Yoshikawa G，et al. Subdural hematoma associated with dural metastasis - case report[J]. Neurol Med Chir(Tokyo)，2005，45(10)：519-522.

[74] Posner JB，Chernik NL. Intracranial metastases from systemic cancer. Advances in Neurology[M]. New York：Raven Press，1978，579-592.

[75] Laigle - Donadey F，Taillibert S，Mokhtari K，et al. Dural metastases[J]. J Neurooncol，2005，75(1)：57-61.

[76] Lee SJ，Bae JH，Lee AW，et al. Clinical characteristics of metastatic tumors to the ovaries[J]. J Korean Med Sci，2009，24(1)：114-119.

[77] De Waal YR，Thomas CM，Oei AL，et al. Secondary ovarian malignancies：frequency，origin，and characteristics[J]. Int J Gynecol Cancer，2009，19(7)：1160-1165.

[78] Guzel A，Gulec UK，Paydas S，et al. Preoperative evaluation，clinical characteristics and prognostic factors of nongenital metastatic ovarian tumors nongenital：Review of 48 patients[J]. Eur J Gynaecol Oncol，2012，33(5)：493-497.

[79] Al - Agha OM，Nieastri AD. An in - depth look at Krukenberg tumor：an ovarian review[J]. Arch Pathot Lab Med，2006，130(11)：1725-1730.

[80] Kobayashi O，Sugiyama Y，Cho H，et al. Clinical and pathological study of gastric cancer with ovarian metastasis[J]. Int J Clin Oncol，2003，8(2)：67-71.

[81] Saif MW，Siddiqui IA，Sohail MA. Management of ascites due to gastrointestinal malignancy[J]. Ann Saudi Med，2009，29(5)：369-377.

[82] Tasleem RA，Chowdhary ND，Kadri SM，et al. Metastasis of solid tumours in bone marrow：a study from Kashmir, India[J]. J Clin Pathol，2003，56(10)：803.

[83] Tyagi R，Singh A，Garg B，et al. Be ware of Bone Marrow：Incidental Detection and Primary Diagnosis of Solid Tumours in Bone Marrow Aspiration and Biopsies：A Study of 22 Cases[J]. Iran J Pathol，2018，13(1)：78-84.

[84] Kucukzeybek BB，Calli AO，Kucukzeybek Y，et al. The prognostic significance of bone marrow metastases：evaluation of 58 cases[J]. Indian J Pathol Microbiol，2014，57(3)：396-399.

[85] Kar R，Jacob S，Basu D，et al. Non - haematopoietic malignancies metastasing to the bone marrow：A 5 year record - based descriptive study from a tertiary care centre in South India

[J]. Indian J Cancer, 2014, 51(1): 30-34.

[86] Moid, De Palma L. Comparison of relative value of bone marrow aspirates and bone marrow trephine biopsies in the diagnosis of solid tumor metastasis and Hodgkin lymphoma: institutional experience and literature review[J]. Arch Pathol Lab Med, 2005, 129(4): 497-501.

[87] Zhou MH, Wang ZH, Zhou HW, et al. Clinical outcome of 30 patients with bone marrow metastases[J]. J Cancer Res Ther, 2018, 14(Supplement): S512-S515.

[88] Huang YS, Chou WC, Chen TD, et al. Prognostic factors in adult patients with solid cancers and bone marrow metastases[J]. Asian Pac J Cancer Prev, 2014, 15(1): 61-67.

[89] Chandra S, Chandra H, Saini S. Bone marrow metastasis by solid tumors – probable hematological indicators and comparison of bone marrow aspirate, touch imprint and trephine biopsy[J]. Hematology, 2010, 15(5): 368-372.

[90] Mohanty SK, Dash S. Bone marrow metastasis in solid tumors[J]. Indian J Patho Microbiol, 2003, 46(4): 613-616.

[91] 陈朴, 王蓓丽, 郭玮, 等. 106例骨髓转移癌临床及细胞形态学特点分析[J]. 检验医学, 2013, 28(7): 595-598.

[92] Frisch B, Lewis SM, Burkhardt R, et al. Biopsy pathology of bone and bone marrow[M]. London: Chapman and Hall Medical, 1985: 243-275.

[93] Xiao L, Luxi S, Ying T, et al. Diagnosis of unknown non hematological tumors by bone marrow biopsy: a retrospective analysis of 10, 112 samples[J]. J Cancer Res Clin Oncol, 2009, 135(5): 687-693.

[94] 弓长丽, 孟莹, 刁斌斌. 老年骨髓转移癌72例临床及血液学分析[J]. 中国老年学杂志, 2011, 31(4): 695-696.

[95] Kaaks R, Sookthai D, Hemminki K, et al. Risk factors for cancers of unknown primary site: results from the prospective EPIC cohort[J]. Int J Cancer, 2014, 135(10): 2475-2481.

[96] Hemminki K, Chen B, Melander O, et al. Smoking and body mass index as risk factors for subtypes of cancer of unknown primary[J]. Int J Cancer, 2015, 136(1): 246-247.

[97] Hemminki K, Försti A, Sundquist K, et al. Cancer of unknown primary is associated with diabetes[J]. Eur J Cancer Prev, 2016, 25(3): 246-251.

[98] Hemminki K, Sundquist K, Sundquist J, et al. Risk of cancer of unknown primary after hospitalization for autoimmune diseases[J]. Int J Cancer, 2015, 137(12): 2885-2895.

[99] Hemminki K, Bevier M, Hemminki A, et al. Survival in cancer of unknown primary site: population-based analysis by site and histology[J]. Ann Oncol, 2012, 23(7): 1854-1863.

[100] Elrassy E, Kattan J, Pavlidis N. A new entity of abdominal squamous cell carcinoma of unknown primary[J]. Eur J Clin Invest, 2019, 49(7): e13111.

[101] Hemminki K, Ji J, Sundquist J, et al. Familial risks in cancer of unknown primary: tracking the primary sites[J]. J Clin Oncol, 2011, 29(4): 435-440.

[102] Losa F, Iglesias L, Pané M, et al. 2018 consensus statement by the Spanish Society of Pathology and the Spanish Society of Medical Oncology on the diagnosis and treatment of cancer of unknown primary[J]. Clin Transl Oncol, 2018, 20(11): 1361-1372.

[103] Naresh KN. Dometastatic tumours from an unknown primary reflect angiogenic incompetence of the tumor at the primary site? - a hypothesis[J]. Med Hypotheses, 2002, 59(3): 357-360.

[104] Komuro H, Imaizumi S. Congenital mediastinal dumb bell neuroblastoma with spontaneous regression of liver metastases[J]. Pediatr Surg Int, 1998, 12(1): 86-88.

[105] Lopez-Lzazro M. The migration ability of stem cells can explain the existence of cancer of unknown primary site. Rethinking metastasis[J]. Oncoscience, 2015, 2(5): 467-475.

[106] Rassy E, Assi T, Pavlidis N. Exploring the biological hall marks of cancer of unknown primary: where do we stand today? [J]. Br J Cancer, 2020, 122(8): 1124-1132.

[107] Klein CA. The Metastasis Cascade[J]. Science, 2008, 321(5897): 1785-1787.

[108] Lefebvre JL, Coche-Dequeant B, Van JT. Cervical lymph nodes from an unknown primary tumor in 190 patients[J]. Am J Surg, 1990, 160(4): 443-446.

[109] 张智显, 马俊峰, 付登礼. 不明原发灶颈部转移癌的诊断和治疗[J]. 医学综述, 2010, 16(10): 1492-1494.

[110] 张延龄. 原发灶不明的肿瘤患者的处理[J]. 国外医学外科学分册, 2002, 29(5): 282-285.

[111] 戴惠, 吴剑, 林权冰. 原发灶不明的颈部淋巴结转移癌治疗失败原因分析[J]. 实用医学杂志, 2006, 22(20): 2404-2405.

[112] 郭伟剑, 张廷. 原发灶不明的转移性肝癌的诊治体会[J]. 实用癌症杂志, 1997, 12(4): 283-284.

[113] 李绍明, 林沸腾, 谢树贤, 等. 不明原发灶转移癌的治疗探讨(附13例报告)[J]. 中国肿瘤临床与康复, 2002, 9(3): 107-108.

[114] 林奔, 邓燕明. 来源隐匿转移癌的诊治探讨[J]. 实用癌症杂志, 2006, 21(3): 312-313.

第六章
可疑 CUP 检查与诊断

第一节 可疑 CUP 一般检查

一、病史询问

既往肿瘤病史、组织活检史或肿瘤病灶切除史、退行性病变史及家族肿瘤病史等，对可疑 CUP 进一步明确原发肿瘤诊断尤为重要。

有研究报道[1]，CUP 患者存在家族易感性倾向及 CUP 与其他一些肿瘤存在一定关联，CUP 通常发生于肺癌、结直肠癌、原发性肝癌、卵巢癌等患者的亲属中，这些肿瘤家族聚集表明可能有共同的遗传学基础。

二、临床表现

CUP 通常表现为全身广泛转移，具有较强的侵袭性。虽然某些转移模式提示了可能的原发肿瘤，但 CUP 可转移到任何部位，超过 50% 的 CUP 患者可出现多个部位受累[2]。因此，不应依赖已知的转移模式来确定可疑 CUP 患者的原发肿瘤。

绝大多数不明原发肿瘤患者常常缺乏原发肿瘤的表现，仅表现出转移灶症状或全身症状(如食欲减退、体重减轻、恶病质等)，少数是通过常规检查或意外发现。

有学者报道[3-4]，转移灶的临床表现为疼痛者占 60%，肝转移或其他腹部表现者占 40%，淋巴结肿大者占 20%，骨痛或病理骨折者占 15%；以呼吸系统症状、中枢神经系统症状为表现者占 15%，体重减轻者占 5%；其他少见表现如皮肤软组织肿块、不明原因恶液质、不明原因发热、游走性血栓性静脉炎占 5%，还有少数患者无任何临床表现。

(一)脑转移

脑转移灶伴明显周围水肿的患者可出现颅内高压症状与体征，如头晕、头痛、呕吐等。

(二) 骨转移

疼痛为骨转移肿瘤侵犯骨皮质所致，多为持续性、进行性加重，有的疼痛剧烈，药物难以缓解；严重的脊柱转移瘤可伴有脊髓和神经根的压迫而出现截瘫。

骨转移患者常因骨痛、肿块、病理性骨折、功能障碍，甚至截瘫等就诊。

(三) 骨髓转移

骨髓转移癌最常见临床症状为骨痛、脊髓压迫和病理性骨折、出血，还有一些不典型症状，如不明原因发热、乏力、消瘦、肝脾肿大等。

骨髓转移癌与单纯的实体肿瘤不同，肿瘤细胞可在骨髓腔内迅速播散，广泛浸润，导致造血细胞破坏及骨髓纤维化，除原发肿瘤症状外，往往更多见血液系统症状。

血液系统改变多见于血细胞减少，包括一系或二系血细胞减少，最常见的是贫血，其次是血小板减少症[5]，还可能存在如弥散性血管内凝血（DIC）和微血管病变性溶血性贫血（MHA）等改变。

除血液系统改变，常见生化结果异常，如高血钙、碱性磷酸酶及乳酸脱氢酶明显升高、轻度至中度胆红素升高、谷草转氨酶和谷丙转氨酶升高。

(四) 恶性浆膜腔积液

恶性浆膜腔积液包括心包腔、胸腔、腹腔积液，其临床表现、体征与积液生长速度、积液量密切相关，少量积液可无任何症状，大量积液可出现心包填塞、呼吸困难、腹部膨隆等。

腹膜种植转移可表现为板状腹、腹腔积液，肠系膜种植转移可发生多节段性肠梗阻。

三、体格检查

体格检查应认真仔细、全面系统，除常规体格检查外，泌尿生殖系流和直肠检查是重点检查部位。女性患者应进行乳房和子宫附件等盆腔区域的检查，男性患者应行前列腺检查。

有阳性体征的患者可侧重检查特定部位，如腋窝淋巴结肿大的女性患者，乳腺检查应视为重点；颈部淋巴结肿大患者，可侧重头颈部及胸部检查。

第二节 可疑 CUP 影像学检查

在对可疑 CUP 患者进行多学科诊断评估时，影像学检查发挥着不可替代的作用[6]。对于可疑 CUP 常规影像学检查而言，X 线、B 超、CT、MRI、骨扫描（ECT）等是寻找原发肿瘤首选检查方法。

原发肿瘤不明的骨转移影像学表现对于发现其原发肿瘤具有重要价值，骨 X 线片、CT 和 MRI 是确认其转移的常规影像学检查手段[7-8]。转移卵巢肿瘤影像学特征是 60%～70% 的患者为卵巢双侧占位，Lee 等[9]报道，如果怀疑患者是转移卵巢肿瘤，75% 的患者可通过术前影像学检查、血清标志物检测而明确原发肿瘤。

一、常规影像学检查

（一）X 线检查

X 线检查是原发性骨肿瘤与转移骨肿瘤诊断最常用方法之一，大部分骨转移肿瘤表现为溶骨性破坏。Scutellari 等[10]报道，溶骨性改变占 52%，其次为成骨性、混合型；在曹来宾等[11]报道的 988 例骨转移肿瘤 X 线表现中，溶骨性改变占 83.5%，混合型占 9.3%，成骨性改变占 5.2%。

建议对疼痛性病变和（或）骨扫描阳性病变和（或）负重部位有骨折可能的病变进行诊断性影像学检查。

可疑 CUP 女性患者通常需进行乳房 X 线检查。

（二）CT 检查

目前，CT 检查已被广泛用于可疑 CUP 患者原发灶的寻找及分期，对位于肺、胰腺、结肠或肾脏等部位的原发肿瘤具有较高的灵敏度，且十分有利于肺、肝、淋巴结及骨等转移灶的发现。一项对纳入 879 例可疑 CUP 患者进行 CT 检查的研究结果显示[12]，CT 检查明确胰腺癌诊断率为 86%、结直肠癌为 36%、肺癌为 74%，总体诊断准确率为 55%。

在对于可疑 CUP 患者进行初始影像学基线检查时，建议胸部、腹部及盆腔 CT 平扫加增强。

(三) MRI 检查

对于颅脑、乳腺、肝脏、胰腺、脊髓及骨骼肌肉系统原发性肿瘤及转移性肿瘤的影像学检查，一般首选 MRI，具有较强的敏感性与较高的诊断准确率。

对于孤立性腋窝淋巴结转移腺癌的女性患者，乳腺钼靶和超声检查均为阴性时，MRI 可检出 75% 的原发乳腺癌[13]。Olson 等[14]对 40 例乳房 X 线未发现原发肿瘤的腋窝淋巴结转移的妇女进行乳房 MRI 扫描检查，28 例发现乳房原发肿瘤，其余 12 例 MRI 扫描阴性，研究结果表明，乳房 MRI 扫描可识别那些只有腋窝淋巴结转移的原发隐匿性乳腺癌。

多参数核磁共振成像(MP-MRI)由 3 个独立的成像参数(T2 加权成像、弥散加权成像和动态对比增强成像)组成，可清晰显示组织及其化学构成。T1 加权高分辨率各相同性容积检查(THRIVE)是一种三维超快破坏梯度磁共振成像序列，与传统的二维脊柱回波磁共振成像相比，它能提供更详细的解剖信息和更高的空间分辨率。在一项对 73 例可疑 CUP 和颈淋巴结转移的患者进行的回顾性研究中[15]，72.9% 的患者通过 3D-THRIVE MRI 明确了原发肿瘤，而自旋回波 MRI 和对比增强 CT 的这一比例分别为 49.2% 和 36.4%；3D-THRIVE MRI 的诊断准确率(71.2%)高于自旋回波 MRI(53.4%)和 CT(46.4%；$P = 0.001$)。

二、PET/CT 检查

据相关文献报道[16-17]，对于可疑 CUP 患者而言，常规影像学检查方法仅能发现 20%~35% 的原发肿瘤，即使尸检亦只能明确 30%~82% 的原发肿瘤。

PET/CT 将解剖学与功能学影像检查相结合，有学者认为其可明显提高原发肿瘤的检出率[18-19]。近年来，PET/CT 检查在可疑 CUP 诊断中的研究报道较多，多数学者认为[20-34]，PET/CT 检查在可疑 CUP 中寻找原发肿瘤、临床分期、治疗方案制订以及随访等方面具有重要价值。有研究报道[35-39]，在 25%~75% 的可疑 CUP 患者中，PET/CT 联合检查可确定原发肿瘤部位。

一项关于 PET/CT 在可疑 CUP 患者中应用的荟萃分析和系统综述中发现[40]，在 11 项研究的 433 例可疑 CUP 患者中，有 37% 的可疑 CUP 患者明确了原发肿瘤,其敏感性和特异性均为84%。在另一项针对56例可疑CUP患者的前瞻性研究中[27],PET/CT检测原发肿瘤的灵敏度和准确性明显高于CT/MRI(分别为69%和77%对比41%和48%;$P<0.04$)。李亚军等[41]对31例常规影像学检查难以确诊的可疑CUP患者行PET/CT全身显像,29例(93.5%)患者明确了原发肿瘤。

一项Meta分析结果显示[42],44%的可疑CUP患者经PET/CT明确了原发肿瘤,敏感性为97%,特异性为68%。Rusthoven等[43]对4项研究的107例可疑CUP患者进行了Meta分析,结果显示,PET/CT检查出了29例患者(27.1%)常规影像学检查未发现的原发肿瘤和远处转移病灶。

Gutzeit等[44]对45例CUP者比较了CT、PET、PET+CT及PET/CT融合显像的诊断敏感性、特异性和准确性,结果显示,敏感性分别为19%、28%、31%和35%,特异性为73%、65%、81%和83%,准确性为73%、65%、81%和83%。

(一)颈部淋巴结转移癌

有研究报道[45],在PET/CT应用之前CUP占头颈部肿瘤的比例为2%~9%,而使用PET/CT之后下降至1%~2%。

Roh等[46]报道,PET/CT寻找颈部淋巴结转移患者原发肿瘤的灵敏度(87.5%)明显高于CT(43.7%)。Freudenberg等[47]的研究表明,CT、PET、PET+CT及PET/CT对21例可疑CUP颈部淋巴结转移患者原发肿瘤的检出率分别为23%、52%、52%和57%,假阳性率分别为14%、14%、4.8%和0%,假阴性率分别为38%、14%、14%、和9.5%。Lee等[27]的前瞻性研究结果表明,PET/CT较增强CT或MRI对伴有颈部转移的CUP肿瘤患者原发肿瘤的诊断更为敏感。

赵春雷等[48]的研究显示,在42例可疑CUP颈部转移癌患者中,PET/CT显像对6例(14%)患者提高了单独PET和单独CT定位、定性的准确性。

(二)腹膜转移癌

腹膜转移癌(peritoneal metastases,PM),几乎可源于任何原发性肿瘤,以卵巢和胃肠道来源多见,其中卵巢约占71%、胃约占17%、结肠约占10%,乳腺癌是引起PM最常见的腹部外原发性肿瘤[49]。Krishnamurthy等[50]认为,PET/CT有助于排除腹膜外疾病。

第六章　可疑CUP检查与诊断

Schmidt等[51]研究发现，全身PET/CT可检测到MDCT和MRI未明确的膈上病变，全身PET/CT可提供更多信息，其检测卵巢癌PM的灵敏度为95%，特异性为96%。但Lopez-Lopez等[52]的研究发现，PET/CT对PM检测的灵敏度低于单独CT检查，认为PET/CT对腹膜外转移性病变的评估更有价值。

有研究报道[53-55]，PET/CT对发现腹部原发肿瘤的敏感性优于CT。Fan等[56]指出，PET/CT作为一种强有力的影像学工具，对临床上怀疑恶性肿瘤或恶性病变原发灶不明的肝硬化伴腹水患者的病因诊断有重要价值。

Burglin等[57]的Meta分析显示，宫颈外转移CUP患者经PET/CT检查，原发肿瘤检出率为31%~39%，敏感性为81%~87%，特异性为83%~88%。

另外，PET/CT检查可以为可疑CUP患者组织活检提供较精准的定位。Wartski等[58]的研究显示，PET/CT发现原发肿瘤的26例CUP患者中，17例患者在PET/CT引导下再一次行全消化道内镜活检，13例（50%）组织学证实为恶性肿瘤。郑容等[18]报道了54例可疑CUP患者，13例（24.1%）在PET/CT结果的引导下行内镜及其他常规影像学检查发现，7例为炎性改变，6例为生理性摄取。

值得一提的是，在可疑CUP患者中经常规影像学检查后再行PET/CT检查，可能改变治疗方案。Seve等[59]对10项PET/CT研究的221例CUP患者进行了Meta分析，结果表明，34.7%的CUP患者更改了治疗方案。Wang等[60]对不明原发肿瘤的研究结果显示，PET/CT检查改变了33.8%的可疑CUP患者的治疗方案。

虽然，PET/CT在可疑CUP中寻找原发肿瘤、准确临床分期、治疗方案制订等方面具有重要价值；但PET/CT对0.4~1cm的病灶进行重建时空间分辨力降低，对极微小的肿瘤存在假阴性[61]。Mevio等[62]认为，PET较CT、MRI无明显优势，PET/CT的检测结果依赖于病灶对FDG摄取量，肿瘤大小、肿瘤细胞活性、是否有出血坏死等均会影响到FDG的摄取量，从而出现假阴性。Kwee等[40]报道，全身^{18}F-FDG PET/CT只能在约1/3的CUP病例中确定原发肿瘤。

有学者分析了PET/CT对部分原发肿瘤不能检出的原因进行了分析，主要有以下几点[17-18,63-64]。

(1) 原发肿瘤太小,超出了 PET/CT 的敏感性和分辨率。

(2) 因肿瘤血管生成不良而导致原发肿瘤细胞凋亡,肿瘤消退。

(3) 原发肿瘤所处周围组织高摄取或排泄 ^{18}F-FDG,当肿瘤极小时,常被生理性摄取掩盖而难以发现。

(4) 一些特殊病理类型的原发肿瘤对 ^{18}F-FDG 的摄取低或不摄取,从而导致检出及诊断困难。

(5) 有的原发肿瘤位于转移肿瘤之间(如肺内原发癌伴肺内转移、肝内原发癌伴肝内转移等),转移灶与原发灶难以分辨。

(6) 原发肿瘤未能形成。

另外,Olson 等[14]认为,与 CT、MRI 比较,PET/CT 在局部组织的分辨能力和解剖定位方面有一定的局限性。陈应瑞等[65]的研究发现,PET/CT 对原发肿瘤在头颈部的 CUP 其诊断价值优于 CT、MRI,但在胸部肿瘤中二者却无明显差异。Yanagawa 等[66]对 24 例 CUP 骨转移患者的研究发现,在查找原发肿瘤方面,PET/CT 较常规检查方法并无明显优势。

因此,目前对于可疑 CUP 患者初始检查选择 PET/CT 尚存在争议[46,67],因目前还缺乏大型前瞻性随机对照研究的验证,在现有指南中尚未被推荐作为 CUP 初始检查的首选手段。

NCCN 指南建议,只有对造影剂增强有禁忌证的可疑 CUP 患者才使用 PET/CT 代替 CT/MRI 进行初步评估。ESMO 指南建议,对于单发或偶发转移性 CUP 患者、怀疑头颈部肿瘤颈部淋巴结转移的 CUP 患者可进行 PET/CT 检查[68-70]。

表 6-1 可疑 CUP 患者影像学检查建议

病理学类型	转移肿瘤部位	影像学检查建议
腺癌及未特殊说明的癌	显著的、孤立的颈部淋巴结	颈部、胸部 CT
	锁骨上淋巴结	颈部、胸部、腹部、盆腔 CT
		乳房 X 线检查(适用于乳腺组织完整的患者,包括男性乳腺增生症患者)
		如果缺乏乳腺癌组织病理学诊断证据,需进行乳腺 MRI 和(或)乳腺超声检查

续表

病理学类型	转移肿瘤部位	影像学检查建议
腺癌及未特殊说明的癌	腋窝淋巴结	颈部、胸部、腹部、盆腔CT
		乳房X线检查(适用于乳腺组织完整的患者,包括男性乳腺增生症患者)
		如果缺乏乳腺癌组织病理学诊断证据,需进行乳腺MRI和(或)乳腺超声检查
	纵隔	胸部、腹部、盆腔CT
		乳房X线检查(适用于乳腺组织完整的患者,包括男性乳腺增生症患者)
		如果缺乏乳腺癌组织病理学诊断证据,需进行乳腺MRI和(或)乳腺超声检查
		睾丸超声:如果β-hCG或AFP升高(有睾丸者)
	胸膜多发结节或胸腔积液	胸部、腹部、盆腔CT
		乳房X线检查(适用于乳腺组织完整的患者,包括男性乳腺增生症患者)
		如果缺乏乳腺癌组织病理学诊断证据,需进行乳腺MRI和(或)乳腺超声检查
	腹膜或腹水	胸部、腹部、盆腔CT
		乳房X线检查(适用于乳腺组织完整的患者,包括男性乳腺增生症患者)
		如果缺乏乳腺癌组织病理学诊断证据,需进行乳腺MRI和(或)乳腺超声检查
	腹膜后肿块	胸部、腹部、盆腔CT
		乳房X线检查(适用于乳腺组织完整的患者,包括男性乳腺增生症患者)
		如果缺乏乳腺癌组织病理学诊断证据,需进行乳腺MRI和(或)乳腺超声检查
		<65岁,睾丸超声(有睾丸者)
	腹股沟淋巴结	胸部、腹部、盆腔CT

续表

病理学类型	转移肿瘤部位	影像学检查建议
腺癌及未特殊说明的癌	肝脏	胸部、腹部、盆腔 CT
		乳房 X 线检查（适用于乳腺组织完整的患者，包括男性乳腺增生症患者）
		如果缺乏乳腺癌组织病理学诊断证据，需进行乳腺 MRI 和（或）乳腺超声检查
	骨	胸部、腹部、盆腔 CT
		骨扫描
		乳房 X 线检查（适用于乳腺组织完整的患者，包括男性乳腺增生症患者）
		如果缺乏乳腺癌组织病理学诊断证据，需进行乳腺 MRI 和（或）乳腺超声检查
	脑	胸部、腹部、盆腔 CT
		乳房 X 线检查（适用于乳腺组织完整的患者，包括男性乳腺增生症患者）
		如果缺乏乳腺癌组织病理学诊断证据，需进行乳腺 MRI 和（或）乳腺超声检查
	多部位	胸部、腹部、盆腔 CT
		乳房 X 线检查（适用于乳腺组织完整的患者，包括男性乳腺增生症患者）
		如果缺乏乳腺癌组织病理学诊断证据，需进行乳腺 MRI 和（或）乳腺超声检查
鳞状细胞癌	头颈部	颈部、胸部 CT
	锁骨上	颈部、胸部、腹部、盆腔 CT
	腋窝	胸部 CT
	腹股沟	腹部、盆腔 CT
	骨	胸部、腹部、盆腔 CT
		骨扫描

第六章 可疑CUP检查与诊断

表 6-2 PET/CT 检查判断标准

分类	标准
阳性判断标准	早期显像 SUVmax > 2.5，或延迟显像局部病灶放射活性至少高于早期显像 20%
	PET 与 CT 图像二者均为阳性或其中任一个为阳性表现时，PET/CT 诊断为阳性
	PET 与 CT 图像二者均为阴性时，诊断为阴性
真阳性(true positive，TP)	PET/CT 发现原发肿瘤部位，后经组织病理学和(或)长期随访证实
真阴性(true negative，TN)	PET/CT 未发现原发肿瘤部位，组织病理学及长期随访均未发现原发灶
假阳性(false positive，FP)	PET/CT 发现原发肿瘤部位，但被组织病理学或长期随访结果否定
假阴性(false negative，FN)	PET/CT 未发现原发肿瘤部位，但经组织病理学和(或)长期随访原发肿瘤得以明确

注：长期随访，指随访时间≥6个月

第三节 可疑 CUP 内镜检查

临床常用内镜主要鼻咽镜、喉镜、支气管镜、胃镜、结直肠镜、小肠镜、阴道镜、膀胱镜等，在可疑 CUP 患者中，内镜检查作用有限，除非有相关临床症状或影像学检查提示原发肿瘤可能，一般不推荐将内镜作为常规检查。

一般而言，通常根据患者临床症状、影像学检查结果而选择相应内镜检查，发现可疑病灶，则需活检。如高度怀疑原发性头颈部肿瘤，可行鼻咽镜和喉镜等检查；若患者存在肺部症状，且影像学检查提示肺部占位，可行支气管镜检查；高度怀疑消化道原发肿瘤时，可选择胃镜和肠镜等检查；若患者尿血、尿液细胞学检查可疑，或影像学检查发现膀胱占位，可行膀胱镜检查等。

第四节 可疑 CUP 肿瘤标志物检测

虽然血液中各种肿瘤标志物(如 CEA、AFP、CA125、CA19-9、CA72-4、CA15-3、PSA 等)的升高与其原发肿瘤类型有一定关系,但特异性、敏感性均不是很强,在确定原发肿瘤部位方面的价值有限,通常不能作为诊断依据[71-74]。

然而,对于一些特殊的可疑 CUP 患者,肿瘤标志物的检测对原发肿瘤的寻找具有一定的参考价值。一般而言,甲胎蛋白(alpha-fetoprotein, AFP)升高,可能提示原发性肝细胞癌[75-78];对于未分化或低分化肿瘤的男性患者,人绒毛膜促性腺激素 β 亚基(β-human chorionic gonadotrophin, β-hCG)和 AFP 水平升高往往提示可能存在性腺外生殖细胞肿瘤[79]。Maeda-Taniguchi 等[81]指出,血清肿瘤标志物是术前寻找转移卵巢肿瘤原发灶的重要手段。

表 6-3 可疑 CUP 患者肿瘤标志物检测建议

病理学类型	转移肿瘤部位	建议
腺癌及未特殊说明的癌	锁骨上淋巴结	年龄 >40 岁(有前列腺或前列腺切除的患者),PSA 检测
	腋窝淋巴结	年龄 >40 岁(有前列腺或前列腺切除的患者),PSA 检测
	纵隔	年龄 >40 岁(有前列腺或前列腺切除的患者),PSA 检测
		β-hCG、AFP 检测
	胸膜多发结节或胸腔积液	年龄 >40 岁(有前列腺或前列腺切除的患者),PSA 检测
		CA125 检测
	腹膜或腹水	年龄 >40 岁(有前列腺或前列腺切除的患者),PSA 检测
		CA125 检测,子宫和(或)卵巢存在者
	腹膜后肿块	年龄 >40 岁(有前列腺或前列腺切除的患者),PSA 检测
		年龄 <65 岁:β-hCG、AFP 检测
	腹股沟淋巴结	年龄 >40 岁(有前列腺或前列腺切除的患者),PSA 检测
		CA125 检测,子宫和(或)卵巢存在者
	肝脏	AFP 检测
	骨	有前列腺或前列腺切除的患者,PSA 检测
	多部位	有前列腺或前列腺切除的患者,PSA 检测

第六章 可疑CUP检查与诊断

第五节 病理学检查

组织病理学检查结果是 CUP 诊断的金标准,仔细的大体标本观察和组织学检查对明确 CUP 原发肿瘤是十分重要的[82]。

在对可疑 CUP 全面、系统影像学检查后,明确了原发肿瘤所在位置,通常需对原发肿瘤进行组织活检,除内镜活检外,还可在 B 超或 CT 引导下进行穿刺活检,如甲状腺、乳腺、肺、肝、腹腔、肾、皮肤、体表软组织、骨等部位的原发肿瘤;若无法取得组织标本,细胞蜡块加免疫组化(immunohistochemistry,IHC)可作为其诊断依据。

一、组织或细胞标本

外科手术的最主要目的是获取足够的组织病理学诊断标本,除手术切除标本外,临床上更常见的标本是粗针穿刺活检、细针穿刺细胞学或脱落细胞学标本制作细胞蜡块等。

一旦获得肿瘤转移部位的活检标本,病理学检查首先应明确肿瘤细胞的基本类型,尽可能确定肿瘤原发部位;可通过常规 HE 染色观察肿瘤细胞的形态结构特征,如砂粒体和乳头状形态多见于卵巢癌、甲状腺癌,印戒细胞多见于胃肠道腺癌等。

二、骨髓涂片和(或)骨髓活检

骨髓涂片和(或)骨髓活检是实体肿瘤骨髓转移诊断的金标准[83],是诊断实体肿瘤骨髓转移最简单、快速、敏感的方法。

骨髓涂片和(或)骨髓活检中发现恶性肿瘤细胞,则提示存在骨髓转移,但并不是所有骨髓转移一次骨穿就能找到肿瘤细胞,因骨髓转移是多灶性的,且骨髓转移常导致骨髓广泛纤维化、肿瘤细胞过多,易"干抽"致无法获取骨髓。

活检与抽吸阳性率差异明显,骨髓活检阳性的骨髓涂片检出率仅为 74.3%,即单独使用抽吸涂片,则约有 25% 的转移性肿瘤仍未被发现[84-85]。因此,骨髓涂片阴性不能排除骨髓受累,诊断时骨髓涂片与骨髓活检需相结合,必要时多次、多部位穿刺以提高检出率[86]。

骨髓转移癌细胞的形态特点如下：

(1)大多数肿瘤细胞在骨髓涂片中成簇、成团出现，少数可散在分布。

(2)肿瘤细胞体积常常较大，有鹤立鸡群之感，具有三大、三深特点，三大指胞体大(大小不等，相差悬殊，常成团分布)、胞核大(核浆比值增加，可见多核型癌细胞)、核仁大；三深指胞质深(深浅不一，系 RNA 和蛋白质旺盛所致)、胞核深(染色质粗细、深浅不一，系 DNA 和蛋白质合成旺盛所致)、核仁深(DNA 合成旺盛)。

一般而言，单从细胞形态学改变很难推测原发肿瘤的类型，有经验的检验医生可大致识别出鳞癌和腺癌[87]。

三、脱落细胞学检查与细胞蜡块技术

在可疑 CUP 患者伴有浆膜腔积液时，鉴别良恶性积液极为重要，而恶性浆膜腔积液是指浆膜腔积液中经病理检查发现恶性肿瘤细胞(如腺癌细胞)或经浆膜组织活检病理诊断为恶性肿瘤。

标本送检量建议尽可能采集 100mL 以上的浆膜腔积液送检，浆膜腔积液离体后 30min 内送到病理科处理。

细胞蜡块制备即对细胞悬浮液进行离心处理后，得到浓缩度十分高的细胞与微小的组织块，而后经固定、脱水、透蜡及石蜡包埋等处理后，获得可长期保存的细胞蜡块。

目前认为，细胞蜡块是最理想的脱落细胞制备技术，其石蜡切片中细胞集中，一定程度上保留了原有组织结构，背景着色低、染色清楚，细胞能实现集中分布，结果易于判断，且可同时制作多张切片，以利于抗体组合应用及基因检测[88-89]。

有学者指出[90]，利用细胞蜡块技术而明确肿瘤类型对寻找原发肿瘤具有较大的临床价值。

虽然采用单一抗体检测积液细胞蜡块的诊断价值不高，但联合抗体检查可明显提高临床诊断的敏感度与特异性[91-92]。

Napsin A 是已被国内外公认的一种判断肺癌组织的免疫标记物，其在肺腺癌内的敏感度、特异度分别为 83%~90%、90%~98%，与 TTF-1 相比，其准确度、特异性更高；且 Napsin A 的染色更强、更具弥漫性，当 TTF-1 弱染色、局灶染色或很难清楚解释染色结果时，Napsin A 表现出十分重要的作用，一般联合应用 TTF-1 用于鉴别诊断肺腺癌[93]。

Villin 仅在带有刷状缘的细胞上表达，胃肠、胰腺及胆管肿瘤内的表达水平均处于较高水平[94]；CK5/6 于间皮细胞及间皮肿瘤内均呈现出高表达特征，若 CK5/6 显阳性，结合他类免疫标记物不表达的实际情况，可将其初步诊断为腺癌细胞。

四、液体活检

狭义的液体活检即对肿瘤患者血液样本中来源于肿瘤的细胞、核酸或蛋白等物质进行分析，目前已有大量基于液体活检的肿瘤标记物被发现并尝试应用于肿瘤早筛、治疗评估和复发监测等领域。

液体活检技术在判断 CUP 的组织起源上仅有少许研究报道[95]。Lu 等[96]认为，对循环肿瘤细胞(circulating tumor cell，CTC)的分选结合 CK7、CK20 等标记物的免疫荧光染色可协助 CUP 组织起源的判断。Best 等[97]利用对 228 例可疑 CUP 肿瘤患者肿瘤细胞来源的血小板(tumor-educated platelets)进行转录组学测序，对组织起源的中位预测准确率达到 73%，可识别出 6 种组织起源的肿瘤。Cohen 等[98]报道，基于细胞游离 DNA(cell-free DNA，cfDNA)和蛋白标记物的泛肿瘤早期筛查工具 Cancer SEEK 在筛查阳性(即患有肿瘤)患者的组织起源判断上达到 83% 的准确度。

五、转移部位肿瘤的主要病理类型

不同的时间段、不同的研究者对 CUP 细胞亚型分类存在一定差异，但总体差异不明显。1986 年，Meyers[99]将 CUP 的病理类型分为腺癌、未分化小细胞癌、未分化大细胞癌 3 种。1994 年，Abbruzzese 等[100]分析了安德森癌症研究中心收治的 657 例 CUP，按腺癌、鳞癌、低分化癌划分，结果显示，腺癌为 58.2%、低分化癌为 29.4%、鳞癌为 5.8%，其他(包括未分化癌和特殊或未被认识的肿瘤)为 6.6%。2005 年，Pavlidis 等[101]将 CUP 病理类型分为中高分化腺癌、低分化癌、鳞癌与未分化癌。2011 年，Natoli 等[102]将 CUP 病理类型分为腺癌、低分化癌、鳞癌与神经内分泌癌。2018 年，ESMO 指南基于光镜检查和 IHC 结果[103]，将 CUP 分为 4 种主要的组织病理类型，即高分化或中分化腺癌(60%)、低分化癌或腺癌(30%)、鳞状细胞癌(5%)和未分类的肿瘤(5%)，后者包括神经内分泌肿瘤、生殖细胞肿瘤、黑色素瘤或肉瘤等。2020 年，Rassy 等[104]指出，CUP 通常可分为高或中分化腺癌、低分化腺癌或未分化腺癌、鳞状细胞癌和未分化癌等类型。

CUP具有高度异质性，从相关文献报道看[105-106]，CUP最常见的病理类型为转移性腺癌，约50%的CUP病例可归类为分化良好至中度分化的腺癌，约30%为分化不良的腺癌或未分化癌，约15%为鳞癌，5%为未分化肿瘤。Pavlidis等[107]报道，病理类型中约60%的CUP为高-中分化腺癌，25%~30%为低分化腺癌或低分化癌，鳞癌仅占5%，未分化神经内分泌癌亦仅占5%。Krämer等[108]的研究显示，CUP患者中约50%为中高分化腺癌，约30%为低分化或未分化癌，约15%为鳞癌，约5%为未分化肿瘤。王成锋等[109]报道了1273例不明原发肿瘤，病理类型分析结果显示，腺癌71.8%、鳞癌10.4%、腺鳞癌0.3%、肉瘤4.2%、肉瘤样癌与神经内分泌样癌0.3%、黑色素瘤3.7%、假性黏液瘤4.4%、恶性间质瘤0.5%、不能确定病理类型者4.4%。

在肿瘤骨转移中，原发肿瘤肺癌多见，腺癌是其主要病理类型，其次为病理类型不明、鳞癌、小细胞癌、腺鳞癌及大细胞癌。叶骉飞等[110]报道的408例恶性肿瘤骨转移患者中，有228例为肺癌骨转移，其肺癌病理类型为腺癌39.91%、病理类型不明26.32%、鳞癌24.56%、小细胞癌5.26%、腺鳞癌3.07%、大细胞癌0.88%。

第六节 免疫组化检测

据Rougraff等[111]报道，单纯依靠常规组织病理学检查，有60%的可疑CUP原发肿瘤部位不能确定。

基于大多数原发肿瘤与转移肿瘤的蛋白表达谱存在一致性，免疫组化检测可提供肿瘤谱系、细胞类型等信息，辅助确定CUP的病理类型、肿瘤原发部位等[112-118]。

Laprovitera等[106]指出，在CUP的病理诊断中，最为关键的步骤是结合肿瘤组织学（或细胞学）基本形态特征进行IHC染色评估。一项Meta分析显示[119]，在不告知肿瘤原发部位的情况下，采用免疫组化标记物能准确识别已查明原发灶的转移癌的比例为65.6%。

IHC作为定位分析的首选方法，具有定性灵敏度高、定位直接准确的特点，是确定肿瘤谱系的主要方法[120-121]。

第一步，用IHC推测原发肿瘤时，其染色通常以递进方式进行。首先

第六章 可疑CUP检查与诊断

通过 IHC 检测角蛋白-AE1/AE3（cytokeratin AE1/AE3，CK AE1/AE3）、淋巴细胞共同抗原（common leukocyte antigen，CLA）、S100、黑色素瘤抗原-45（human melanoma black-45，HMB-45）和波形蛋白（vimentin）等标记物初步判断组织学起源，以确定肿瘤属于癌、淋巴瘤、软组织肉瘤或黑色素瘤。

广谱角蛋白（如 AE1/AE3、OSCAR）可确定上皮表型，分化簇 45（CD45）可确定血液淋巴来源的肿瘤（注意未成熟 B 细胞肿瘤中 CD45 表达下调），黑色素瘤则为 SOX10 和（或）S100；软组织肉瘤没有单一的筛查免疫标志物。

第二步，通过第一步部分标记物缩小范围，确定肿瘤细胞亚型，如腺癌、鳞癌、神经内分泌肿瘤、生殖细胞肿瘤或间皮瘤等。

细胞角蛋白-7（cytokeratin 7，CK7）和 CK20 的表达状态可提示不同器官来源腺癌的判断，p63 和 CK5/6 在鳞癌中表达；p16 蛋白可作为鳞癌的免疫组化标记物用于鉴别头颈部原发肿瘤[122]；突触素（synaptophsin，Syn）、嗜铬粒蛋白 A（chromogranin A，CgA）和神经元特异性烯醇化酶（neuron-specific enolase，NSE）是神经内分泌肿瘤的标记物；AFP、人绒毛膜促性腺激素（human chorionic gonadotropin，hCG）和八聚体结合转录因子 4（octamer-binding transcription factor-4，OCT4）是生殖细胞肿瘤的标记物；Wilm 瘤基因-1（Wilm's tumor gene 1，WT-1）和间皮素（mesothelin）是间皮瘤的标记物。Vimentin（波形蛋白）可用于鉴别肉瘤、淋巴瘤或黑素瘤。根据临床医生、病理科医生判断，NTRK 蛋白检测可作为广泛 IHC 检测的一部分（阳性检测应通过 NGS 确认）[123-124]。

第三步，通过进一步的免疫组化标记物的组合，可推测原发肿瘤部位。对于 CUP 免疫组化标记物选择多采用 2 种以上联合，相较单一的免疫标记物，Dennis 等[125]报道，采用包含 10 个免疫组化标记物的组合鉴别腺癌的原发肿瘤部位，诊断率达 88%。

一般而言，对于有腋窝淋巴结转移的女性患者应行雌激素受体（estrogen receptor，ER）和孕激素受体（progesterone receptor，PR）等检测，对于女性纵隔肿瘤患者应行 AFP 联合 β-hCG 检测，女性腹膜或腹股沟转移性腺癌患者需行 CA125 检测；对于正中线恶性肿瘤转移的可疑 CUP 患者，应行 AFP 和 β-hCG 检测。

ER、PR 阳性常提示乳腺癌、卵巢癌和子宫内膜癌等，前列腺特异性抗原(PSA)、前列腺酸性磷酸酶(prostate acid phosphatase, PAP)阳性通常提示前列腺癌，肠上皮标记物尾型同源框转录因子-2(caudal-related homeobox 2, CDX2)结合 CK7 和 CK20 的表达情况可以提示胰腺、胆道和肠道肿瘤。

对于癌细胞，细胞角蛋白 CK7 和 CK20 染色模式可提示原发肿瘤部位[126]，如 CK20 阳性、CK7 阴性，强烈支持结直肠源性肿瘤；CK20 阴性、CK7 阳性，多见于肺、乳腺、胆管、胰腺、卵巢和子宫内膜等部位来源的肿瘤[127]。

只有 60% 的分化不良和转移性肺腺癌的甲状腺转录因子 1(TTF-1)染色阳性[128]。在 CK7 阳性、TTF-1 阴性但怀疑肺原发癌的情况下，应考虑 SWI/SNF 相关、基质相关、肌动蛋白依赖的染色质调节因子 A 亚家族成员 4(SMARCA4)染色，因许多 TTF-1 阴性的肺腺癌显示 SMARCA4 核染色缺失。

Napsin A(天冬氨酸蛋白酶 A)在 80%~90% 的肺腺癌中表达阳性[129]，在肺腺癌的诊断工作中，Napsin A 可与 TTF-1 一起用于检测，但当 TTF-1 阴性时，Napsin A 的价值有限。

TFF(乳腺癌雌激素诱导蛋白)，乳腺癌和结直肠癌均可过表达 TFF-1，TFF-3 可鉴别乳腺癌和卵巢浆液性癌，其表达与肠分化密切相关。

Heppar 1 的表达主要限于肝细胞(良性和恶性)中，Heppar 1 在大多数胆管癌中呈阴性，在肝转移腺癌中具有点状阳性特征。通过形态学和 Heppar1 检测通常能给出肝细胞癌(hepatocellular carcinoma, HCC)的诊断[130]。

ER、GCDFP-15、MGB 被认为是乳腺特异性免疫标记物，GCDFP-15 和 MGB 灵敏度分别为 35%~55% 和 65%~70%[131]。Halperin 等[132]报道，62.5% 双原发癌和原发卵巢癌可通过检测子宫内膜和卵巢组织的 ER、PR 含量与转移卵巢肿瘤进行鉴别。

值得一提的是，IHC 图谱的预测价值会随着对特定肿瘤强烈提示模式的识别而提高，然而，IHC 检测的局限性包括影响组织抗原性的因素、观察者之间和观察者内部的判读差异、组织异质性和活检样本不足。尽管如此，病理学家仍可利用操作和染色良好的 IHC 面板，可在约 75% 的样本中确定 CUP 的原发部位[133]。

另外，不同的低分化肿瘤可以有着相同的表达标记，对确定单一的原发肿瘤部位仍具有挑战性[134-135]。Economopoulou 等[136]报道,光镜检查结合 IHC 只能确定约 30% CUP 的肿瘤组织起源。Hainsworth 等[137]亦指出,如果 CUP 以胰腺癌、胃癌、胆管癌、尿路上皮癌等为原发部位时,IHC 染色进行鉴别诊断的特异性较低,即使增加更多的 IHC 染色指标也并不能提高鉴别诊断的准确性。

目前,随着靶向治疗、免疫治疗的广泛应用,IHC 检测可为 CUP 患者制定最佳治疗方案提供重要参考依据[138],如 HER-2、ALK、ROS1、BRAF V600E、pan-NTRK、MMR(MLH1、MSH2、MSH6、PMS2)、PD-L1 等。

一、细胞角蛋白

细胞角蛋白(cytokeratin,CK)是上皮细胞中维持组织连续性和完整性的、分子量不同的一种细胞骨架蛋白,分为 20 多种不同的亚型。

CK 是一种常用的肿瘤 IHC 标记物,目前被广泛用于推测腺癌的原发部位[118]。其中,CK7 和 CK20 较为常用,在甲状腺癌、肺癌、乳腺癌及卵巢癌中 CK7 呈阳性,在胃肠道、泌尿道上皮和 Merkel 细胞中 CK20 常呈阳性[131]。

CK7 在肺癌、卵巢癌、子宫内膜癌和乳腺癌中有表达,而在低位胃肠道肿瘤未发现表达[127];CK20 是一种低分子 CK,在胃肠道上皮、泌尿道上皮和 Merkel 细胞中表达。

CK20 阳性和 CK7 阴性强烈支持结直肠原发肿瘤,75%~95% 的结直肠肿瘤呈现此染色模式;而在肺癌仅有 9%~15% CK20 呈阳性。CK20 阴性和 CK7 阳性将鉴别诊断缩小至肺癌、乳腺癌、胆管癌、胰腺癌、卵巢癌和子宫内膜癌。

原发性卵巢上皮性肿瘤大多数表达为 CK20 阴性和 CK7 阳性,而原发灶是结直肠癌的转移性卵巢肿瘤多数表达为 CK7 阴性和 CK20 阳性,联合使用 CEA、CA125、CDX2 或 Villin 等相关抗体则诊断准确性更高。

有报道称[139],高达 12% 的子宫的子宫内膜样腺癌和卵巢子宫内膜样腺癌可同时发生,且两者的免疫表型有非常多重叠的地方,多数都表现为 CK7 阳性和 CK20 阴性。

二、GATA3

GATA3 是乳腺癌和尿路上皮癌高度敏感和特异的标记物,在导管和小叶型乳腺癌中的表达率为92%~100%，低GATA3表达被认为与乳腺癌预后不良有关[140]。

GATA3联合S100可作为尿路上皮癌和卵巢Brenner肿瘤的免疫组化标记物。

三、TTF-1

TTF-1是一种38kD的含有同源结构域的核蛋白，在甲状腺、中脑和呼吸道上皮胚胎发生过程的转录活化中起着重要作用[141]。几乎在所有甲状腺癌和70%~90%的肺腺癌中表达[129,142]，肺类癌、非典型类癌、小细胞癌中TTF-1的表达具有高度特异性，也可用于鉴别肺癌和恶性间皮瘤[143]。

四、GCDFP 15

GCDFP 15(巨囊性病纤维状蛋白)是一种单体蛋白，分子量为15kD，亦被称为催乳素可诱导蛋白、糖蛋白-17(glycoprotein-17)、分泌性肌动蛋白结合蛋白，是分化标记物，存在于皮肤、唾液腺、支气管腺和精囊腺中，在乳腺癌中特异性表达[144]。

五、URO Ⅲ

URO Ⅲ是鉴别膀胱上皮细胞表面特异性标记物[145]。Parker等[146]对112例泌尿道上皮肿瘤的石蜡包埋标本进行研究，发现URO Ⅲ染色阳性者占57%，血栓调节蛋白(thrombomodulin, TM)染色阳性者占69%，高分子量CK阳性者占80%，CK20阳性者占48%，且这4个标记物的表达具有随肿瘤的恶性程度和阶段不同而变化，在所有的小细胞癌均呈阴性的特点。

表6-4 可疑CUP潜在免疫标记物确定肿瘤细胞系

肿瘤标记物物	最可能的细胞系
Pan-keratin(AE1/AE3 & CAM5.2)	癌
CK5/6, p63/p40	鳞状细胞癌
S100, SOX10	黑色素瘤和肉瘤
LCA ± CD20 ± CD3 ±	淋巴瘤
OCT3/4 ± SALL4 ±	生殖细胞肿瘤
WT1, calretinin, mesothelin, D2-40	间皮瘤

第六章 可疑CUP检查与诊断

表 6-5 肿瘤特异性标记物及其染色模式、相关原发肿瘤

标记物	肿瘤	染色模式
Arginase-1	肝癌	核/细胞质
Calretinin	间皮瘤、性索间质瘤、肾上腺皮质瘤	核/细胞质
CDX2	结直肠、其他胃肠道、胰胆道	核
D2-40	间皮瘤，淋巴管内皮细胞标志物	膜
EBV	鼻咽部	核
ER/PR	乳腺、卵巢、子宫内膜	核
GATA3	乳腺、膀胱、唾液腺	细胞质
Glypican-3	肝细胞	细胞质
HepPar-1	肝细胞	细胞质
HPV	子宫颈、外阴、阴道、阴茎、肛门、口咽	核（DNA）；核/细胞质（RNA ISH）
Inhibin	性索-基质、肾上腺皮质	细胞质
Melan-A	肾上腺皮质、黑色素瘤	核
Napsin A	肺癌	细胞质
NKX3-1	前列腺癌	细胞质
PAP	前列腺	膜质
PAX8	甲状腺、肾脏、卵巢、子宫内膜、子宫颈、胸腺	核膜
PSA	前列腺	细胞质
RCC marker	肾脏	膜质
SF-1	肾上腺皮质、性索间质	核
SATB2	结肠直肠癌、骨肉瘤和其他胃肠道肿瘤	细胞质
Thyroglobulin	甲状腺	细胞质
TTF-1	肺、甲状腺	核
Uroplakin Ⅲ	尿道	膜质
Villin	胃肠道（刷状缘上皮）	顶部
WT1	卵巢浆液性癌、间皮瘤、威尔姆斯瘤	核

表 6-6 常见原发肿瘤免疫标记选择

肿瘤部位或类型	CK7, CK20	其他阳性标记	其他有用标记
涎腺癌	CK7+/CK20-	CK5/6, p63	GATA3, AR, HER-2
甲状腺癌（滤泡癌或乳头状癌）	CK7+/CK20-	TTF1, PAX8, CK19±	甲状腺球蛋白
甲状腺癌（髓样癌）	CK7+/CK20-	TTF1, PAX8, CK19±	降钙素,突触素,嗜铬粒蛋白,单克隆癌胚抗原
肺腺癌	CK7+/CK20-	TTF1, Napsin A	
乳腺癌	CK7+/CK20-	GATA3, GCDFP-15(BRST2)±, Mammaglobin±	ER/PR±
食管癌,胃癌	CK7+/CK20±	CDX-2±, Villin±	
小肠癌,阑尾癌,大肠癌	CK7-/CK20+	CDX2, Villin, SATB2	
肝细胞癌	CK7-/CK20-	Arginase-1, HepPar-1, Glypican-3, CD10 and polyclonal, CEA±（小管周围型）	MOC31-（与肝内胆管癌相鉴别）,白蛋白原位杂交-（也适用于肝内胆管癌）
胰胆管癌,包括肝内胆管癌	CK7+/CK20±	CDX2±, CK19	SMAD4缺失±（胰腺癌,肝外胆管癌和结肠直肠癌）,白蛋白原位杂交-（也适用于肝内胆管癌）
卵巢黏液性癌	CK7+/CK20±	PAX8±, CDX2±	SATB2-
卵巢浆液性癌	CK7+/CK20-	PAX8, WT1	
宫颈内膜腺癌	CK7+/CK20-	p16+（弥漫性强染色）, PAX8±	p53（异常）, p16（弥漫 强烈）Vimentin, ER/PR±, 人类乳头瘤病毒原位杂交
子宫内膜腺癌	CK7+/CK20-	Vimentin, PAX8	ER/PR±, p16-（与宫颈内膜癌和子宫浆液性癌相鉴别）

续表

肿瘤部位或类型	CK7,CK20	其他阳性标记	其他有用标记
肾上腺皮质癌	CK7-/CK20-	SF-1,Melan A,Inhibin	
肾细胞癌	CK7±/CK20-	PAX2,PAX8,EMA±,碳酸酐酶Ⅸ(CA9)±,Vimentin±,CD10±(膜)	
尿路上皮癌	CK7+/CK20±	GATA3,p63 或 p40,CK5/6±,34βE12,S100P,尿溶蛋白 2	
鳞状细胞癌	CK7-/CK20-	CK5/6,p63 或 p40,34βE12	p16(强弥漫性染色)和/或 HPV 原位杂交(HPV 相关性癌症)
神经内分泌癌,包括小细胞癌	CK7±/CK20±(默克尔细胞癌中的"点状"模式)	CgA,Syn,CD56	TTF1±,CDX-2±,有丝分裂率和/或 Ki-67(用于分级)
非肉芽肿性生殖细胞瘤	CK7-/CK20-	SALL4,OCT3/4±	CD30,Glypican-3,PLAP(进一步亚型分型)
间皮瘤	CK7+/CK20-	Calretinin,WT1,CK5/6,D2-40,Mesothelin	p63±,CEA,MOC31-,BerEP4-,TTF-1-(与肺腺癌相鉴别)

表 6-7 CUP 免疫组化检测步骤

检测步骤	免疫标记物	原发肿瘤判定
第一步：确定肿瘤大类型	AE1/AE3	癌
	LCA	淋巴瘤
	S100, HMB-45	黑色素瘤
	S100, vimentin	软组织肉瘤
第二步：确定肿瘤亚型	CK7/CK20	腺癌
	PLAP, OCT4, HCG	生殖细胞肿瘤
	CgA, Syn, CD56	神经内分泌癌
	CK5/CK6, p63	鳞癌
第三步：确定肿瘤原发部位	PSA, PAP	前列腺癌
	TTF1	肺癌
	CDX2, CK20	结肠癌
	CDX2, CK20, CK7	小肠癌
	ER, CA125, mesothelin, WT1	卵巢癌
	mammaglobulin, ER	乳腺癌

第七节 可疑 CUP 分子基因检测

据报道[138]，在可疑的不明原发肿瘤患者中，通过影像学检查、常规病理学检查及免疫组化检测，最终仅 30% 的患者可明确原发肿瘤部位。

有研究发现[95,137]，转移部位肿瘤细胞的基因表达谱与其原发部位肿瘤的基因表达谱存在相似性，提示肿瘤在其发生、发展、转移过程中，始终保留其组织起源的基因表达特征。因此，通过对比转移肿瘤组织样本与已知来源的肿瘤分子特征的相似性，一般可推测出转移肿瘤最可能的组织起源[147-148]。

近年来的研究发现[149]，CUP 常伴有多种染色体异常和多种基因过表达，如表皮生长因子受体（EGFR）、c-kit/PDGFR、RAS、BCL2、HER2、p53 等，以及血管生成基因激活（占 CUP 肿瘤的 50%~89%）、癌基因过表达（占 CUP 肿瘤的 10%~30%）、上皮-间质转化（epithelial-mesenchymal transition，EMT）标记物升高（占 CUP 肿瘤的 16%）、缺氧相关蛋白激活

（占CUP肿瘤的25%）和细胞内信号分子激活（占CUP肿瘤的20%～35%）。

一项对252例CUP患者进行基因组测序的研究发现[150]，CUP最常见的基因改变是抑癌基因p53（49.6%）、CDKN2A（19.0%）和NOTCH1（14.1%）的缺失，以及致癌基因KRAS（23.4%）、FGFR4（14.9%）和PIK3CA（10.7%）的激活。Gatalica等[151]对389例CUP患者的石蜡包埋组织样本进行了592个基因突变、52个融合基因和免疫标记物的分析，共检测出了70个致癌或可能致癌的基因突变，其中最常见的突变基因是TP53（53.6%）、KRAS（21.7%）。Stella等[152]对47例肿瘤转移患者标本间质-上皮转化（mesenchymal-epithelial transition factor，MET））因子进行检测，并通过IHC方法确定原发肿瘤部位，24例被确定了原发肿瘤，23例为CUP；7例患者发现MET体细胞突变，均在CUP队列；CUP中MET突变率（30%）明显高于实体瘤（约4%）。

Ross等[153]，通过高通量测序检测了303例CUP患者转移灶肿瘤组织TMB、MSI，使用IHC检测了PD-L1表达，11.6%的转移灶肿瘤组织具有高肿瘤突变负荷（TMB-high），14%的转移灶肿瘤组织存在PD-L1过表达，1%的转移灶肿瘤组织具有高度微卫星不稳定性（MSI-high）。

另外，染色体易位t（15；19）导致的BRD4-NUT癌基因已在中线结构癌和肿瘤原发部位不明确的儿童和年轻成人中发现[154]。

一、推测CUP组织起源

近年来，有关不明原发肿瘤的分子基因检测的研究报道众多，总体而言，基因突变谱、microRNA、DNA甲基化等组学特征对CUP起源判断有一定的临床应用价值。

"癌症基因组图谱（The Cancer Genome Atlas，TCGA）"描述了多种类型肿瘤的基因组和基因表达变化，而"泛癌症图谱（Pan-Cancer Atlas）"则主要研究不同类型肿瘤之间基因表达的差异性和相似性[155-156]，这些研究成果可为进一步明确可疑CUP的起源提供更大的帮助。

基因表达谱（gene expression profiling，GEP）分析技术是基于信使RNA（mRNA）、DNA或microRNA（miRNA）平台，通过对获取的CUP组织进行实时反转录酶聚合酶链式反应（real-time polymerase chain reaction，RT-PCR）、基因芯片或二代测序（next generation sequencing，NGS）检测，进一

步利用生物信息学方法提取基因特征表达分子作为判断原发肿瘤的特异性"分子指纹",并建立相应数学模型进行推测与判断[138,157-159],可同时分析10~2000个基因,并能区分6~50种不同的肿瘤类型,用于推测肿瘤组织起源的准确率为85.0%~94.4%[160-161]。多项研究表明[162-173],对肿瘤转移灶石蜡包埋的肿瘤活检组织、肿瘤细胞蜡块或血液等样本进行GEP、NGS等分子检测及人工智能分析可进一步提高IHC推测CUP肿瘤起源部位的敏感性和准确性。Mileshkin等[174]的前瞻性队列研究表明,联合基因突变谱分析与CUP Guide基因表达谱检测有助于更精准的进行原发肿瘤溯源诊断。Posner等[175]报道,DNA谱和RNA谱分析可发现33%的原发肿瘤部位,作者认为,DNA突变谱分析是信息更为丰富的诊断方法。一项大型前瞻性、非随机Ⅱ期临床研究在252例CUP患者中通过92基因检测,有247例标本检测结果提示了组织起源,仅5例患者的基因表达谱未明确分类[176]。

目前,有研究者使用基因表达水平、miRNA水平、lncRNA水平等特征构建肿瘤溯源模型,并取得了较高的原发肿瘤诊断准确率。

Schipper等[177]通过全基因组测序构建了一个名为CUP-PA的分类器,该分类器涵盖29种肿瘤类型,临床验证结果表明,可指导68%的CUP患者进行原发肿瘤的判断。Wei等[157]通过公开的肿瘤数据库收集来自26种不同组织类型的3244个肿瘤样本的转录组测序(RNA Sequencing, RNAseq)表达数据,使用特征提取的方式选择每种肿瘤的特征分子构建的模型,其CUP总体判断准确率为90.5%,敏感度和特异度分别为92.0%和97.7%。Xu等[178]建立了一个154基因模型,涵盖22种肿瘤,通过在1248例低分化肿瘤、未分化肿瘤或转移性肿瘤的标本中进行验证,结果显示,对CUP组织起源的推测具有92%的准确率、99.6%的特异性和86.5%的敏感性。

Tothill等[179]选择了79个基因,基于支持向量机(Support Vector Machine,SVM)建立了一个13种肿瘤的分类器,达到了89%的精确度。王奇峰等[168]使用支持向量机,基于94个基因建立了对22种肿瘤的分类模型,在206个样本的测试集上达到了88.4%的精确度。

有研究者采用肿瘤mRNA荧光定量PCR并结合人工智能的体外诊断方法[180],在包含21种肿瘤的5434例肿瘤样本中进行验证,结果表明,推测肿瘤起源的准确率为94.6%,与病理诊断进行比较,总体准确率为

第六章　可疑CUP检查与诊断

90%，对低分化癌或未分化癌、鳞癌的判断准确率分别为90.0%、84.4%。Talantov等[138]选取了10个来自肺癌、结肠癌、胰腺癌、乳腺癌、前列腺癌和卵巢癌的组织特异表达基因，对260个原发肿瘤已知的转移癌样本进行了RT-PCR检测，在48个样本组成的独立测试集上取得了76%的准确率。Hainsworth等[181]报道，采用RT-PCR方法对CUP患者进行了92个基因检测，98%患者可确定组织器官来源。一项涉及104例CUP患者的研究中[135]，通过RT-PCR来检测10个特定基因标志物的表达，结果显示，61%的可疑CUP患者明确了肿瘤来源。

目前，CUP中NGS技术仍处在探索阶段[182-183]。CUP组织学亚型不同，其突变谱亦不同。腺癌和低分化癌亚型在涉及信号转导通路的基因中表现出突变，而鳞癌的突变多涉及细胞周期和DNA修复[106]。CUP腺癌中HER-2、EGFR、BRAF发生率（80%、8%、6%）高于非腺癌（4%、3%、4%），腺癌中受体酪氨酸激酶（receptor tyrosine kinase，RTK）/RAS通路活化改变亦高于非腺癌（72%和39%）[184]。

Varghese等[185]分析了333例CUP患者的临床资料及分子特征，150例患者进行了NGS检测，最常见的突变基因为TP53、KRAS、细胞周期依赖性激酶抑制因子2A（cell cycle dependent kinase inhibitionfactor 2A，CDKN2A），Kelch样环氧氯丙烷相关蛋白-1（Kelch-like ECH-associated protein-1，KEAP1）与SWI/SNF相关基质结合的肌动蛋白依赖的染色质调控因子超家族A成员4（SM/SNF related, matrix associated, actindependent regulator of chromatin, subfamily a, member 4，SMARCA4）。

DNA甲基化图谱可为肿瘤组织分型鉴定、确定CUP组织起源提供重要线索[186-187]。Moran等[188]基于38种已知肿瘤类型的2790例肿瘤样本DNA甲基化的特点建立了肿瘤分类系统，216例可疑CUP患者中188例（87%）确定了原发肿瘤来源。Stackpole等[189]通过检测血液中的游离DNA（cell-free DNA，cfDNA）靶向甲基化情况，区分不同分期的结肠癌、肝癌、肺癌、胃癌等4种恶性肿瘤，且对CUP组织起源推测的准确度为85%~89%。

Liu等[190]开展了一项基于6689例参与者的大样本研究显示，Grail-CCGA通过检测甲基化程度对不同分期的50多种肿瘤进行定位，灵敏度为54.9%，特异度高达99.3%。Losa等[191]通过检测多个基因的表达水平和检测肿瘤相关的特定DNA甲基化水平等表观遗传学，与已知原发肿瘤的遗传或表观遗传特征进行相似性评分,其诊断符合率为82%~97%。Fernandez等[192]首先确定来自1628例患者样本(424例正常组织,1054肿瘤样本,150非肿瘤病变)包含1505个CpG位点的DNA甲基化图谱,其后分析了42例CUP患者DNA甲基化图谱,29例(69%)可明确肿瘤类型,后经临床病理验证后的准确率为78%。

通过对循环肿瘤细胞(circulating tumor cell,CTC)进行分选,并结合CK7和CK20等标记物的免疫荧光染色,可辅助判定CUP的组织起源[96]。一项针对442例CUP患者的研究表明,80%的患者循环肿瘤DNA(circulating tumor DNA,ctDNA)中可检测到基因变异[193]。

游离DNA(cell free DNA,cfDNA)片段特征(如拷贝数变异、片段大小、片段末端序列特征、核小体印记等)可提供CUP起源信息,用NGS检查cfDNA在CUP诊断中具有一定的潜力,既可判断肿瘤起源[194]。Cohen等[98]采用Cancer-SEEK的多组学检测方法,针对卵巢癌、肝癌、胃癌等8种肿瘤,通过检测cfDNA与循环蛋白,灵敏度为70%,特异度可达99%;在判断肿瘤起源中,综合前两位判定结果的中位准确率为83%。

基因微阵列分析技术在CUP进一步明确原发肿瘤方面亦有报道,Tissue-of-Origin试剂盒采用基因微阵列技术[195],可检测2000个基因探针杂交的GEP信息,包括膀胱癌、乳腺癌等15种肿瘤中的58个肿瘤亚型,推测原发肿瘤的准确率达88.5%。

Pillai等[196]对462例低分化或未分化肿瘤转移灶标本构建了微阵列数据库,采用2000个基因分类模型对肿瘤原发部位进行鉴定,结果显示,总体一致性为89%,多部位重复性为89.3%。但Dolled-filhart等[161]认为,微阵列技术检测在CUP诊断中有很大的局限性。

miRNA具有高度稳定性及高度的组织特异性,根据转移灶肿瘤组织的miRNA表达谱可有效地推测原发肿瘤部位[197]。Skilde等[198]报道,miRNA分析技术在推测原发肿瘤方面的准确率达88%。Rosenfeld等[165]基于48个miRNA来确定CUP的组织来源建立了22种肿瘤分类器,在独立测试集上达到了89%的精确度。

Varadhachary等[199]基于miRNA的肿瘤溯源可用于大多数转移性肿瘤,使用48个miRNA对25种肿瘤建立了决策树和K近邻分类器,结果显示,84%的样本明确了原发肿瘤。Ferracin等[167]使用47个miRNA建立了10种肿瘤的分类器,在独立测试集上达到了86%的精确度。

尽管针对 CUP 组织、器官起源有较多、较新的分子基因检测研究报道，但大样本的前瞻性研究较少，且价格昂贵，临床尚难以广泛开展，故目前多数指南不建议常规使用基因测序来推测 CUP 原发肿瘤部位。

二、指导 CUP 系统治疗方案制订

近年来，有研究报道[105,200-201]，分子基因检测可能有助于制订 CUP 系统治疗方案，在 30%～85% 的 CUP 患者中发现了具有潜在治疗意义的突变。

一项大型前瞻性研究对 4200 例 CUP 患者进行了基因检测[184]，并分析了潜在的靶向治疗位点以评估患者对相关靶向治疗的反应性，结果显示，在 95% 的标本中至少存在 1 个基因突变，其中 85% 的患者存在多个潜在的靶向治疗靶点。Gatalica 等[200] 使用 IHC、基因测序和原位杂交方法检测 1806 例 CUP 患者疗效标志物的改变，结果显示，96% 的患者存在潜在药物获益的生物标志物；其中，最常见的蛋白过表达为拓扑异构酶（topoisomerase，Topo）1 和 Topo2α 表达（分别为 55% 和 64%），激素受体表达率为 20%，甲基鸟嘌呤甲基转移酶（meth-ylguanine methyltransferase，MGMT）和酪氨酸磷酸酶基因（gene of phosphatase and tensin homolog deletedon chromosome ten，PTEN）缺失表达率分别为 40% 和 52%。

Varadhachary 等[135] 使用 RT-PCR 检查了 120 例 CUP 患者中 10 个特征性基因表达，结果显示，与含有紫杉醇类和铂类的 CUP 经验性化学治疗方案相比，具有结肠癌特征的 CUP 患者对结肠癌标准治疗方案的反应更好。

但欧洲 GEFCAPI 04 随机 III 期试验直接比较了基于 GEP 结果的系统治疗与顺铂联合吉西他滨经验性化学治疗的临床疗效[202]，有 243 例患者入组，结果显示，两组患者的中位无进展生存期（PFS）和 OS 相似。且另一项针对 194 例 CUP 患者的前瞻性 II 期研究结果亦显示[181]，临床特征、治疗反应与分子基因检测结果基本一致。

因此，目前尚没有充分证据表明在 CUP 患者中使用以分子检测结果为指导的肿瘤部位特异性治疗可改善疗效和远期生存，对指导 CUP 治疗决策的临床益处有待于进一步验证。

表6-8 对于CUP中最常见高度可疑原发肿瘤的分子基因检测建议

高度可疑原发肿瘤	推荐检测的基因	可选择的靶向治疗药物
肺癌（腺癌、鳞癌）	EGFR（突变）	阿法替尼，厄洛替尼，达克替尼，吉非替尼，奥希替尼，阿美替尼，伏美替尼
	ALK（基因重排）	阿来替尼，布加替尼，色瑞替尼，克唑替尼，劳拉替尼
	ROS1（基因重排）	色瑞替尼，克唑替尼，恩曲替尼，瑞波替尼
	BRAF V600E（突变）	达拉非尼+曲美替尼，康奈非尼+贝美替尼，达拉非尼，维莫非尼
	NTRK1/2/3（基因融合）	拉罗替尼，恩曲替尼
	MET（外显子14跳突）	卡马替尼，克唑替尼，特泊替尼
	RET（基因重排）	塞普替尼，普拉替尼，卡博替尼
	HER-2（突变）	Fam - trastuzumab deruxtecan - nxki，Ado - trastuzumab emtansine（T - DM1），DS - 8201
乳腺癌	HER-2（过表达或扩增阳性）	曲妥珠单抗，帕妥珠单抗，拉帕替尼，Fam - trastuzumab deruxtecan - nxki，Ado - trastuzumab emtansine（T - DM1），DS - 8201
结直肠腺癌	KRAS/NRAS/BRAF（野生型）	西妥昔单抗，帕尼单抗
	KRAS G12C（突变）	索托拉西布或阿达格拉西布+西妥昔单抗或帕尼单抗
	HER-2（扩增阳性）	曲妥珠单抗，帕妥珠单抗，拉帕替尼，Fam - trastuzumab deruxtecan - nxki
卵巢癌	BRCA（突变）	奥拉帕利

第八节 诊 断

在临床实践中，对CUP的诊断目前仍是一个巨大挑战[82]，但通常应发挥多学科协作的积极作用。英国NICE颁布的指南将CUP的诊断过程中分为如下3个关键步骤，值得借鉴。

第一步：原发灶未定肿瘤（malignancy of undefined primary origin，MUO），即经初步检查暂时未发现明确的原发肿瘤。

下篇　不明原发肿瘤
第六章　可疑CUP检查与诊断

第二步：暂定原发灶不明肿瘤（provisional CUP），即虽经初步组织学/细胞学诊断为暂未发现原发肿瘤的转移性上皮来源癌或神经内分泌肿瘤，但未经过专家进一步讨论判定。

第三步：确定不明原发肿瘤（confirmed CUP），即经过组织学最终确认的转移性上皮来源癌或神经内分泌肿瘤，且经过全面、系统检查及专家进一步研究判定，仍未确定肿瘤来源。

一般而言，在完成病理和临床诊断检查后，CUP的诊断取决于多学科团队对临床表现、病理学、免疫组化和影像学检查结果的解读，以确定肿瘤相关信息是原发肿瘤还是与CUP相符的转移肿瘤。为此，最重要的诊断工具是合理的临床推理[203]。

影像学检查需明确肿瘤大小、位置、影像学特征，以及向邻近结构的侵袭模式，血行转移灶、淋巴转移灶的分布。具体而言，沿着预先形成的淋巴通路转移的肿瘤可能被淋巴转移的非典型位置所包围，其中最接近的相邻淋巴结群通常是最严重的。

在没有可明确识别的原发肿瘤特异性基因组改变的情况下，必须判断其中一个可见病灶是否可能代表原发肿瘤。

一、尽力明确原发肿瘤

CUP诊断首先需仔细寻找隐匿原发灶，然而，一些CUP存活者可能会患上最初隐藏的原发肿瘤导致转移疾病或发生第二原发肿瘤。据报道[204]，有几种类型的第二原发肿瘤的发生风险较高，其中男性生殖器官与消化道肿瘤的发生风险最高。此外，非霍奇金淋巴瘤和皮肤鳞癌的发病风险亦很高。

对于可疑CUP而言，通常需要对转移灶组织标本进行组织病理学和免疫组化检查，首先应采用基于形态模式的方法来区分上皮癌、圆形细胞肿瘤、梭形细胞肿瘤和未分化癌，以确定实体肿瘤组织和肿瘤细胞来源；对于未分化肿瘤或细胞谱不明确的细胞，要进行初步的IHC筛查[148]，如对于男性患者，需使用前列腺特异性膜抗原（PSMA）和（或）NKX3.1作为标记物来排除转移性前列腺癌；对于女性患者，应使用GATA3来筛查乳腺癌，使用SOX10来筛查三阴性乳腺癌。

在分析包括肝脏转移腺癌在内的活组织切片时，初始IHC检测应包括CK7、CK20、尾型同源染色体2（CDX2）和TTF-1[女性还需加上GATA3

和(或)SOX10],以筛查乳腺癌、肺癌、胃肠道癌和(或)胰胆管转移性肿瘤。

至少80%的结直肠癌(CRC)表现出典型的CK7阴性、CK20阳性、CDX2阳性免疫表型,CK20和CDX2染色通常呈弥漫性阳性且较强;偶见上消化道腺癌和罕见的胰胆管腺癌也表现出结直肠癌免疫表型,在这种情况下,特殊的富AT序列结合蛋白2(SATB2)阳性对于下消化道来源的肿瘤具有相当的特异性[205]。

由于缺乏特异性标记物,通过IHC对肝内胆管癌(CCA)进行鉴别诊断仍然很困难。BRCA1相关蛋白1(BAP1)或富含AT交互结构域的蛋白1A(ARID1A)的免疫组化缺失可支持诊断,但最终决定只能结合临床和放射学检查结果[203]。

为了鉴别神经内分泌肿瘤,需对具有实性、小梁状、回旋状或规则腺状生长形态、均匀的细胞核和粗条纹("盐和胡椒")染色质的肿瘤进行突触素和(或)INSM1染色;同样,对于类似肺小细胞癌或大细胞神经内分泌肿瘤的高级别肿瘤,亦应进行突触素和(或)INSM1染色。CDX2和ISLET1阳性可能提示神经内分泌肿瘤的原发部位分别在消化道和胰腺。

间皮瘤通常CK阳性,可能会被误诊为癌,因此在进行CUP检查时需特别注意。源自胸膜、心包和腹膜的活组织检查应考虑间皮瘤,在这些病例中应进行钙结合蛋白免疫染色,阳性时应辅以WT-1、CK5/6、D2-40和BAP1(丢失)。

间叶组织肿瘤的广谱上皮标记物表达在大多数情况下是局灶性的。不过,在上皮样形态的病例中,这些标记物的表达可能是弥漫性的,CK强阳性(如滑膜肉瘤、上皮样肉瘤)往往会导致被错误地归类为癌;CK阳性还可能见于小圆形蓝细胞肉瘤(如纤维肉瘤、尤因肉瘤)[206],无论广泛型上皮标记是否阳性,在纵隔、腹膜后和软组织中均应考虑肉瘤的可能性,尤其是在出现梭形细胞形态的情况下。

另外,血液淋巴肿瘤(如浆细胞瘤、无细胞大细胞淋巴瘤和套细胞淋巴瘤)亦可表达广谱角蛋白[207]。

(一)病史询问与体格检查

前已述及,详细的病史、家族史询问对推测原发肿瘤有一定作用。

在病史询问中,需注意患者既往是否有恶性肿瘤切除史,既往组织活检结果；在确定诊断时，需排除多原发肿瘤（multiple primary neoplasmas，MPNs）的可能。家族史很可能提示遗传性非息肉病性结肠癌或乳腺癌易感性。

在临床实践中，原发肿瘤的线索常常在重复细致的体格检查时被发现。全面体格检查通常包括鼻腔、口腔、咽部、喉部、胸部（包括乳腺）、腹部、盆腔、直肠、阴道、肛门、阴囊、会阴及四肢等部位。

浅表淋巴结的全面触诊检查在体格检查中尤为关键，往往可为寻找原发肿瘤提供重要线索。

颈部淋巴结比较表浅，易于发现，临床上诸多患者因为无意间发现颈部肿块就医，其中部分被诊断为原发肿瘤不明的颈部淋巴结转移癌。

颈部中上组淋巴结往往以转移性鳞状细胞癌或未分化癌多见，原发肿瘤多来源于头颈部，而口咽、舌根及扁桃体是头颈部原发肿瘤比较常见的隐匿部位，增强以上部位的诊断性活检可提高早期癌的检出率。

颈部下组淋巴结大部分为转移性腺癌，原发肿瘤大多来源于肺、乳腺、胃肠道及其他脏器等[208]。

锁骨上淋巴结转移，原发肿瘤多见于锁骨以下的脏器；腋窝淋巴结转移，原发肿瘤多来源于乳腺、肺；腹股沟淋巴结转移，多见于外生殖器、肛管直肠、下肢、会阴部皮肤等部位的原发肿瘤。

但左侧锁骨上淋巴结肿大、脐周淋巴结肿大等可能对表现有低分化癌的患者给出胃肠道检查的提示。

（二）影像学检查

X线、超声、CT、MRI、PET/CT等影像学检查对于可疑CUP患者寻找原发肿瘤是必须的，必要时进行颅脑、脊髓、骨与软组织MRI检查，以及全身骨扫描、甲状腺放射性核素现象。

Olson等[14]报道，MRI对于仅有腋下淋巴结转移的隐匿性乳腺癌的发现率高达70%。

一般而言，在病史询问、体格检查、症状体征、常规实验室检查（如粪便或尿液隐血试验）及影像学检查基础上，应针对性选择内镜检查[209]。

（三）病理学检查

对肿瘤转移灶组织病理学、细胞学病理检查（如浆膜腔积液、尿液等）被证实是明确原发肿瘤的有效方法，准确率为51%[82]。

对获取转移灶活检组织,需进行常规组织病理学检查及免疫组化检测。

值得注意的是,转移性卵巢肿瘤的病理特征与原发性卵巢癌具有相似之处,普通光学显微镜下,来源于结肠、胰腺、阑尾和子宫颈腺体的转移性卵巢肿瘤与原发性卵巢黏液性腺癌组织学相似,FIGO Ⅲ期、Ⅳ期原发性卵巢黏液性腺癌与结肠腺癌转移至卵巢误诊率高达57%。

来源于子宫内膜癌的卵巢转移癌与卵巢子宫内膜样腺癌、子宫内膜癌及卵巢癌的双原发癌在临床症状及组织学病理学极其相似。

(四)分子基因检测

一般而言[210-212],通过详细询问患者病史、家族史,仔细体格检查、实验室检查、影像学检查、转移灶组织病理学检查、免疫组化检查等进行初步判断,如果通过以上方法仍未明确肿瘤原发部位,可进一步选择分子基因检测,尽可能明确原发肿瘤[213]。

值得一提的是,Gallagher等[214]指出,对于那些一般状态较差的患者,过多的检查没必要,因这些检查消耗了患者体能,且这类患者往往生存期不长,原发肿瘤的明确需要较长时间,对改善患者预后意义不大。NCCN指南、ESMO指南认为可疑CUP患者辅助检查的一个重要原则是合理检查,避免过度,如对于病情进展迅速和身体状况较差者,寻找原发肿瘤在短期内意义不大,而支持治疗是最佳选择。

二、CUP诊断标准

多数学者认为[215],在经过询问病史、体格检查,实验室检查、常规影像学(X线、B超、CT、MRI)和(或)内窥镜检查、转移灶组织或细胞病理学检查、免疫组化检测等,仍未能发现原发肿瘤,即可诊断为不明原发肿瘤;PET/CT、分子基因检测结果不作为常规诊断标准。

CUP诊断的具体标准主要有如下3条:

(1)转移灶经组织、细胞病理学证实为恶性肿瘤。

(2)首发部位无法明确肿瘤来源。

(3)经详尽的病史采集、体格检查、实验室检查、影像学检查、内镜检查等均未发现原发肿瘤。

第六章 可疑CUP检查与诊断

三、几种常见原发肿瘤与可疑 CUP 鉴别诊断的逻辑推理

(一) 肺癌

CUP 与非小细胞肺癌（NSCLC）的鉴别诊断是一个难题，因 40% 的肺癌 TTF1 阴性，出现肺部肿瘤性病变的患者可能是从未知的原发肿瘤转移到肺部，或其中一个肺部病变本身就是原发肿瘤，通常是非小细胞肺癌，并伴有肺外转移和肺转移。其鉴别要点是基于肺部肿块的病理、影像学特征、肺门和纵隔淋巴结受累情况以及远处转移的模式，脑、骨、肝、肾上腺和胸膜是 NSCLC 最常见的转移部位。

1. TTF-1 阴性 NSCLC 与 CUP

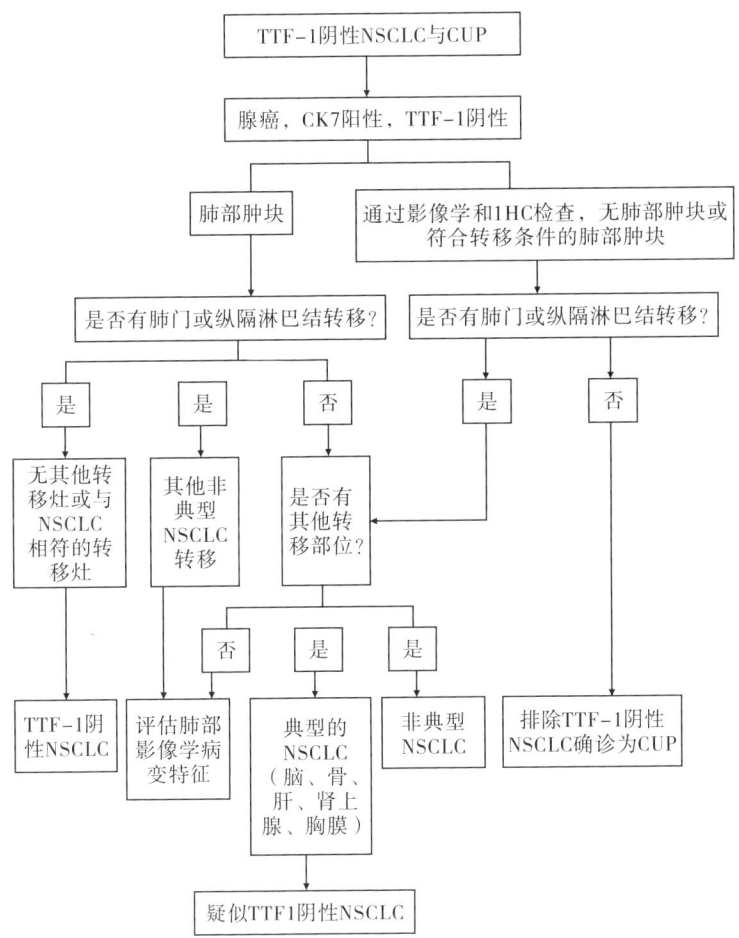

图 6-1　TTF-1 阴性 NSCLC 与 CUP 鉴别诊断的逻辑推理

2. TTF-1 阳性 NSCLC 与 CUP

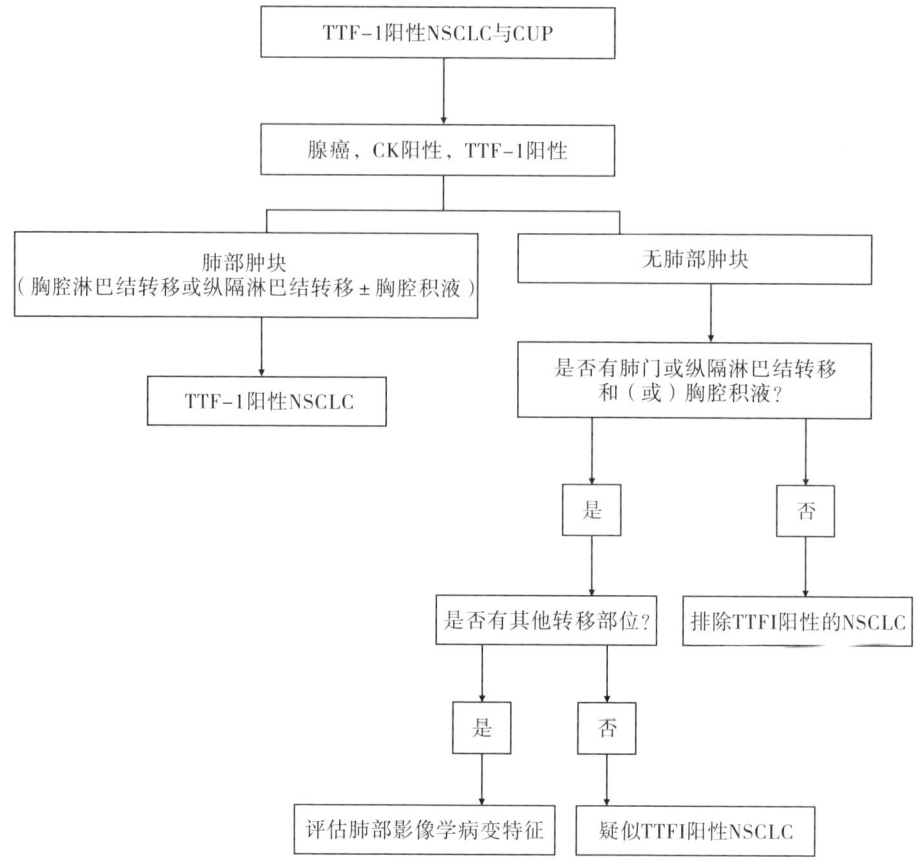

图 6-2 TTF-1 阳性 NSCLC 与 CUP 鉴别诊断的逻辑推理

(二)肝内胆管细胞癌

临床上,当肝内病变的组织学病理学诊断为腺癌时,区分原发性肝内胆管细胞癌(CCA)(伴有或不伴有其他肝内转移灶)和未知肝外原发肿瘤导致的肝转移(伴有或不伴有其他肝外转移灶)通常是比较困难的[216-217]。一般而言,区分伴有肝转移的 CUP 与肝内 CCA 的方法是根据 IHC、影像学形态、肝脏病灶的大小和数量以及总体转移模式而进行判断。

下篇 不明原发肿瘤

第六章 可疑CUP检查与诊断

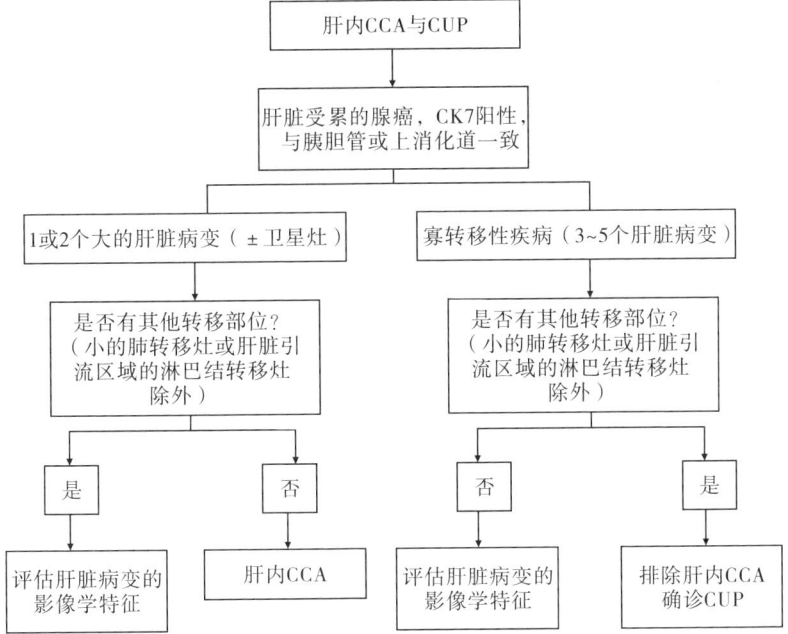

图6-3 肝内CCA与CUP鉴别诊断的逻辑推理

（三）乳腺癌

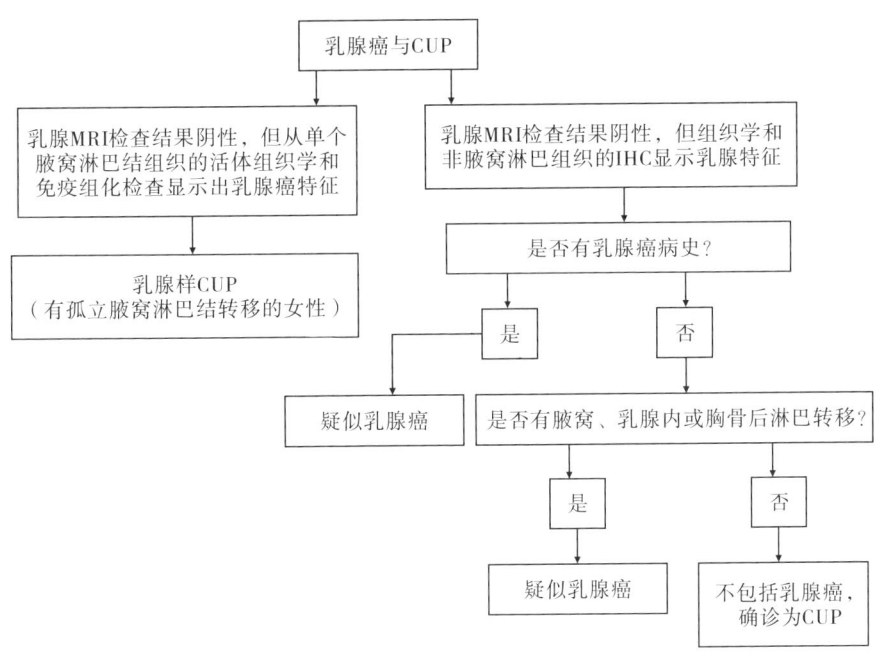

图6-4 乳腺癌与CUP鉴别诊断的逻辑推理

(四)原发性卵巢癌

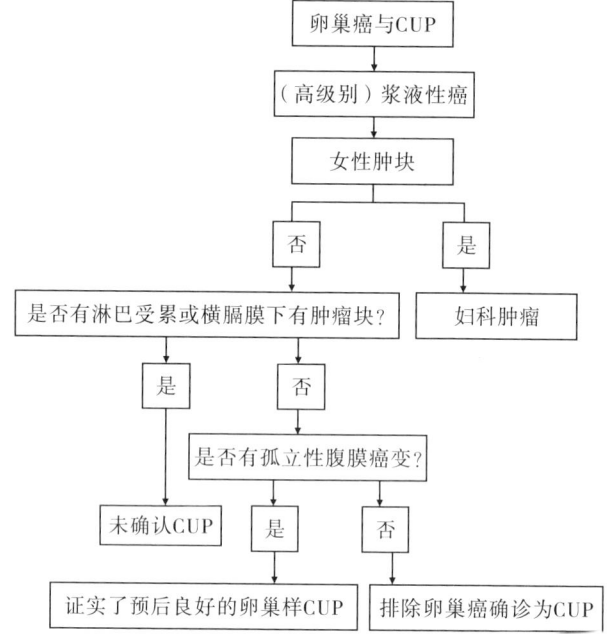

图6-5 原发性卵巢癌与CUP与鉴别诊断的逻辑推理

(五)肾细胞癌

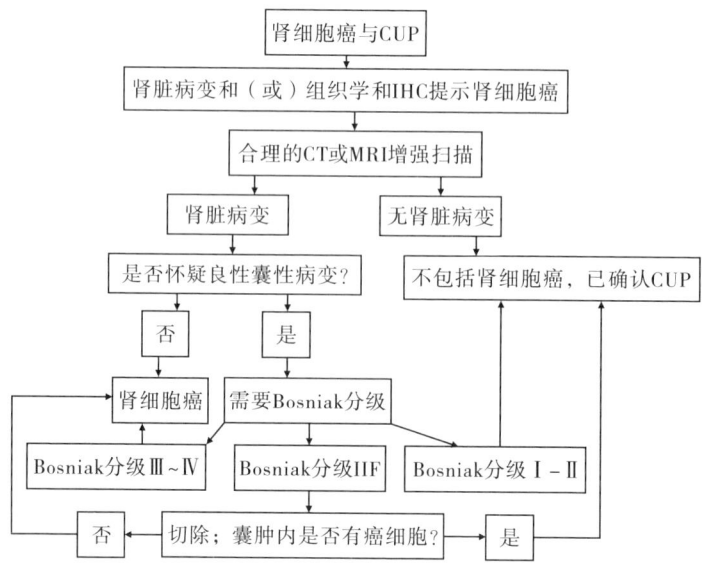

图6-6 肾细胞癌与CUP鉴别诊断的逻辑推理

附：肾囊性病变 Bosniak 分级标准

分级	标准
Bosniak Ⅰ级	轮廓分明，薄(≤2mm)光滑的壁；均匀的流体(-9~20HU)，无隔膜或钙化，壁可能会增强
Bosniak Ⅱ级	六种类型，均具有薄壁(≤2mm)且轮廓分明： 囊性肿块，薄(≤2mm)和少数(1~3)分隔；分隔和囊壁可能会增强；可能有任何类型的钙化。 平扫 CT 均质密度-9~20HU。 平扫 CT 均匀高密度(≥70HU)肿块。 肾脏增强扫描时，CT 值>20HU 的均质的没有强化的肿块。可能有任何类型的钙化。 肾脏增强扫描时，门静脉期 CT 为 21~30HU 的均质肿块。 均匀的低密度，太小而无法表述
Bosniak ⅡF级	两种类型： 囊性肿块伴有许多(≥4个)光滑的分隔，(≤2mm)分隔可增强。 囊性肿块具有光滑的轻微增厚(3mm)增强的壁，或光滑的轻微增厚的分隔(3mm)可伴强化
Bosniak Ⅲ	一个或多个增强的厚壁(≥4mm)或增强的不规则(≤3mm)的壁或分隔
Bosniak Ⅳ	一个或多个增强的壁结节(≥4mm)

四、几种特殊转移灶的诊断

(一)恶性胸腔积液

胸腔积液细胞学诊断恶性胸腔积液时，在第一次采样的灵敏度仅为65%，在连续3次送检后可达90%[218]。

在一项大样本的研究中[219]，内科胸腔镜对恶性胸腔积液的诊断率为88.9%，而闭式胸膜活检的诊断率为61.7%($P<0.05$)。Yap 等[220]报道，电视辅助胸腔镜(VATS)对恶性胸腔积液的诊断准确率可达到94%。

(二)恶性腹腔积液

对于大多数恶性腹腔积液患者而言，传统影像学检查即可发现原发肿瘤，然而，有少数患者，即使进行这些检查，原发肿瘤仍难以明确。

腹部超声和 PET/CT 对恶性腹腔积液原发肿瘤的检出率分别为62.5%、79.5%，PET/CT 结合超声对诊断卵巢来源恶性腹腔积液的灵敏度、特异度分别为98.1%、89.1%；超声对＞5cm肿瘤的诊断准确度最高，为77.0%；PET/CT在检测3～5cm肿瘤的准确度最高，为84.2%，二者结合可提高对不同大小病变的诊断准确率[221]。

腹腔镜检查可用于不明原因腹腔积液患者的评估，通过进行活组织检查，其诊断准确率为91%，但因其为有创侵入性检查，较少用于腹腔积液初步评估[222]。

对于女性附件肿块伴有腹腔积液、CA125＞1000u/L、可疑腹膜癌的患者，超声引导下的穿刺活检可明确诊断，可避免不必要的腹腔镜手术[223]。

Han等[224]研究表明，PET/CT结合腹腔积液中的肿瘤标记物诊断恶性腹腔积液的敏感性、特异性和准确性分别为97.7%、80.0%和90.4%，单独PET/CT诊断恶性腹腔积液的敏感性、特异性和准确性分别为92.3%、83.6%和88.7%；PET/CT联合腹腔积液CA125或CEA检测，可提高不明原发肿瘤腹腔积液的诊断。

(三) 腹膜转移癌

肿瘤腹膜转移(peritoneal metastases, PM)的不同表现，如腹膜微结节、结节、斑块状、网膜饼状、肿块及腹腔积液形成等增加了组织活检的难度。

Laghi等[225]认为，CT由于空间分辨率不足，对肠系膜根部、小网膜、左膈下和肠系膜表面＜5mm的病变及＜1cm的转移灶的灵敏度较低，可能低估12%～33%的腹膜癌指数(peritoneal cancer index, PCI)。

确诊腹膜癌的金标准是活检组织病理检查，与剖腹探查相比，腹腔镜检查评估腹膜癌的侵袭性相对小，在诊断的准确度上，无明显差异[226]。Long等[227]的研究表明，经脐内窥镜手术(transumbilical endoscopic surgery, TUES)是一种可行、经济且微创进入腹腔的方法，TUES联合活检，可安全有效地明确诊断。

另外，血清肿瘤标记物CA125水平在卵巢癌相关性腹膜癌变中最高，高于结核性腹膜炎和非卵巢癌相关性腹膜炎，CEA在非卵巢癌相关的腹膜癌变中升高更为显著[228]。

(四) 骨髓转移癌

根据文献报道[229-232]，将骨髓转移癌的诊断要点总结如下：
(1) 出现原因不明的贫血、发热、消瘦、骨痛等。

第六章　可疑CUP检查与诊断

（2）病理性骨折。

（3）同位素骨扫描或 ^{18}F FDG–PET/CT 中无法解释的"热点"。

（4）无法解释的生化异常，如高钙血症，血清乳酸脱氢酶与碱性磷酸酶升高。

（5）无法解释的血细胞减少，如红细胞、血小板减少。

（6）发生微血管内溶血性贫血（MAHA）、弥散性血管内凝血（DIC）。

（7）红细胞分布宽度（RDW）升高，平均血小板体积（MPV）降低。

（8）外周血涂片发现幼红细胞、幼粒细胞。

（9）多部位骨髓穿刺涂片或骨髓活检发现恶性细胞。

骨髓转移癌X线呈现溶骨性损害或骨密度显著增高，类似多发性骨髓瘤及原发骨肿瘤等改变，临床易与多发性骨髓瘤、原发性骨髓纤维化及骨结核病等相混淆。

因癌细胞浸润骨髓可造成骨髓腔内细胞填塞或骨髓造血抑制细胞数过少，转移癌细胞释放的因子及毒素导致骨髓坏死及细胞退化，在穿刺时出现的"干抽"，或抽取时困难，或抽出物呈血水样或坏死物质，可作为骨髓转移癌诊断的参考指标。

参考文献

[1] Hemminki K, Sundquist K, Sundquist J, et al. Location of metastases in cancer of unknown primary are not random and signal familial cluste–ring[J]. Sci Rep, 2016, 6：22891.

[2] Chorost MI, Lee MC, Yeoh CB, et al. Unknown primary[J]. J Surg Oncol, 2004, 87(4)：191–203.

[3] Hans Christiansen, Robert Michael Hermann, Alexios Martin, et al. Neck Lymph Node Metastases from an Unknown Primary Tumor Neck lymph node metastases from an unknown primary tumor retrospective study and review of literature[J]. Strahlenther Onkol, 2005, 181(6)：355–362.

[4] Konstantinos S, Polyzoidis A, George Miliara S, et al. Brain metastasis of unknown primary：A diagnostic and therapeutic dilemma[J]. Cancer Treat Rev, 2009, 35(3)：221–227.

[5] Kamby C, Guldhammer B, Vejborg I, et al. The presence of tumor cells in bone marrow at the time of first recurrence of breast cancer[J]. Cancer, 1987, 60(6)：1306–1312.

[6] Kim KW, Krajewski KM, Jagannathan JP, et al. Cancer of unknown primary sites：what radiologists need to know and what oncologists want to know[J]. AJR Am J Roentgenol, 2013,

[7] Chen X, Jacobson AF. Nonosseous uptake on bone scan inadenocarcinoma of unknown primary origin[J]. Clin Nucl Med, 2000, 25(9): 751-752.

[8] Cooke KS, Kirpekar M, Abiri MM, et al. Skeletal metastasis from poorly differentiated carcinoma of unknown origin[J]. Radiographics, 1997, 17(2): 542-544.

[9] Lee SJ, Bae JH, Lee AW, et al. Clinical characteristics of metastatic tumors to the ovaries[J]. J Korean Med Sci, 2009, 24(1): 114-119.

[10] Scutellari PN, Addonisio G, Righi R, et al. Diagnostic imaging of bone metastases[J]. Radiol Med(Torino), 2000, 100(6): 429-435.

[11] 曹来宾, 王安明, 徐爱德, 等. 1047例骨转移瘤的影像学诊断[J]. 中华放射学杂志, 1997, 31(8): 547-551.

[12] Abbruzzese JL, Abbruzzese MC, Lenzi R, et al. Analysis of a diagnostic strategy for patients with suspected tumors of unknown origin[J]. J Clin Oncol, 1995, 13(8): 2094-2103.

[13] Bleicher RJ, Morrow M. MRI and breast cancer: role in detection, diagnosis, and staging[J]. Oncology (Williston Park), 2007, 21(12): 1521-1528.

[14] Olson JA Jr, Morris EA, Van Zee KJ, et al. Magnetic resonance imaging facilitates breast conservation for occult breast cancer[J]. Ann Surg Oncol, 2000, 7(6): 411-415.

[15] Yoo MG, Kim J, Bae S, et al. Detection of clinically occult primary tumours in patients with cervical metastases of unknown primary tumours: comparison of three-dimensional THRIVE MR, two-dimensional spin-echo MRI, and contrast-enhanced CT[J]. Clin Radiol, 2018, 73(5): 410.e9-410.e15.

[16] Pelosi E, Pennone M, Deandreis D, et al. Role of whole body positron emission tomography/computed tomography scan with ^{18}F-fluorodeoxyglucose in patients with biopsy proven tumor metastases from unknown primary site[J]. Q J Nucl Med Mol Imaging, 2006, 50(1): 15-22.

[17] Naani C, Rubello D, Castellucci P, et al. Role of ^{18}F-FDG PET/CT imaging for the detection of an unknown primary tumour: preliminary results in 21 patients[J]. Eur J Nucl Med Mol Imaging, 2005, 32(5): 589-592.

[18] 郑容, 吴宁, 李静, 等. ^{18}F-FDG PET/CT显像在寻找转移性肿瘤原发灶中的应用. 中国临床医学影像杂志, 2008, 19(3): 164-167.

[19] Rodel R, Straehler Pohl HJ, Palmedo H, et al. PET/CT imaging in head and neck tumours[J]. Radiologe, 2004, 44(11): 1055-1059.

[20] 陈刚, 管樑. ^{18}F-FDG PET/CT在寻找转移瘤原发灶中的临床标准应用[J]. 中国标准化, 2021, 589(16): 184-186.

[21] Miller FR, Hussey D, Beeram M, et al. Positron emission tomography in the management of unknown primary head and neck carcinoma[J]. Arch Otolaryngol Head Neck Surg, 2005,

131(7)：626-629.

[22] Paul SA, Stoeckli SJ, von Schulthess GK, et al. FDG PET and PET/CT for the detection of the primary tumour in patients with cervical non-squamous cell carcinoma metastasis of an unknown primary[J]. Eur Arch Otorhinolaryngol, 2007, 264(2)：189-195.

[23] Schoder H, Yeung HW. Positron emission imaging of head and neck cancer, including thyroid carcinoma[J]. Semin Nucl Med, 2004, 34(3)：180-197.

[24] 刘红红, 兰晓莉, Anand Gungadin, 等. ^{18}F-FDG PET/CT 对原发灶不明颈部淋巴结转移癌的诊断及预后价值[J]. 中华核医学与分子影像杂志, 2016, 36(1)：48-53.

[25] Pak K, Kim SJ, Kim IJ, et al. Clinical implication of $^{(18)}$F-FDG PET/CT in carcinoma of unknown primary[J]. Neoplasma, 2011, 58(2)：135-139.

[26] Moller AK, Loft A, Berthelsen AK, et al. A prospective comparison of ^{18}F-FDG PET/CT and CT as diagnostic tools to identify the primary tumor site in patients with extracervical carcinoma of unknown primary site[J]. Oncologist, 2012, 17(9)：1146-1154.

[27] Lee JR, Kim JS, Roh JL, et al. Detection of occult primary tumors in patients with cervical metastases of unknown primary tumors：comparison of $^{(18)}$F-FDG PET/CT with contrast-enhanced CT or CT/MR imaging-prospective study[J]. Radiology, 2015, 274(3)：764-771.

[28] Park GC, Roh JL, Cho KJ, et al. ^{18}F-FDG PET/CT vs. human papilloma virus, p16 and Epstein-Barr virus detection in cervical metastatic lymph nodes for identifying primary tumors[J]. Int J Cancer, 2017, 140(6)：1405-1412.

[29] Avci NC, Hatipoglu F, Alacacioglu A, et al. FDG PET/CT and conventional imaging methods in cancer of unknown primary：an approach to over scanning[J]. Nucl Med Mol Imaging, 2018, 52(6)：438-444.

[30] Wong WL, Sonoda LI, Gharpurhy A, et al. ^{18}F-fluorodeoxyglucose positron emission tomography/computed tomography in the assessment of occult primary head and neck cancers：an audit and review of published studies[J]. Clin Oncol, 2012, 24(3)：190-195.

[31] Rudmik L, Lau HY, Matthews ATW, et al. Clinical utility of PET/CT in the evaluation of head and neck squamous cell carcinoma with an unknown primary：a prospective clinical trial [J]. Head Neck, 2011, 33(7)：935-940.

[32] 张倩, 李亚明, 李雪娜. ^{18}F-FDGPET/CT 显像在不明原发灶淋巴结转移癌中的应用价值[J]. 中国临床医学影像杂志, 2011, 22(6)：412-414.

[33] Chen YH, Yang XM, Li SS, et al. Value of fused positron emission tomography CT in detecting primaries in patients with primary unknown cervical lymph node metastasis[J]. J Med Imaging Radiat Oncol, 2012, 56(1)：66-74.

[34] 赵铭, 王娟, 田蓉蓉, 等. ^{18}F-FDG PET/CT 在寻找不明原发灶肿瘤患者原发灶中的价值[J]. 中国医学影像学杂志, 2012, 20(6)：468-470.

[35] Breuer N, Behrendt FF, Heinzel A, et al. Prognostic relevance of ^{18}F-FDG PET/CT in carcinoma of unknown primary[J]. Clin Nucl Med, 2013, 39(2): 131-135.

[36] Hu M, Zhao W, Zhang PL, et al. Clinical applications of ^{18}F-fluorodeoxyglucose positron emission tomography/computed tomography in carcinoma of unknown primary[J]. Chin Med J (Engl), 2011, 124(7): 1010-1014.

[37] Imperiale A, Rust E, Gabriel S, et al. ^{18}F-Fluorodihydroxyphenylalanine PET/CT in patients with neuroendocrine tumors of unknown origin: relation to tumor origin and differentiation[J]. J Nucl Med, 2013, 55(4): 367-372.

[38] Tamam MO, Mulazimoglu M, Guveli TK, et al. Prediction of survival and evaluation of diagnostic accuracy whole body ^{18}F-fluoro-2-deoxyglucose positron emission tomography/computed tomography in the detection carcinoma of unknown primary origin[J]. Eur Rev Med Pharmacol Sci, 2012, 16(15): 2120-2130.

[39] RodelR, Straehler Pohl HJ, Palmedo H, et al. PET/CT imaging in head and neck tumors[J]. Radiologe, 2004, 4(11): 1055-1059.

[40] Kwee TC, Kwee RM. Combined FDG-PET/CT for the detection of unknown primary tumors: systematic review and meta-analysis[J]. Eur Radiol, 2009, 19(3): 731-744.

[41] 李亚军, 高硕, 陈秋松, 等. ^{18}F-FDG PET/CT 显像探测原发肿瘤病灶的临床价值[J]. 中华核医学杂志, 2005, 25(1): 37-38.

[42] Mackenzie K, Watson M, Jankowska P, et al. Investigation and management of the unknown primary with metastatic neck disease: United Kingdom National Multidisciplinary Guidelines[J]. J Laryngol Otol, 2016, 130(S2): S170-S175.

[43] Rusthoven KE, Koshy M, Paulino AC. The role of fluorodeoxyglucose positron emission tomography in cervically mph node metastases from an unknown primary tumor[J]. Cancer, 2004, 101(11): 2641-2649.

[44] Gutzeit A, Antoch G, Kuhl H, et al. Unknown Primary Tumors: Detection with Dual-Modality PET/CT-Initial experience[J]. Radiology, 2005, 234(1): 227-234.

[45] 宋建华, 赵晋华, 邢岩, 等. ^{18}F-FDG PET/CT 对原发不明颈部淋巴结转移癌患者原发灶检出的价值[J]. 中华核医学与分子影像杂志, 2013, 33(6): 417-420.

[46] Roh JL, Kim JS, Lee JH, et al. Utility of combined $^{(18)}$F-fluorodeoxyglucose-positron emission tomography and computed tomography in patients with cervical metastases from unknown primary tumors[J]. Oral Oncol, 2009, 45(3): 218-224.

[47] Freudenberg LS, Fischer M, Antoch G, et al. Dual Modality of ^{18}F-Fluorodeoxyglucose-Positron Emission Tomography/Computed Tomography in Patients with Cervical Carcinoma of Unknown Primary[J]. Med Princ Pract, 2005, 14(3): 155-160.

[48] 赵春雷, 李天然, 陈自谦, 等. 全身^{18}F-FDG PET/CT 在原发灶不明的颈部转移癌中的应用价值[J]. 中国医学影像技术, 2006, 22(11): 1745-1748.

[49] Coakley FV, Choi PH, Gougoutas CA, et al. Peritoneal metastases: detection with spiral CT in patients with ovarian cancer[J]. Radiology, 2002, 223(2): 495-499.

[50] Krishnamurthy S, Balasubramaniam R. Role of Imaging in Peritoneal Surface Malignancies [J]. Indian J Surg Oncol, 2016, 7(4): 441-452.

[51] Schmidt S, Meuli RA, Achtari C, et al. Peritoneal carcinomatosis in primary ovarian cancer staging: comparison between MDCT, MRI, and ^{18}F-FDG PET/CT[J]. Clin Nucl Med, 2015, 40(5): 371-377.

[52] Lopez-Lopez V, Cascales-Campos PA, Gil J, et al. Use of $(^{18})$F-FDG PET/CT in the preoperative evaluation of patients diagnosed with peritoneal carcinomatosis of ovarian origin, candidates to cytoreduction and hipec. A pending issue[J]. Eur J Radiol, 2016, 85(10): 1824-1828.

[53] Alberini JL, Belhocine T, Hustinx R, et al. Whole-body positron emission tomography using fluorodeoxy glucose in patients with metastases of unknown primary tumors (UPT syndrome) [J]. Nucl Med Common, 2003, 24(10): 1081-1086.

[54] Jungehulsing M, Scheidhauer K, Damm M, et al. 2[^{18}F]-fluoro-2-deoxy-D-glucose positron emission tomography is a sensitive tool for the detection of occult primary cancer (carcinoma of unknown primary syndrome) with head and neck lymphnode manifestation[J]. Otolaryngol Head Neck Surg, 2000, 123(3): 294-301.

[55] Vankadari K, Mittal BR, Kumar R, et al. Detection of Hepatic Encephalopathy on ^{18}F-FDG PET/CT Brain Images in a Patient With Decompensated Liver Cirrhosis[J]. Clin Nucl Med, 2018, 43(12): e486-e487.

[56] Fan HB, Wang AJ, Yang DL, et al. Use of ^{18}F-FDG PET/CT to locate primary malignancies in patients with hepatic cirrhosis and malignant ascites[J]. Chin J Cancer Res, 2013, 25(5): 500-504.

[57] Burglin SA, Hess S, Hilund-Carlsen PF, et al. ^{18}F-FDG PET/CT for detection of the primary tumor in adults with extracervical metastases from cancer of unknown primary: A systematic review and meta-analysis[J]. Medicine(Baltimore), 2017, 96(16): e6713.

[58] Wartski M, Stanc EL, Gontier E, et al. In search of an unknown primary tumor presenting with cervical metastases: Performance of hybrid FDG-PET-CT[J]. Nucl Med Commun, 2007, 28(5): 365-371.

[59] Seve P, Billotey C, Broussolle C, et al. The role of 2-deoxy-2-F-[^{18}]fluoro-D-glucose positron emission tomography in disseminated carcinoma of unknown primary site[J]. Cancer, 2007, 109(2): 292-299.

[60] Wang G, Wu Y, Zhang W, et al. Clinical value of whole-body ^{18}F-fluorodeoxyglucose positron emission tomography/computed tomography in patients with carcinoma of unknown primary[J]. J Med Imaging Radiat Oncol, 2013, 57(1): 65-71.

[61] Fletcher JW, Djulbegovic B, Soares HP, et al. Recommendations on the use of ^{18}F – FDG PET in oncology[J]. J Nucl Med, 2008, 49(3): 480 – 508.

[62] Mevio E, Gorini E, Sbrocca M, et al. The role of positron emission tomography (PET) in the management of cervical lymph nodes metastases from an unknown primary tumour[J]. Acta Otorhinolaryngol Ital, 2004, 24(6): 342 – 347.

[63] 李剑明, 辛军, 王晓明, 等. ^{18}F – FDG PET/CT 全身显像在寻找肿瘤原发灶中的临床价值[J]. 中国肿瘤临床, 2007, 34(17): 1001 – 1003, 1007.

[64] 陈钊, 郑容, 吴宁. ^{18}F – FDG PET/CT 的主要局限性和相应处理措施[J]. 中国医学影像技术, 2006, 22(2): 320 – 323.

[65] 陈应瑞, 李伟雄, 辜梅新, 等. ^{18}F – 脱氧葡萄糖显像在原发灶不明转移癌中的应用[J]. 中华放射肿瘤学杂志, 2002, 11(2): 130 – 132.

[66] Yanagawa T, Shinozaki T, Iizuka Y, et al. Role of 2 – deoxy2 – F – 18 fluoro – D – glucose positron emission tomography in the management of bone and soft – tissue metastases[J]. J Bone Joint Surg Br, 2010, 92(3): 419 – 423.

[67] Gutzeit A, Antoch G, Kühl H, et al. Unknown primary tumors: detection with dual – modality PET/CT – initial experience[J]. Radiology, 2005, 234(1): 227 – 234.

[68] Lievens Y, Guckenberger M, Gomez D, et al. Defining oligometastatic disease from a radiation oncology perspective: an ESTRO – ASTRO consensus document[J]. Radiother Oncol, 2020, 148: 157 – 166.

[69] Albertson M, Chandra S, Sayed Z, et al. PET/CT evaluation of head andneck cancer of unknown primary[J]. Semin Ultrasound CT MR, 2019, 40(5): 414 – 423.

[70] Maghami E, Ismaila N, Alvarez A, et al. Diagnosis and management of squamous cell carcinoma of unknown primary in the head and neck: ASCO guideline[J]. J Clin Oncol, 2020, 38(22): 2570 – 2596.

[71] Losa F, Fernfindez I, Etxaniz O, et al. ESMO – GECOD clinical guideline for unknown primary cancer(2021)[J]. Clin Transl Oncol, 2022, 24(4): 681 – 692.

[72] Molina R, Bosch X, Auge JM, et al. Utility of serum tumor markers as an aid in the differential diagnosis of patients withclinical suspicion of cancer and in patients with cancer of unknown primary site[J]. Tumour Biol, 2012, 33(2): 463 – 474.

[73] Varadhachary GR, Raber MN. Cancer of unknown primary site[J]. N Engl J Med, 2014, 371(8): 757 – 765.

[74] Fizazi K, Greco FA, Pavlidis N, et al. Cancers of unknown primary site: ESMO Clinical Practice Guidelines for diagnosis, treatment and follow – up[J]. Ann Oncol, 2015, 26(Suppl 5): V133 – V138.

[75] Stenman UH. Biomarker development, from bench to bedside[J]. Crit Rev Clin Lab Sci, 2016, 53(2): 69 – 86.

[76] Dolscheid-Pommerich RC, Keyver-Paik M, Hecking T, et al. Clinical performance of LOCI-based tumor marker assays for tumor markers CA 15-3, CA 125, CEA, CA 19-9 and AFP in gynecological cancers[J]. Tumour Biol, 2017, 39(10): 1-11.

[77] Yu Z, Wang R, Chen F, et al. Five novel oncogenic signatures couldbe utilized as AFP-related diagnostic biomarkers for hepatocellular carcinoma based on next-generation sequencing[J]. Dig Dis Sci, 2018, 13(2): 1-13.

[78] Losa F, Iglesias L, Pané M, et al. 2018 consensus statement by the Spanish Society of Pathology and the Spanish Society of Medical Oncology on the diagnosis and treatment of cancer of unknown primary[J]. Clin Transl Oncol, 2018, 20(11): 1361-1372.

[79] Alberti C. Carcinoma of unknown primary (CUP); some considerations about pathogenesis and diagnostic strategy, particularly focusing on CUPS pertaining to the Urology[J]. G Chir, 2012, 33(1-2): 41-46.

[80] Diederich S, Padge B, Vossas U, et al. Application of a single needle type for all image-guided biopsies: results of 100 consecutive core biopsies in various organs using a novel triaxial, end-cut needle[J]. Cancer Imaging, 2006, 6(4): 3-50.

[81] Maeda-Taniguchi M, Ueda Y, Miyake T, et al. Metastatic mucinous adenocarcinoma of the ovary is characterized by advanced patient age, small tumor size, and elevated serum CA125[J]. Gynecol Obstet Invest, 2011, 72(3): 196-202.

[82] Al-Brahim N, Ross C, Carter B, et al. The value of post mortem examination in cases of metastasis of unknown origin-20-year retrospective data from a tertiary care center[J]. Ann Diagn Pathol, 2005, 9(2): 77-80.

[83] Moid F, De Palma L. Comparison of relative value of bone marrow aspirates and bone marrow trephine biopsies in the diagnosis of solid tumor metastasis and Hodgkin lymphoma: institutional experience and literature review[J]. Arch Pathol Lab Med, 2005, 129(4): 497-501.

[84] Xiao L, Luxi S, Ying T, et al. Diagnosis of unknown non-hematological tumors by bone marrow biopsy: a retrospective analysis of 10, 112 samples[J]. J Cancer Res Clin Oncol, 2009, 135(5): 687-693.

[85] Sharma S, Murari M. Bone marrow involvement by metastatic solid tumors[J]. Indian J Pathol Microbiol, 2003, 46(3): 382-384.

[86] Bearden JD, Ratkin GA, Coltman CA. Comparison of the diagnostic value of bone marrow biopsy and bone marrow aspiration in neoplastic disease[J]. J Clin Pathol, 1974, 27(9): 738-740.

[87] 莫东华, 莫汉有, 王晓桃. 100例骨髓转移瘤骨髓组织病理学的观察[J]. 临床肿瘤学杂志, 2007; 10(12): 773-774.

[88] 王文军, 张伟, 陈玉娟, 等. 细胞蜡块免疫标记在浆膜腔积液腺癌细胞病理学诊断中

的临床价值[J]. 山西医科大学学报, 2014, 45(4): 288-290.

[89] 陈一峰, 陈婷, 陈玮姗, 等. 胸水细胞蜡块在肺癌诊断和 EGFR 基因检测中的应用研究[J]. 中国现代医学杂志, 2018, 28(29): 43-46.

[90] 尚芳芳, 赵辉, 王强, 等. 液基薄层细胞检测联合细胞块技术诊断胸腹水肿瘤[J]. 实用医药杂志, 2016, 33(4): 302-304.

[91] 赵业, 张继新, 梁丽, 等. 细胞块技术在胸腔积液病理诊断评估中的应用[J]. 中国组织工程研究, 2018, 22(12): 1934-1938.

[92] 徐晓艳, 杜华, 宝鲁日, 等. 非小细胞肺癌活检标本中 CK7、TTF-1、NapsinA、CK5/6 及 p63 的表达及其意义[J]. 诊断病理学杂志, 2015, 22(11): 688-691.

[93] 张功学, 丁凯, 齐峰, 等. 胸腔积液细胞块免疫组织化学检测对疑似肺癌患者的诊断价值. 新乡医学院学报, 2018, 35(2): 129-132.

[94] 李勇, 詹仁溥, 曹文瑜, 等. 胸腹水细胞块技术的临床应用研究[J]. 中国基层医药, 2017, 24(24): 3727-3729.

[95] Conway AM, Mitchell C, Kilgour E, et al. Molecular characterisation and liquid biomarkers in Carcinoma of Unknown Primary (CUP): taking the 'U' out of CUP[J]. Br J Cancer, 2019, 120(2): 141-153.

[96] Lu SH, Tsai WS, Chang YH, et al. Identifying cancer origin using circulating tumor cells [J]. Cancer Biol Ther, 2016, 17(4): 430-438.

[97] Best MG, Sol N, Kooi I, et al. RNA-Seq of tumor-educated platelets enables blood-based pan-cancer, multiclass, and molecular pathway cancer diagnostics[J]. Cancer Cell, 2015, 28(5): 666-676.

[98] Cohen JD, Li L, Wang Y, et al. Detection and localization of surgically resectable cancers with a multi-analyte blood test[J]. Science, 2018, 359(6378): 926-930.

[99] Meyers FJ, Lewis JP. A focused approach to patients with cancer of unknown primary site [J]. West J Med, 1986, 145(3): 403-404.

[100] Abbruzzese JL, Abbruzzese MC, Hess KR, et al. Unknown primary carcinoma: natural history and prognostic factors in 657 consecutive patients[J]. J Clin Oncol, 1994, 12(6): 1272-1280.

[101] Pavlidis N, Fizazi K. Cancer of unknown primary (CUP)[J]. Crit Rev Oncol Hematol, 2005, 54(3): 243-250.

[102] Natoli C, Ramazzotti V. Unknown primary tumors[J]. Biochim Biophys Acta, 2011, 1816 (1): 13-24.

[103] Losa F, Soler G, Casado A, et al. ESMO clinical guideline on unknown primary cancer (2017)[J]. Clin Transl Oncol, 2018, 20(1): 89-96.

[104] Rassy E, Pavlidis N. Progress in refining the clinical management of cancer of unknown primary in the molecular era[J]. Nat Rev Clin Oncol, 2020, 17(9): 541-554.

[105] Binder C, Matthes KL, Korol D, et al. Cancer of unknown primary Epidemiological trends and relevance of comprehensive genomic profiling[J]. Cancer Med, 2018, 7(9): 4814-4824.

[106] Laprovitera N, Riefolo M, Ambrosini E, et al. Cancer of Unknown Primary: Challenges and Progress in Clinical Management[J]. Cancers(Basel), 2021, 13(3): 451-462.

[107] Pavlidis N, Pentheroudakis G. Cancer of unknown primarysite[J]. The Lancet, 2012, 379(9824): 1428-1435.

[108] Krämer A, Bochtler T, Pauli C, et al. Cancer of unknown primary: ESMO clinical practice guideline for diagnosis, treatment and follow-up[J]. Ann Oncol, 2023, 34(3): 228-246.

[109] 王成锋, 田艳涛, 张建伟. 不明原发灶肿瘤1273例报告[J]. 中国微创外科杂志, 2007, 7(11): 1072-1074.

[110] 叶骉飞, 王斌, 代丽, 等. 408例恶性肿瘤骨转移临床特征分析[J]. 中国肿瘤临床, 2013, 40(4): 217-220.

[111] Rougraff BT, Kneisl JS, Simon MA. Skeletal metastases of unknown origin: A prospective study of a diagnostic strategy[J]. J Bone Joint Surg Am, 1993, 75(9): 1276-1281.

[112] Selves J, Long-Mira E, Mathieu MC, et al. Immunohisto-chemistry for Diagnosis of Metastatic Carcinomas of Unknown Primary Site [J]. Cancers (Basel), 2018, 10(4): 108.

[113] Oien KA. Pathologic evaluation of unknown primary cancer[J]. Semin Oncol, 2009, 36(1): 8-37.

[114] Varadhachary GR, Greco FA. Overview of patient management and future directions in unknown primary carcinoma[J]. Semin Oncol, 2009, 36(1): 75-80.

[115] Wick MR. Immunohistochemical approaches to the diagnosis of undifferentiated malignant tumors[J]. Ann Diagn Pathol, 2008, 12(1): 72-84.

[116] Bender RA, Erlander MG. Molecular classification of unknown primary cancer[J]. Semin Oncol, 2009, 36(1): 38-43.

[117] Monzon FA, Koen TJ. Diagnosis of metastatic neoplasms: molecular approaches for identification of tissue of origin[J]. Arch Pathol Lab Med, 2010, 134(2): 216-224.

[118] Conner JR, Hornick JL. Metastatic carcinoma of unknown primary: diagnostic approach using immunohistochemistry[J]. Adv Anat Pathol, 2015, 22(3): 149-167.

[119] Anderson GG, Weiss LM. Determining tissue of origin for metastatic cancers: meta-analysis and literature review of immunohistochemistry performance [J]. Appl Immunohistochem Mol Morphol, 2010, 18(1): 3-8.

[120] Oien KA, Dennis JL. Diagnostic work-up of carcinoma of unknown primary: from immunohistochemistry to molecular profiling[J]. Ann Oncol, 2012, 23(2): 71-77.

[121] Greco FA. Cancer of unknown primary site: evolving understanding and management of patients[J]. Clin Adv Hematol Oncol, 2012, 10(8): 518-524.

[122] Zaun G, Schuler M, Herrmann K, et al. CUP Syndrome-Metastatic Malignancy with Unknown Primary Tumor[J]. Dtsch Arztebl Int, 2018, 115(10): 157-162.

[123] Drilon A, Laetsch TW, Kummar S, et al. Efficacy of larotrectinib in TRK fusion-positive cancers in adults and children[J]. N Engl J Med, 2018, 378(8): 731-739.

[124] Doebele RC, Drilon A, Paz-Ares L, et al. Entrectinib in patients with advanced or metastatic NTRK fusion-positive solid tumours: integrated analysis of three phase 1-2 trials[J]. Lancet Oncol, 2020, 21(2): 271-282.

[125] Dennis JL, Hvidsten TR, Wit EC, et al. Markers of adenocarcinoma characteristic of the site of origin: development of a diagnostic algorithm[J]. Clin Cancer Res, 2005, 11(10): 3766-3772.

[126] 周晓军, 陈旭东. 免疫组化在来源不明转移性腺癌鉴别诊断中应用[J]. 临床与实验病理学杂志, 2005, 21(5): 515-519.

[127] Rubin BP, Skarin AT, Pisick E, et al. Use of cytokeratin 7 and 20 in determining the origin of metstatic carcinoma of unknown primary, with special emphasison lung cancer[J]. Eur J Cancer Prev, 2001, 10(1): 77-82.

[128] Noh S, Shim H. Optimal combination of immunohistochemical markers for sub-classification of non-small cell lung carcinomas: a tissue microarray study of poorly differentiated areas[J]. Lung Cancer, 2012, 76(1): 51-55.

[129] Stelow EB, Yaziji H. Immunohistochemistry, carcinomas of unknown primary, and incidence rates[J]. Semin Diagn Pathol, 2018, 35(2): 143-152.

[130] Lau SK, Prakash S, Geller SA, et al. Comparative immunohistochemical profile of hepatocellular carcinoma, cholangio carcinoma, and metastatic adene carcinoma[J]. Hum Pathol, 2002, 33(12): 1175-1181.

[131] Lin F, Liu H. Immunohistochemistry in undifferentiated neoplasm/tumor of uncertain origin[J]. Arch Pathol Lab Med, 2014, 138(12): 1583-1610.

[132] Halperin R, Zehavi S, Hadas E, et al. Simultaneous carcinoma of the endometrium and ovary vs endometrial carcinoma with ovarian metastases: a clinical and immunohistochemical determination[J]. Int J Gynecol Cancer, 2003, 13(1): 32-37.

[133] Kandalaft PL, Gown AM. Practical applications in immunohistochemistry: carcinomas of unknown primary site[J]. Arch Pathol Lab Med, 2016, 140: 508-523.

[134] Ettinger DS, Agulnik M, Cates JM, et al. NCCN clinical practice guidelines occult primary[J]. J Natl Compr Canc Netw, 2011, 9(12): 1358-1395.

[135] Varadhachary GR, Talantov D, Raber MN, et al. Molecular profiling of carcinoma of unknown primary and correlation with clinical evaluation[J]. J Clin Oncol, 2008, 26(27):

4442 - 4448.

[136] Economopoulou P, Mountzios G, Pavlidis N, et al. Cancer of unknown primary origin in the genomic era: Elucidatingthe dark box of cancer[J]. Cancer Treat Rev, 2015, 41(7): 598 - 604.

[137] Hainsworth JD, Greco FA. Gene expression profiling in patients with carcinoma of unknown primary site: from translational research to standard of care[J]. Virchows Arch, 2014, 464(4): 393 - 402.

[138] Talantov D, Baden J, Jatkoe T, et al. A quantitative reverse transcriptase-polymerase chain reaction assay to identify metastatic carcinoma tissue of origin[J]. J Mol Diagn, 2006, 8(3): 320 - 329.

[139] Grosso G, Raspagliesi F, Baiocchi G, et al. Endometrioid carcinoma of the ovary: a retrospective analysis of 106 cases[J]. Tumori, 1998, 84(5): 552 - 557.

[140] Selves J, Long - Mira E, Mathieu MC, et al. Immunohistochemistry for diagnosis of metastatic carcinomas of unknown primary site[J]. Cancers (Basel), 2018, 10(4): 108 - 117.

[141] Tan D, Li O, Deeb G, et al. Thyroid tran scription facmr - 1 expression prevalence and its clinical implications in non - small cell lung cancer: a high - throughput tissue microarray an d immunohistochemistry study[J]. Hum Pathol, 2003, 34(6): 597 - 604.

[142] Chang YL, Lee YC, Liao WY, et a1. The utility and limitation of thyroid transcription factor - 1 protein in primary and metastatic pulmonary neoplasms[J]. Lung Cancer, 2004, 44(2): 149 - 157.

[143] Kuakpaetoon T. Immunohistochemistry of Cytokeratin 7, Cytokeratin 20 and Thyroid Transcription Factor - 1 in Metastatic Carcinoma of Cervical Lymph Node Biopsy for Identification of Pulmonary Origin in Rajavithi Hospital[J]. J Med Assoc Thai, 2017, 100(Suppl 1): S172 - S176.

[144] Satoh F, Umemura S, Osamum RY. Immunohistochemical analysis of GCDFP - 15 and GCDFP - 24 inmammary and non - mammary tissue[J]. Breast Cancer, 2000, 7(1): 49 - 55.

[145] Kaufmann O, Volmerig J, Dietel M. Uroplakin III is a highly specific and moderately sensitive immunohistechemical marker for primary and metastatic urothelial carcinomas[J]. Am J Clin Pathol, 2000, 113(5): 683 - 687.

[146] Parker DC, Folpe AL, Bell J, et a1. Potential utility of uroplakin III, thrombomodulin, high molecular weight cytokemtin, and cytokeratin 20 in non invasiv, invasive, and metastatic urothel(transitional cell) carcinomas[J]. Am J Surg Pathol, 2003, 27(1): 1 - 10.

[147] Hayashi H, Kurata T, Takiguchi Y, et al. Randomized Phase II Trial Comparing Site-

Specific Treatment Based on Gene Expression Profiling With Carboplatin and Paclitaxel for Patients With Cancer of Unknown Primary Site[J]. J Clin Oncol, 2019, 37(7): 570-579.

[148] Horlings HM, Vanlaar RK, Kerst JM, et al. Gene expression profiling to identify the histogenetic origin of metastatic adenocarcinomas of unknown primary[J]. J Clin Oncol, 2008, 26(27): 4435-4441.

[149] Losa F, Iglesias, Pane M, et al. 2018 consensus statement by the Spanish Society of Pathology and the Spanish Society of Medical Oncology on the diagnosis and treatment of cancer of unknown primary[J]. Clin Transl Oncol, 2018, 20(11): 1361-1372.

[150] Bochtler T, Reiling A, Endris V, et al. Integrated clinicomolecular characterization identifies RAS activation and CDKN2A deletion to predict prognosis in cancer of unknown primary[J]. Int J Cancer, 2020, 146(11): 3053-3064.

[151] Gatalica Z, Xiu J, Swensen J, et al. Comprehensive analysis of cancers of unknown primary for the biomarkers of response to immune checkpoint blockade therapy[J]. Eur J Cancer, 2018, 94: 179-186.

[152] Stella GM, Benvenuti S, Gramaglia D, et al. MET mutations in cancers of unknown primary origin (CUPs)[J]. Hum Mutat, 2011, 32(1): 44-50.

[153] Ross JS, Sokol ES, Moch H, et al. Comprehensive Genomic Profiling of Carcinoma of Unknown Primary Origin: Retrospective Molecular Classification Considering the CUPISCO Study Design[J]. Oncologist, 2021, 26(3): E394-E402.

[154] French CA, Kutok JL, Faquin WC, et al. Midline carcinoma of children and young adults with NUT rearrangement. J Clin Oncol, 2004, 22(20): 4135-4139.

[155] Cooper LA, Demicco EG, Saltz JH, et al. Pan-Cancer insights from The Cancer Genome Atlas: the pathologist's perspective[J]. J Pathol, 2018, 244(5): 512-524.

[156] Zhang Y, Wang P, Li X, et al. GABC: A comprehensive resource and Genome Atlas for Breast Cancer[J]. Int J Cancer, 2021, 148(4): 988-994.

[157] Wei IH, Shi Y, Jiang H, et al. RNA-Seq accurately identifies cancer biomarker signatures to distinguish tissue of origin[J]. Neoplasia, 2014, 16(11): 918-927.

[158] Ahmed AA, Abedalthagafi M. Cancer diagnostics: The journey from histomorphology to molecular profiling[J]. Oncotarget, 2016, 7(36): 58696-58708.

[159] Monzon FA, Lyons-Weiler M, Buturovic LJ, et al. Multicenter validation of a 1,550-gene expression profile for identification of tumor tissue of origin[J]. J Clin Oncol, 2009, 27(15): 2503-2508.

[160] Sun W, Wu W, Wang Q, et al. Clinical validation of a 90-gene expression test for tumor tissue of origin diagnosis: a large-scale multicenter study of 1417 patients[J]. J Transl Med, 2022, 20(1): 114.

[161] Dolled-Filhart MP, Rimm DL. Gene expression array analysis to determine tissue of origin

of carcinoma of unknown primary: cutting edge or already obsolete? [J]. Cancer Cytopathol, 2013, 121(3): 129-135.

[162] Weiss LM, Chu P, Schroeder BE, et al. Blinded comparator study of immunohistochemical analysis versus a 92-gene cancer classifier in the diagnosis of the primary site in metastatic tumors[J]. J Mol Diagn, 2013, 15(2): 263-269.

[163] Ma XJ, Patel R, Wang X, et al. Molecular classification of human cancers using a 92-gene real-time quantitative polymerase chain reaction assay[J]. Arch Pathol Lab Med, 2006, 130(4): 465-473.

[164] Tothill RW, Kowalczyk A, Rishin D, et al. An expression-based site of origin diagnostic method designed for clinical application to cancer of unknown origin[J]. Cancer Res, 2005, 65(10): 4031-4040.

[165] Rosenfeld N, Aharonov R, Meiri E, et al. MicroRNAs accurately identify cancer tissue origin[J]. Nat Biotechnol, 2008, 26(4): 462-469.

[166] Varaghachary GR, Spector Y, Abbruzzese JL, et al. Prospective gene signature study using microRNA to identify the tissue of origin in patients with carcinoma of unknown primary[J]. Clinical Cancer Research: An Official Journal of the American Association for Cancer Res, 2011, 17(12): 4063-4070.

[167] Ferracin M, Pedriali M, Veronese A, et al. MicroRNA profiling for the identification of cancers with unknown primary tissue-of-origin[J]. J Pathol, 2011, 225(1): 43-53.

[168] 王奇峰, 徐清华, 陈金影. 一种新型肿瘤组织起源分子标志物的建立与评价[J]. 中国癌症杂志, 2016, 26(10): 801-812.

[169] Moran S, Martinez-Cardus A, Sayols S, et al. Epigenetic profiling to classify cancer of unknown primary: a multicentre, retrospective analysis[J]. Lancet Oncol, 2016, 17(10): 1386-1395.

[170] Bochtler T, Loffler H, Kramer A. Diagnosis and management of metastatic neoplasms with unknown primary[J]. Semin Diagn Pathol, 2018, 35(3): 199-206.

[171] Lu MY, Chen TY, Williamson DFK, et al. AI-based pathology predicts origins for cancers of unknown primary[J]. Nature, 2021, 594(7861): 106-110.

[172] Tothill RW, Li J, Mileshkin L, et al. Massively-parallel sequencing assists the diagnosis and guided treatment of cancers of unknown primary[J]. J Pathol, 2013, 231(4): 413-423.

[173] Loffler H, Pfarr N, Kriegsmann M, et al. Molecular driver alterations and their clinical relevance in cancer of unknown primary site[J]. Oncotarget, 2016, 7(28): 44322-44329.

[174] Mileshkin LR, Sivakumaran T, Etemadmoghadam D, et al. Clinical impact of tissue of origin testing and mutation profiling in the solving unknown primary Cancer (SUPER)

national prospective study: Experience of the first two years[J]. J Clin Oncol, 2019, 37 (Suppl 15): 3072.

[175] Posner A, Prall OW, Sivakumaran T, et al. A comparison of DNA sequencing and gene expression profiling to assist tissue of origin diagnosis in cancer of unknown primary[J]. J Pathol, 2023, 259(1): 81-92.

[176] Hainsworth JD, Greco FA. Cancer of unknown primary site: new treatment paradigms in the era of precision medicine[J]. Am Soc Clin Oncol Educ Book, 2018, (38): 20-25.

[177] Schipper LJ, Samsom KG, Snaebjornsson P, et al, Complete genomic characterization in patients with cancer of unknown primary origin in routine diagnostics[J]. ESMO Open, 2022, 7(6): 100611.

[178] Xu Q, Chen J, Ni S, et al. Pan-cancer transcriptome analysis reveals a gene expression signature for the identification of tumor tissue origin[J]. Mod Pathol, 2016, 29(6): 546-556.

[179] Tothill RW, Kowalczyk A, Rischin D, et al. An expression-based site of origin diagnostic method designed for clinical application to cancer of unknown origin[J]. Cancer Res, 2005, 65(10): 4031-4040.

[180] Ye Q, Wang Q, Qi P, et al. Development and clinical validation of a 90-Gene expression assay for identifying tumor tissue origin[J]. J Mol Diagn, 2020, 22(9): 1139-1150.

[181] Hainsworth JD, Rubin MS, Spigel DR, et al. Molecular gene expression profiling to predict the tissue of origin and direct site-specific therapy in patients with carcinoma of unknown primary site: a prospective trial of the Sarah Cannon research institute[J]. J Clin Oncol, 2013, 31(2): 217-223.

[182] Mullauer L. Next generation sequencing: clinical applications in solid tumours[J]. Memo, 2017, 10(4): 244-247.

[183] Murugaesu N, Wilson GA, Birkbak NJ, et al. Tracking the genomic evolution of esophageal adenocarcinoma through neoadjuvant chemotherapy[J]. Cancer Discov, 2015, 5(8): 821-831.

[184] Ross JS, Wang K, Gay L, et al. Comprehensive genomic profiling of carcinoma of unknown primary site: new routes to targeted therapies[J]. JAMA Oncol, 2015, 1(1): 40-49.

[185] Varghese AM, Arora A, Capanu M, et al. Clinical and molecular characterization of patients with cancer of unknown primary in the modern era[J]. Ann Oncol, 2017, 28(12): 3015-3021.

[186] Moran S, Martinez-Cardus A, Boussios S, et al. Precision medicine based on epigenomics: the paradigm of carcinoma of unknown primary[J]. Nat Rev Clin Oncol, 2017, 14(11): 682-694.

[187] Koch A, Joosten SC, Feng Z, et al. Analysis of DNA methylation in cancer: location

revisited[J]. Nat Rev Clin Oncol, 2018, 15(7): 459-466.

[188] Moran S, Martínez-Cardús A, Sayols S, et al. Epigenetic profiling to classify cancer of unknown primary: a multicentre, retrospective analysis[J]. Lancet Oncol, 2016, 17(10): 1386-1395.

[189] Stackpole ML, Zeng W, Li S, et al. Cost-effective methylome sequencing of cell-free DNA for accurately detecting and locating cancer[J]. Nat Commun, 2022, 13(1): 5566.

[190] Liu MC, Oxnard GR, Klein EA, et al. Sensitive and specific multi-cancer detection and localization using methylation signatures in cell-free DNA[J]. Ann Oncol, 2020, 31(6): 745-759.

[191] Losa F, Fernandez I, Etxaniz O, et al. ESMO-GECOD clinical guideline for unknown primary cancer(2021)[J]. Clin Transl Oncol, 2022, 24(4): 681-692.

[192] Fernandez AF, Assenov Y, Martin-Subero JI, et al. A DNA methylation fingerprint of 1628 human samples[J]. Genome Res, 2012, 22(2): 407-419.

[193] Kato S, Krishnamurthy N, Banks KC, et al. Utility of Genomic Analysis In Circulating Tumor DNA from Patients with Carcinoma of Unknown Primary[J]. Cancer Res, 2017, 77(16): 4238-4246.

[194] Weipert C, Kato S, Saam J, et al. Utility of circulating cell-free DNA (cfDNA) analysis in patients with carcinoma of unknown primary (CUP) in identifying alterations with strong evidence for response or resistance to targeted therapy[J]. J Clin Oncol, 2020, 38(15): 105.

[195] Bridgewater J, Vanlaar R, Floore A, et al. Gene expression profiling may improve diagnosis in patients with carcinoma of unknown primary[J]. Br J Cancer, 2008, 98(8): 1425-1430.

[196] Pillai R, Deeter R, Rigl CT, et al. Validation and reproducibility of a microarray-based gene expression test for tumor identification informal in-fixed, paraffin-embedded specimens[J]. J Mol Diagn, 2011, 13(1): 48-56.

[197] Laprovitera N, Riefolo M, Porcelline E, et al. MicroRNA expression profiling with a droplet digital PCR assay enables molecular diagnosis and prognosis of cancers of unknown primary[J]. Mol Oncol, 2021, 15(10): 2732-2751.

[198] Skilde R, Vincent M, Mller AK, et al. Efficient identification of miRNAs for classification of tumor origin[J]. J Mol Diagn, 2014, 16(1): 106-115.

[199] Varadhachary GR, Spector Y, Abbruzzese JL, et al. Prospective gene signature study using microRNA to identify the tissue of origin in patients with carcinoma of unknown primary[J]. Clin Cancer Res, 2011, 17(12): 4063-4070.

[200] Gatalica Z, Millis SZ, Vranic S, et al. Comprehensive tumor profiling identifies numerous biomarkers of drug response in cancers of unknown primary site: analysis of 1806 cases[J].

Oncotarget, 2014, 5(23): 12440-12447.

[201] Ross JS, Sokol ES, Moch H, et al. Comprehensive genomic profiling (CGP) of carcinoma of unknown primary origin (CUP): Retrospective molecular classification of potentially eligible patients (pts) for targeted or immunotherapy treatment (tx) using the prospective CUPISCO trial's criteria[J]. Ann Oncol, 2019, 30(3): e394-e402..

[202] Fizazi K, Maillard A, Penel N, et al. A phase Ⅲ trial of empiric chemotherapy with cisplatin and gemcitabine or systemic treatment tailored by molecular gene expression analysis in patients with carcinomas of an unknown primary (CUP) site (GEFCAPI 04)[J]. Ann Oncol, 2019, 30(suppl 5): v851-934.

[203] Pauli C, Bochtler T, Mileshkin L, et al. A challenging task: identifying patients with cancer of unknown primary (CUP) according to ESMO guidelines: the CUPISCO trial experience[J]. Oncologist, 2021, 26(5): e769-e779.

[204] Shu X, Liu H, Ji J, et al. Subsequent cancers in patients diagnosed with cancer of unknown primary (CUP): etiological insights?[J]. Ann Oncol, 2012, 23(1): 269-275.

[205] Lugli A, Tzankov A, Zlobec I, et al. Differential diagnostic and functional role of the multi-marker phenotype CDX2/CK20/CK7 in colorectal cancer stratified by mismatch repair status[J]. Mod Pathol, 2008, 21(11): 1403-1412.

[206] Bahrami A, Gown AM, Baird GS, et al. Aberrant expression of epithelial and neuroendocrine markers in alveolar rhabdomyosarcoma: a potentially serious diagnostic pitfall[J]. Mod Pathol, 2008, 21(7): 795-806.

[207] Adams H, Schmid P, Dirnhofer S, et al. Cytokeratin expression in hematological neoplasms: a tissue microarray study on 866 lymphoma and leukemia cases[J]. Pathol Res Pract, 2008, 204(8): 569-573.

[208] Bree R. The real additional value of FDG-PET in detecting the occult primary tumour in patients with cervical lymph node metastases of unknown primary tumour[J]. Eur Arch Otorhinolaryngol, 2010, 267(11): 1653-1655.

[209] Fizazi K, Greco FA, Pavlidis N, et al. Cancers of unknown primary site: ESMO Clinical Practice Guidelines for diagnosis, treatment and follow-up[J]. Ann Oncol, 2011, 22(6): vi64-vi68.

[210] Briasoulis E, Pavlidis N. Cancer of unknown primary origin[J]. Oncologist, 1997, 2(3): 142-152.

[211] 洪亮. 原发灶不明转移癌的临床诊断[J]. 国际肿瘤学杂志, 2008, 35(10): 759-762.

[212] Michael J, Nissenblatt MD, Piscataway NJ. Carcinoma with unknown primary tumor (CUP syndrome)[J]. South Med J, 1981, 74(12): 1497-1502.

[213] Krämer A, Bochtler T, Pauli C, et al. Cancer of unknown primary: ESMO clinical practice guideline for diagnosis, treatment and follow-up[J]. Ann Oncol, 2023, 34(3): 228-246.

[214] Gallagher CJ, Reznek RH. Cancer of unknown primary site[J]. Clin Med, 2008, 8(4): 451-454.

[215] Bugat R, Bataillard A, Lesimple T, et al. Summary of the standards, options and recommendations for the patients with carcinoma of unknown primary site[J]. Br J Cancer, 2003, 89(Suppl1): S59-S66.

[216] Bridgewater J, Galle PR, Khan SA, et al. Guidelines for the diagnosis and management of intrahepatic cholangiocarcinoma[J]. J Hepatol, 2014, 60(6): 1268-1289.

[217] Conway AM, Morris GC, Smith S, et al. Intrahepatic cholangiocarcinoma hidden within cancer of unknown primary[J]. Br J Cancer, 2022, 127(3): 531-540.

[218] 韩雪梅, 陶维华, 王苑玲. 内科胸腔镜与闭式胸膜活检对胸腔积液的诊断价值比较[J]. 广东医学, 2011, 32(7): 903-905.

[219] Loddenkemper R. Thoracoscopy: state of the art[J]. Eur Respir J, 1998, 11(1): 213-221.

[220] Yap KH, Phillips MJ, Lee YC, et al. Medical thoracoscopy: rigid thoracoscopy or flexi-rigid pleuroscopy?[J]. Curr Opin Pulm Med, 2014, 20(4): 358-365.

[221] Liu J, Liu G, Liu X, et al. Clinical Value of Positron emission tomography-computed tomography combined with ultrasound in detection of primary tumors in patients with malignant ascites[J]. Cancer Biother Radiopharm, 2019, 34(3): 203-207.

[222] Amarapurkar D, Bhatt N, Patel N, et al. Diagnostic laparoscopy in the era of modern imaging-retrospective analysis from a single center[J]. Indian J Gastroenterol, 2013, 32(5): 302-306.

[223] Akhtar N, Hayat Z, Nazim F. Genital tuberculosis mimicking carcinoma ovary: can ultrasound guided biopsy be a resolution[J]. J Ayub Med Coll Abbottabad, 2017, 29(3): 496-498.

[224] Han N, Sun X, Qin C, et al. Value of ^{18}F-FDG PET/CT combined with tumor markers in the evaluation of ascites[J]. AJR Am J Roentgenol, 2018, 210(5): 1155-1163.

[225] Laghi A, Bellini D, Rengo M, et al. Diagnostic performance of computed tomography and magnetic resonance imaging for detecting peritoneal metastases: systematic review and meta-analysis[J]. Radiol Med, 2017, 122(1): 1-15.

[226] Bravo R, Jafari MD, Pigazzi A. The utility of diagnostic laparoscopy in patients being evaluated for cytoreductive surgery and hyperthermic peritoneal chemotherapy[J]. Am J Clin Oncol, 2018, 41(12): 1231-1234.

[227] Long Y, Tang A, Tian L, et al. Transumbilical endoscopic surgery in the diagnosis of

ascites of unknown origin[J]. Journal of Central South University Medical Scince, 2019, 44(6): 634-641.

[228] Trapé J, Gurt G, Franquesa J, et al. Diagnostic Accuracy of Tumor Markers CYFRA21-1 and CA125 in the Differential Diagnosis of Ascites[J]. Anticancer Res, 2015, 35(10): 5655-5660.

[229] 骆成玉,赵丹宁,李世拥,等. 大肠癌骨髓微转移的检测及其对治疗的反应[J]. 中国肿瘤临床与康复, 2001, 8(3): 28-29.

[230] Zaeh O, Ltm D. Tumor cell detection in peripheral blood and bone marrow[J]. Curt Opin Onto J, 2006, 18(1): 48-56.

[231] 胡响祥,朱思国,陈风. 骨髓转移癌患者的外周血象特征分析[J]. 临床和实验医学杂志, 2008, 9(7): 1532-1533.

[232] Fehm T, Becker S, Bachmann C, et al. Detection of disseminated tumor cells in patients with gynecological cancers[J]. Gynecol Oncol, 2006, 103(3): 942-947.

第七章

CUP 治疗与预后

第一节 治 疗

一、治疗原则

迄今为止，CUP 治疗尚缺乏充分的循证医学依据[1]，且无标准治疗方案推荐，故多数学者认为，最好由多学科专家讨论，达成一致意见。

英国 NICE 在其《原发灶不明转移癌诊治指南》中指出，当决定给予 CUP 患者进行治疗时，要考虑患者预后因素，尤其是体能状态（PS 评分）、肝转移灶、碱性磷酸酶（ALP）及血清白蛋白水平。

目前，对于 CUP 多主张采取以手术、放射治疗、化学治疗等综合治疗模式。多数 CUP 患者在诊断时已失去手术机会，但对孤立性转移的 CUP 患者，手术治疗或局部放射治疗仍是首选方法。

对于头颈部转移性鳞癌、腋窝淋巴结转移性腺癌及局限于腹股沟淋巴结转移性鳞癌患者，需由相应外科、放射治疗专家评估是否可行淋巴结清扫术和（或）放射治疗；对肝、脑、骨、皮肤或肺内孤立转移病变，请多学科专家讨论是否给予根治性局部治疗或手术切除。

对于可能有脑转移的多发性癌转移患者，请神经肿瘤学科专家讨论，除患者参加临床试验外，一般不给予化学治疗，因目前没有证据表明任何药物治疗可改善患者生存，仅有限的证据提示手术和（或）全脑放射治疗可控制神经系统症状。

对于有症状的、广泛转移的、PS 评分 0~2 分的 CUP 患者，或无症状的侵袭性强的 CUP 患者，可考虑化学治疗。若不具备则告知化学治疗可能的获益和风险，以及不能给患者提供参加临床试验的机会，当决定给予化学治疗时，应考虑其肿瘤的临床和病理特征、药物毒性反应及疗效。一般而言，化学治疗方案的选择应依据转移灶的组织病理学类型。

（一）根据转移性肿瘤组织病理制订治疗方案

1. 转移性腺癌

不明原发肿瘤转移性腺癌，最常见为分化良好与分化中等的腺癌。对于女性腋窝淋巴结转移性腺癌治疗上可同Ⅱ期乳腺癌，采用乳腺癌改良根治术、局部放射治疗、全身化学治疗、内分泌治疗、靶向治疗等；对于女性腹腔转移腺癌治疗上以开腹减瘤术加以铂类为基础的化学治疗；对于男性伴发 PSA 升高的转移性腺癌或成骨性骨转移患者，推荐抗雄激素内分泌治疗。

2. 转移性鳞癌

不明原发肿瘤转移性鳞癌，常见为颈部与锁骨上淋巴结转移性鳞癌，治疗上主要采用手术切除，或放射治疗（剂量和方法类似于原发头颈部肿瘤）；对于腹股沟淋巴结转移性鳞癌，以淋巴结清扫为首选，亦可选择放射治疗联合系统治疗；而其他部位淋巴结转移性鳞癌多来自肺部，可参考非小细胞肺癌系统治疗。

3. 转移性低分化癌

转移性低分化癌，其中 2/3 为分化不良癌，1/3 为分化不良腺癌，通常疾病进展迅速，发现时多已转移至淋巴结、纵隔和腹膜后，通常选择经验性系统治疗。

4. 转移性神经内分泌肿瘤

转移性神经内分泌肿瘤为一组具有侵袭性生物学行为的恶性肿瘤，常见有类癌、小细胞肺癌、胰腺神经内分泌癌、胰岛细胞瘤、肾上腺嗜铬细胞瘤、甲状腺髓样癌以及神经元副神经节瘤等，一般以系统化学治疗联合生物治疗为主。

（二）根据转移性肿瘤发生部位制订治疗方案

1. 淋巴结转移癌

不明原发肿瘤淋巴结转移癌，应结合病理类型、体能状态评分，选择手术/放射治疗或联合化学治疗的综合治疗。

2. 内脏转移癌

不明原发肿瘤内脏转移癌，需根据病理类型、疾病进展速度与机体状况决定治疗策略，其预后一般较差，对于估计可切除的大肿块，应尽可能手术切除。

3. 脑转移癌

不明原发肿瘤脑转移癌，单发者可手术治疗，症状明显者需缓解颅内高压，可考虑开颅术或减压术，放射治疗、化学治疗均可选择，小分子、脂溶性易通过血脑屏障的药物可静脉、口服给药，同时可联合鞘内药物注射。

4. 肺转移癌

不明原发肿瘤肺转移癌，全身化学治疗与局部放射治疗或手术切除治疗相结合可取得较好疗效。

5. 肝转移癌

对于不明原发肿瘤肝转移癌患者，全身状况较好且病灶孤立或局限者，手术是其首选方法；不适于手术者，可选择肝动脉介入药物灌注和(或)栓塞、消融(包括射频、微波、冷冻等)治疗等。

6. 骨转移癌

关于不明原发肿瘤骨转移癌的治疗，目前尚存争议，缺乏明确的治疗指南。预后良好型，如伴成骨性转移和PSA水平升高的男性患者可按转移性前列腺癌治疗，首先进行药物去势，内分泌治疗失败后可考虑化学治疗[2]。预后不良型，相关荟萃分析显示[3-4]，铂类、紫杉醇类等化学治疗药物对此类型患者的治疗并不能有效延长生存期。因此，对于骨转移CUP患者治疗而言，多数学者认为[5-8]，应根据组织学类型、全身体能状况和生存评估，对于伴有孤立、疼痛、承重部位、潜在性骨折的患者，若患者全身状况良好、肿瘤可切除者选择广泛切除，潜在性骨折者可选择外科固定或选择放射治疗；若患者全身状况差，可选择单独放射治疗；对病理性骨折患者可选择外科治疗和椎管减压。

7. 骨髓转移癌

骨髓转移癌患者通常表现为贫血、血小板减少和全血细胞减少，单纯输血等对症支持治疗无法从根本上改善患者生存。研究表明[9-10]，仅对症支持治疗的患者中位生存期仅1个月，而积极的抗肿瘤治疗(如系统治疗)后生存时间可延长至1年。

8. 卵巢转移癌

对于孤立的卵巢转移或局部进展的肿瘤，一般通过手术可延长患者生存，而对伴腹膜有播散的患者应避免积极的手术治疗[11]。

Taylor等[12]报道，若原发肿瘤为结直肠腺癌的卵巢转移患者使用5-

FU、胃腺癌卵巢转移患者使用顺铂联合 5 - FU 的化学治疗,其有效患者的中位生存时间为 20 个月,而无效患者中位生存时间仅 9 个月。

(三)根据转移性肿瘤患者预后制订治疗方案

有学者根据转移性肿瘤的临床和病理学特征,将 CUP 分为预后良好型与预后不良型[13]。临床上,仅有 15%~20% 的 CUP 患者属于预后良好型,80%~85% 的 CUP 患者为预后不良型。有研究报道[14-15],预后良好的 CUP 患者中位生存期为 12 个月,1 年生存率 45%,预后不良的 CUP 患者中位生存期仅 8 个月,1 年生存率仅 11%。

1. 预后良好型 CUP

除单一部位和寡转移性 CUP 外,预后良好型 CUP 与某些已知原发肿瘤有明显相似之处,一般建议这些患者接受针对假定原发肿瘤部位的特定治疗,因与绝大多数 CUP 患者相比,这些患者预后较好[16]。

目前认可的预后良好型 CUP,主要有可接受局部消融治疗的单发转移性疾病(单发或寡转移性 CUP)、有孤立性腋窝淋巴结转移的女性 CUP(乳腺样 CUP)、累及非锁骨上的鳞状细胞癌、浆液性乳头状腺癌、腹膜癌的女性(卵巢样 CUP)、有小细胞癌骨转移和(或)IHC 或血清 PSA 表达的男性(前列腺样 CUP)、具有结直肠 IHC(CK7 阴性、CK20 阳性、CDX2 阳性)或分子特征的腺癌(结肠类 CUP),以及具有肾细胞组织学和免疫组化特征的腺癌(肾样 CUP)。

单一转移或寡转移是指转移灶数量不超过 5 个,且未累及弥漫性器官,如胸膜、心包膜、腹膜或脑膜。这类 CUP 患者通过手术和(或)放射治疗对所有病灶进行局部消融治疗被认为是可行的[17-18],有研究报道[19-20],局部治疗可观察到此类患者长期生存的结果。对于单发脑转移[21-22]、颈部淋巴结转移(不包括锁骨上淋巴结)[23],以及腹股沟、髂淋巴结转移性鳞癌[24],可将局部治疗作为其标准治疗方法。然而,单一转移或寡转移性 CUP 患者在接受消融手术和(或)RT 局部治疗前,应进行 PET/CT 和脑 MRI 检查。

1)头颈部样 CUP

累及非锁骨上颈淋巴结的鳞癌(头颈部 CUP)是指鳞状细胞癌累及非锁骨上颈淋巴结,但影像学检查未发现原发肿瘤。

确定原发肿瘤的方法,应包括内镜检查、对比增强 CT 和(或)最好是

第七章 CUP治疗与预后

头颈部的 MRI 以及 FDG PET。

如果经过这些检查仍无法确定原发肿瘤，则应进行鼻咽、下咽部和口咽部进行内镜检查及活检，同时进行双侧扁桃体切除术。

通常需检测肿瘤组织 p16 表达，如果阳性，还应检测人类乳头瘤病毒（HPV）、EB 病毒（EBV），对于疾病复发或远处转移的患者，可检测 PD-L1 的表达[25]。

一般而言，对于头颈部 CUP 推荐将颈部淋巴结切除和（或）放射治疗±化学治疗作为非远处转移性疾病的一线治疗方案。颈部病变体积小的患者应接受手术或放射治疗±化学治疗，而体积大的患者则应同时接受这两种治疗。头颈部 CUP 综合治疗，5 年生存率为 20%～60%。

2）乳腺样 CUP

女性孤立性腋窝淋巴结转移（乳腺样 CUP）是指女性孤立性腋窝淋巴结转移性腺癌与乳腺癌免疫组化结果相符，且同侧无乳腺癌影像学证据。

在多项回顾性分析中，约 2/3 临床检查阴性和乳腺 X 线检查阴性的患者通过乳腺 MRI 发现了原发肿瘤[26]。因此，在诊断乳腺样 CUP 之前必须进行乳腺 MRI 检查，淋巴结转移标本应检测雌激素受体（ER）、孕激素受体（PR）和人类表皮生长因子受体 2（HER-2）的状态[27]。

乳腺样 CUP 患者应假定为隐匿性原发性乳腺癌，并遵循原发性乳腺癌治疗方案。关于腋窝淋巴结清扫，已达成广泛共识[28]。

采用乳房切除术或放射治疗进行同侧乳房靶向治疗可降低复发风险并提高生存率；然而，关于首选局部治疗是手术治疗还是放射治疗，目前没有一致的意见。就局部复发和无复发生存率而言，腋窝淋巴结清扫后的乳腺放射治疗似乎至少与乳房切除术相当，提示该类患者可以避免手术[29-32]。

在选择放射治疗时，是否应将锁骨上淋巴结或乳腺内区域淋巴结纳入放射治疗范围，目前没有一致的观点[32]。

乳腺样 CUP 患者的系统治疗应与乳腺癌的现行治疗标准保持一致，包括内分泌治疗（如果 ER 或 PR 阳性）、化学治疗（蒽环类或紫杉醇类为基础）、靶向治疗（HER-2 过表达，或扩增阳性），此类患者 5 年生存率为 75%，10 年生存率为 60%[33]。

3）卵巢样 CUP

女性腹膜浆液性乳头状腺癌（卵巢样 CUP）是指（孤立的）女性腹膜浆液性或未分化腺癌，无卵巢、输卵管或子宫原发癌[34]，可能与原发性腹膜浆液性癌相同[35]。

IHC、基因分析发现，卵巢样 CUP 患者通常 CA125 升高和 BRCA1/2 基因突变，与卵巢癌的特征相符[36]。

可采用与Ⅲ/Ⅳ期卵巢癌的治疗方法，即细胞减灭术[37]后进行卡铂+紫杉醇±贝伐单抗，并对治疗有反应的患者进行多聚(ADP-核糖)聚合酶(PARP)抑制剂维持治疗[38]。

卵巢样 CUP 一般对化学治疗较敏感，30%~40%的患者可达到完全缓解(CR)，70%部分缓解(PR)，中位 OS 为 3 年[39]。

4) 结直肠样 CUP

具有结直肠 IHC(CK7 阴性、CK20 阳性、CDX2 阳性)或分子特征的腺癌(结直肠样 CUP)是指腺癌组织学符合消化道原发、腹腔内转移为主、CK7 阴性、CK20 阳性、CDX2 阳性、具有 CRC 特征的 IHC 标志以及结肠镜检查阴性[40-41]。回顾性数据表明[40]，结肠样 CUP 患者接受 FOLFOX 或 FOLFIRI 方案治疗，其反应率和生存率与转移性 CRC 患者相似。对于微卫星稳定(MSS)的肿瘤患者，可采用以 5-FU 为基础的治疗方案(即 FOLFOX 或 FOLFIRI)，对于 KRAS 或 NRAS 未突变的患者，可与抗表皮生长因子受体(EGFR)抗体联合使用[42]；对于 MSI-H 的肿瘤患者，应使用 ICIs[43]。

因 CK20 在 MSI-H 型 CRC 中表达减少或缺失，对于 CK20 阴性、MSI-H 型 CUP 且符合结肠样标准的患者，也可考虑诊断为结肠样 CUP，采用晚期结直肠系统治疗方案[44]。

5) 前列腺样 CUP

男性骨盆、脊柱下部的成骨转移和(或)血清中 PSA 的高浓度或 IHC 表达水平与转移性前列腺癌的结果十分相似，通常建议前列腺样 CUP 的诊断程序和治疗方法应与转移性前列腺癌一致[45]，包括抗雄激素内分泌治疗、化学治疗(当肿瘤对去势治疗抵抗时)、局部放射治疗(骨转移部位疼痛明显、存在病理性骨折风险、脊髓压迫等)及双膦酸盐、地舒单抗等舒缓治疗[2]。

6) 肾样 CUP

临床上有少部分 CUP 患者在没有发现任何肾脏病变的情况下，其转移性肿瘤组织学、免疫组化特征似乎与肾细胞癌相吻合。有研究报道[46-47]，对肾脏特异性治疗的反应支持肾脏原发推定的准确性，应用 TKIs 和 ICIs 治疗可获得较好的远期疗效。

7) 其他预后良好型 CUP

对于孤立性腹股沟淋巴结转移性鳞癌，可通过手术达到根治，术后视情况行局部放射治疗，或辅以术后化学治疗，患者可获得长期无瘤生存[2]。

转移性神经内分泌癌化学治疗方案可参照小细胞肺癌，通常采用以铂类为基础的联合化学治疗，中位生存时间为 15.5 个月[48]。肿瘤生长局限者，新辅助化学治疗缓解率可高达 50%~70%，其中有 25% 完全缓解，10%~15% 的患者可长期生存；或先手术切除后再进行辅助化学治疗。

沿中线分布的低分化或未分化癌多为 20~35 岁男性，其生物学特征类似于性腺外生殖细胞肿瘤，推荐铂类为基础的两药方案，ORR 为 45%~65%，CR 为 20%~25%，中位 OS 为 12 个月[49-50]。

2. 预后不良型 CUP

预后不良型 CUP 是指不属于上述任何预后较好的 CUP 患者，主要包括大部分原发肿瘤不明的转移性腺癌或低分化癌，发生部位通常有内脏转移癌、骨髓转移癌及恶性浆膜腔积液。

根据小样本临床研究数据，尽管这类患者接受了联合化学治疗，但预后不佳[51]。

目前，对这部分 CUP 患者而言，唯一的治疗目标是获得较好的生活质量，但也有罕见治愈病例的报道[52]。

对于预后不良型 CUP 患者的治疗，临床上往往采用经验性化学治疗。一项荟萃分析显示[4]，预后不良型 CUP 患者接受经验性化学治疗后中位生存时间为 8.9 个月，3 年生存率为 12%。

迄今为止，Ⅱ期临床试验评估了由铂类、紫杉醇类、吉西他滨、长春碱或伊立替康组成的治疗方案，但没有证据表明任何方案具有统计学意义上的显著疗效[53-57]。

尽管目前还没有随机试验证明化学治疗优于最佳支持治疗，但一般建议将以铂类药物为基础的两药联合化学治疗作为标准治疗。

据报道[53]，"顺铂+吉西他滨"的疗效优于单用顺铂，但这并没有在一项大型且有足够样本量的Ⅲ期随机试验中进行验证。

在一项随机Ⅱ期试验中[54]，"顺铂+吉西他滨"的疗效优于"顺铂+伊立替康"，且毒性更低。"卡铂+紫杉醇"亦在 CUP 中显示出一定疗效[56]。

一项单臂研究发现[58]，102 例预后不良型 CUP 患者接受"卡铂+多柔比星+依托泊苷"方案化学治疗，ORR 为 26.5%，中位 OS、PFS 分别为 9 个月、4个月。有研究评估了"吉西他滨+卡铂+紫杉醇"联合化学治疗在预后不良型CUP患者中的疗效，ORR为25%，mOS、PFS分别为9个月和6个月[59]。Hainsworth等[60]对"紫杉醇+卡铂+依托泊苷"与"吉西他滨+伊立替康"在198例预后不良型CUP患者中的疗效和毒性进行了比较研究，结果发现，两组在中位生存时间上相近，分别为7.4个月、8.5个月，但"吉西他滨+伊立替康"组患者毒性反应相对更小。因此，一般推荐将两药联合化学治疗方案作为标准治疗，而三药联合化学治疗毒性过大，不推荐使用。

根据其他常见鳞状细胞癌（包括宫颈癌、头颈部癌、非小细胞肺癌和食管癌）的情况推断，对于不同组织学类型的预后不良型CUP，一般也建议采用以铂类药物为基础的两药联合化学治疗。

目前还没有二线化学治疗方案的临床试验数据，在进展中的CUP患者进行化学治疗方案间的转换似乎是合理的；通常情况下，分子靶向药物和ICIs可作为预后不良型CUP二线治疗选择。

目前还没有高级别证据表明，基因表达谱指导治疗可改善预后不良型CUP患者的预后。

鉴于预后不良型CUP患者治疗缺乏高水平的临床证据，故鼓励患者参加临床试验。

二、外科治疗

因CUP特殊的生物学行为，且CUP临床分期通常为Ⅳ期（疑似原发性头颈部肿瘤颈部淋巴结转移性鳞癌、疑似乳腺癌腋窝淋巴结转移性腺癌除外），故手术切除作为CUP局部治疗的应用受到限制，一般可作为减轻瘤负荷、缓解症状（如梗阻、疼痛）、进一步获取组织标本等时应用，而手术指征、切除范围等尚存在争议。

多数学者认为[16,61]，CUP的外科治疗一般主要针对预后良好型，该类患者术前需对其临床特征、转移灶组织病理类型、患者体能状态等进行充分评估，以孤立性或局限性病灶能进行根治性手术为基本原则，否则应放弃外科手术。

对于女性孤立腋窝淋巴结转移性腺癌、原发性颈部淋巴结转移性鳞癌、女性腹膜浆液性乳头状腺癌、腹股沟淋巴结孤立性转移性鳞癌，以及单发、病灶局限且较小的来源不明转移性肿瘤等可考虑采取积极的手术治疗方式，一般可获得较长的生存期。

下篇 不明原发肿瘤
第七章 CUP治疗与预后

表 7-1 CUP 总体治疗原则

分类	转移性肿瘤部位		治疗原则
已明确原发肿瘤	/		参考相应原发肿瘤治疗指南
不明原发肿瘤 腺癌或非特异性癌	头颈部		参考头颈部肿瘤治疗指南
	锁骨上		参考头颈部肿瘤治疗指南
	腋窝		参考乳腺肿瘤治疗指南
	纵隔	<40岁	手术切除；如有临床指征，可考虑放射治疗
		40~50岁	参考睾丸癌治疗指南，或生殖细胞瘤治疗指南
		≥50岁	参考睾丸癌治疗指南，或生殖细胞瘤治疗指南，或参考非小细胞肺癌治疗指南；如有临床指征，可考虑放射治疗
	肺（结节）		参考非小细胞肺癌治疗指南
	胸腔积液	乳腺标记物阳性	如果可以完全切除，考虑手术治疗
		其他	首选临床试验，考虑系统治疗，控制症状
			立体定向放射治疗或立体定向消融放射治疗
			按乳腺肿瘤 CACA 指南治疗
			首选临床试验，考虑系统治疗，控制症状
			高度怀疑肺原发（Ⅳ期），按非小细胞肺癌指南治疗
	腹膜转移/腹腔积液	组织学检查与卵巢癌一致	按卵巢癌指南治疗
		其他	首选临床试验，考虑系统治疗，控制症状

续表

分类	转移性肿瘤部位		治疗原则
不明原发肿瘤	腺癌或非特异性癌	腹膜后肿块 组织学检查与生殖细胞肿瘤一致	参考睾丸癌治疗指南或生殖细胞瘤治疗指南
		腹膜后肿块 非生殖细胞	手术和(或)放射治疗,考虑对特定患者系统治疗
		腹股沟(结节) 单侧	淋巴结清扫;如有临床指征,考虑放射治疗,±系统治疗
		腹股沟(结节) 双侧	双侧淋巴结清扫,考虑临床指征,考虑放射治疗±系统治疗
		肝 不可切除	按转移性肿瘤治疗和(或)考虑局部治疗
		肝 可切除	手术切除±系统治疗;医学上存在手术禁忌症者,按"不可切除"处理
		骨	承重部位孤立性病变、疼痛性病变,可能发生骨折的病变,即将发生骨折的手术的病变(状态良好的患者)和(或)放射治疗
		脑	参考中枢神经系统肿瘤治疗指南
	鳞癌	头颈部	参考头颈部肿瘤治疗指南
		锁骨上	参考头颈部肿瘤治疗指南
		腋窝	手术切除;如有临床指征,可考虑放射治疗±系统治疗
		纵隔	参考非小细胞肺癌治疗指南
		肺(多发性结节)	首选临床试验,考虑系统治疗,控制症状
		胸腔积液	首选临床试验,考虑系统治疗,考虑放射治疗,控制症状
		腹股沟(结节) 单侧	淋巴结清扫;如有临床指征,考虑放射治疗±系统治疗
		腹股沟(结节) 双侧	双侧淋巴结清扫,考虑临床指征,考虑放射治疗±系统治疗

续表

分类		转移性肿瘤部位	治疗原则
不明原发肿瘤	鳞癌	骨	承重部位孤立性病变、疼痛性病变,可能发生骨折的病变;即将发生骨折的患者(状态良好的患者)和(或)放射治疗
		脑	参考中枢神经系统肿瘤治疗指南
		广泛转移	控制症状,首选临床试验,考虑系统治疗

表7-2 CUP不同预后情况治疗方案的选择

预后分型	转移肿瘤部位	倾向性原发肿瘤	治疗建议
预后良好型	颈部转移性鳞癌	头颈部鳞癌	颈淋巴结清扫+局部放射治疗±辅助化学治疗
	腋窝淋巴结转移性腺癌(女性)	乳腺癌	腋窝淋巴结清扫,乳腺切除或乳腺放射治疗+辅助化学治疗±内分泌治疗±靶向治疗
	腹膜浆液性乳头状转移性腺癌	卵巢癌	减瘤手术+紫杉醇/铂类联合化学治疗
	腹股沟淋巴结转移性鳞癌	宫颈癌	腹股沟淋巴结清扫+局部放射治疗±辅助化学治疗
	伴PSA升高的成骨转移性腺癌(男性)	前列腺癌	雄激素阻断治疗
	中线部位的低分化癌	生殖细胞肿瘤	以铂类为基础的联合化学治疗
	伴有结直肠癌免疫组化CK20阳性/CDX2阳性/CK7阴性	结直肠癌	化学治疗±靶向治疗±免疫治疗
	低分化神经内分泌肿瘤	可发生于多个部位	铂类+依托泊苷治疗
	高分化神经内分泌肿瘤	可发生于多个部位	链脲菌素+氟尿嘧啶、舒尼替尼、依维莫司
	孤立性转移灶	某一器官(如肺、肝)	手术和(或)放射治疗±系统治疗

续表

预后分型	转移肿瘤部位	倾向性原发肿瘤	治疗建议
预后不良型	转移性腺癌或低分化癌	无倾向性原发肿瘤	手术和(或)放射治疗±系统治疗(如经验性化学治疗、靶向治疗，若全身状况良好，肿瘤还可选择放射固定、免疫治疗)
	骨转移癌	单纯骨转移	孤立、疼痛、承重部位，进行或潜在性骨折的患者，若全身状况良好，肿瘤可切除的选择广泛切除，进行性骨折的治疗，可选择单独放射治疗；若全身状况差，可选择单独放射治疗，对病理性骨折可选择缓解性外科治疗和椎管减压术；控制疼痛，双膦酸盐类药物，地舒单抗
	骨髓转移	通常为病理类型不明	经验性化学治疗
	恶性胸腹腔积液	多为腺癌	全身系统治疗联合腔内药物灌注
	脑转移	通常为病理类型不明	放射治疗+经验性化学治疗+靶向治疗(如贝伐单抗)

表7-3 CUP外科、放射治疗、内科综合治疗选择建议

治疗方法	腺癌	鳞癌
外科治疗	肺转移性结节可切除者，建议手术切除	部位特殊早期性鳞癌，局部腋窝或腹股沟淋巴结受累的患者，建议手术切除
	肝转移性结节可切除者，建议手术切除	
	非生殖细胞转移组织的腹膜后肿块，建议手术切除	
	腹股沟转移性淋巴结，建议行淋巴结清扫	PS评分良好，建议手术治疗
	PS评分良好且负重部位有可能发生骨折的骨转移患者，建议手术切除	PS评分良好且负重部位有可能发生骨折的骨转移患者，建议手术治疗

第七章 CUP治疗与预后

续表

治疗方法	腺癌	鳞癌
放射治疗	转移性局部病变生长快的患者，建议行根治性放射治疗	
	对有症状的患者，可进行舒缓性放射治疗	
	对于局限性（1~3个）转移灶和肺转移灶，考虑采用SBRT/立体定向消融放射治疗（SABR）转移灶[（48~60）Gy/（4~5）次]	
	单个转移结节，但有结节外浸润，或手术结节清扫不充分，或有多个阳性结节，考虑在淋巴结清扫后行辅助放射治疗	
	对于转移位异侧腹股沟淋巴结转移的患者，可考虑单独放射治疗	
	双侧腹股沟淋巴结转移的患者，局部腺窝或腹股沟区肿块，可考虑放射治疗	
	非生殖细胞组织学的腹膜后转移，可考虑放射治疗	
	PS评分良好且负重严重的骨转移患者，可考虑放射治疗	
	无法控制的疼痛，即将发生病理性骨折或即将发生脊髓压迫的骨转移患者，建议采用低分次放射治疗	
系统治疗	有症状（PS为1~2分）或无症状（PS为0分）的侵袭性肿瘤患者，可考虑接受系统治疗	
	根据转移灶肿瘤组织学类型选择相应系统治疗方案	
	恶性胸腔积液，疑似肺癌、乳腺癌，按Ⅳ期非小细胞肺癌、乳腺癌治疗	
	预后特征良好患者，选择特定的系统治疗方案，如疑似结肠原发癌，选择以氟尿嘧啶为基础的治疗；疑似生殖细胞瘤的治疗，选择以顺铂为基础的治疗	
	BRAF V600E基因突变阳性患者，选择达拉非尼+曲美替尼	
	NTRK基因融合阳性患者，选择恩曲替尼，或拉罗替尼	

· 227 ·

预后不良型患者不推荐常规手术治疗,如包括累及多个器官(如肝、肺、骨、肾上腺等)、低分化癌、多发性脑转移肿瘤(如腺癌或鳞癌)、多发性转移性骨肿瘤(如腺癌或鳞癌)、多发性肺/胸膜转移癌(腺癌、鳞癌,包括形成恶性胸腔积液)、腹膜转移(包括形成恶性腹腔积液)、腹腔广泛种植转移等[14]。

对不明原发肿瘤的脊柱转移的治疗目的主要侧重于缓解疼痛、保护神经功能、预防病理性骨折、保持脊柱稳定性等[62-66]。目前,脊柱转移瘤的主要治疗手段包括止痛等对症治疗、放射治疗、化学治疗以及手术治疗,开放性手术治疗指征为预期生存时间 >3 个月、肿瘤或病理性骨折压迫神经或引起脊柱不稳、肿瘤对放射治疗不敏感、诊断不明确而需病理学确诊[67]。对于一般情况差,不能耐受手术治疗或生存预期 <3 个月的患者,应采取舒缓治疗,如应用止痛药物、双膦酸盐类药物、放射性核素治疗、局部放射治疗等。

孤立性腹膜癌,原则上可采用细胞缩减手术、腹腔热灌注化学治疗(HIPEC)作为局部治疗[68],但疗效不确定。

一项针对结肠癌和腹膜癌患者进行的随机研究显示[69],采用减瘤手术治疗时加用 HIPEC,其疗效不佳且毒性更大。

有研究报道[70-72],腹膜切除的细胞减灭手术可延长 CUP 患者生存时间。因此,对于卵巢样或结肠样 CUP 和孤立性腹膜癌的患者,可以选择腹膜切除术,但不建议进行额外的 HIPEC,因目前还没有关于该方法在 CUP 中应用的数据。

对进行减瘤术的 CUP 人群要仔细、严格地筛选,一般而言,良好的 PS 评分、较低的肿瘤负荷、腹膜癌指数(PCI)、排除任何额外的腹腔外转移的 CUP 患者,可选择减瘤术[73]。

值得注意的是,预后不良型 CUP 患者不推荐进行腹膜切除术。

三、放射治疗

放射治疗亦是 CUP 局部治疗方法之一,在 CUP 舒缓治疗中具有一定的临床应用价值。

一项回顾性研究评估了调强放射治疗在 260 例颈部淋巴结转移的 CUP 患者中的疗效[74],5 年 OS、区域控制和无远处转移生存率分别为 84%、91% 和 94%。Mourad 等[75]对 68 例不明原发肿瘤转移性头颈部鳞癌患者的放射治疗结果进行了回顾性分析，这些患者接受了口咽精准放射治疗，以保留鼻咽、下咽和喉部的黏膜表面，40%的患者接受了IMRT，56%的患者同时接受了化学治疗，结果显示，局部控制率为95.5%，局部复发的中位时间为18个月；放射治疗相关毒性包括Ⅰ级口腔异物感、吞咽困难、颈部僵硬和肢体瘫痪。

Janssen等[76]对28例颈椎转移性CUP患者进行了IMRT，多数患者（71%）同时接受了系统治疗，没有患者出现局部复发，也未报道Ⅱ级或以上不良事件。

一般而言，对于CUP下列情况可选择放射治疗。

（1）淋巴结清扫术后的后续治疗，若肿瘤仅限于单个结节部位但有结节外扩展，或结节清扫不彻底且有多个阳性结节，则可能适于辅助放射治疗。

（2）对于病变局限者，可考虑进行根治性放射治疗。

（3）对于骨病变、非生殖细胞组织学的腹膜后肿块或锁骨上淋巴结转移性鳞癌，可考虑单纯放射治疗。

（4）立体定向消融放射治疗（SABR）可用于局限性（1~3个）转移或肺转移。

（5）对于疼痛无法控制、即将发生病理性骨折或脊髓即将受到压迫的无症状患者，可考虑采用大分割放射治疗。

四、内科治疗

对于已明确的原发肿瘤内科系统治疗原则，按相应原发肿瘤治疗方案进行。

对于最终确诊为CUP患者而言，无论组织病理学何种类型，内科系统治疗对提高患者生存质量、延长患者生存均具有重要意义[77]。

CUP内科系统治疗主要包括化学治疗、靶向治疗及免疫治疗，然而80%~85%的CUP患者对药物治疗敏感性不高，中位生存期一般<1年，体力状态良好和LDH正常的患者平均预期寿命为1年，而两者均不佳者，中位生存期仅为4个月[16]。

一般而言，对与广泛转移患者的内科系统治疗应仅限于有症状且PS为1~2分的患者，或无症状且肿瘤具有明显侵袭性且PS评分为0分的患者。

(一)化学治疗

目前,没有任何特定的化学治疗方案被推荐为标准治疗方案[78],主要根据转移性肿瘤组织病理类型选择化学治疗方案,CUP 主要组织病理类型包括腺癌、鳞癌与神经内分泌癌。

通常而言,CUP 化学治疗多选择广谱细胞毒性药物[79]。目前,多数 CUP 患者使用的是经验性化学治疗,经验性化学治疗多采用以铂类、紫杉醇类、吉西他滨、氟尿嘧啶类为基础的方案。欧洲 ESMO、美国 NCCN 指南推荐的化学治疗方案主要有顺铂+吉西他滨、紫杉醇+卡铂、多西他赛+卡铂、卡培他滨+奥沙利铂、吉西他滨+伊立替康等[16,49]。

对于大多数预后不良型 CUP 患者而言,经验性化学治疗在传统上被认为是标准的一线治疗,但获益并不显著,其 ORR<40%,mOS<11 个月,2 年生存率<20%[80]。Losa 等[49]报道,ORR 为 25%~35%,mOS 为 8~11 个月。

一项研究纳入 683 例 CUP 患者,比较了铂类、紫杉醇类、吉西他滨、伊立替康在 CUP 中的疗效[3],结果显示,不同治疗方案疗效无明显差异。另一项随机Ⅱ期临床研究[81],一线使用紫杉醇+卡铂经验性化学治疗方案,联合或不联合贝利司他(一种组蛋白去乙酰化酶抑制剂)治疗 CUP,共入组 89 例患者(联合组 44 例,不联合组 45 例),联合组 ORR 提高(45% vs. 21%,$P=0.02$),但 mPFS(5.4 个月 vs. 5.3 个月,$P=0.20$)和 mOS(12.4 个月 vs. 9.1 个月,$P=0.85$)延长均无统计学意义。

另外,Hasegawa 等[82]认为,CUP 患者采用器官特异性化学治疗优于经验性化学治疗。

一项前瞻性、单中心研究入组 252 例 CUP 患者,采用 92 基因分类模型判定组织器官来源,247 例(98%)患者明确了组织器官来源,其中 194 例接受器官特异性化学治疗患者的 mOS 为 12.5 个月,较既往经验性化学治疗(mOS 为 9.1 个月)生存延长[83]。Hainsworth 等[41]采用 92 基因分类模型对 1544 例 CUP 患者组织来源进行鉴定,其中 125 例(8%)患者推测原发肿瘤为结直肠癌,可能性>80%,32 例患者接受结直肠癌的化学治疗方案,mOS 为 27 个月,明显高于经验性化学治疗,且与已知的结直肠癌患者生存类似。

但一项针对 CUP 患者的Ⅱ期随机对照临床试验结果显示,基因表达谱

第七章 CUP治疗与预后

指导下的器官特异性化学治疗并未显示出优于经验性化学治疗的疗效[84]。Nishikawa等[85]的研究中，器官特异性化学治疗组和经验性化学治疗组的总生存率亦未显示出统计学差异。Rassy等[86]对已报道的4项针对CUP患者的经验性化学治疗和器官特异性化学治疗疗效对比的前瞻性研究进行的一项Meta分析发现，接受器官特异性化学治疗的CUP患者有获益倾向，但差异尚未达到统计学意义（$P=0.06$）。

综上所言，对于经验性化学治疗与器官特异性化学治疗孰优孰劣，尚需要更多的循证医学证据。

1. 腺癌

对于CUP中分化差的腺癌，以顺铂为基础的化学治疗方案，两项研究报道[87-88]的CR分别为12%、26%，ORR分别为53%、63%。在一项以顺铂为基础的化学治疗方案研究中，具有生殖细胞外特征的肿瘤患者的反应率较高，未分化癌患者的反应率高于分化不良癌患者（79%对35%；$P=0.02$）[88]。

以紫杉醇类药物为基础的化学治疗CUP腺癌患者，1年、2年、3年和4年生存率分别为42%、22%、17%和17%，mOS为10个月[89]。

1）紫杉醇+卡铂

在德国CUP研究组进行的一项随机前瞻性Ⅱ期研究中[55]，"紫杉醇+卡铂"的临床疗效优于"吉西他滨+长春瑞滨"，"紫杉醇+卡铂"治疗患者的中位OS、1年生存率和ORR分别为11.0个月、38%和23.8%，而"吉西他滨+长春瑞滨"治疗患者的中位OS、1年生存率和ORR分别为7.0个月、29%和20%。

2）紫杉醇+卡铂+卡培他滨

一项Ⅱ期研究纳入25例不明原发肿瘤转移性腺癌患者[90]，采用"卡培他滨+紫杉醇+卡铂"治疗，结果显示，ORR为32%，mPFS为5.5个月，mOS为10.8个月。

3）紫杉醇+卡铂±依托泊苷

"紫杉醇+卡铂"常用于治疗非小细胞肺癌和食管癌[91]。多项研究发现[92-93]，"紫杉醇+卡铂±依托泊苷"对原发肿瘤不明的腺癌有效，在希腊合作肿瘤学组的Ⅱ期研究中[93]，"紫杉醇+卡铂"治疗耐受性良好，ORR为38.7%。

一项Ⅲ期随机试验发现[60]，"紫杉醇+卡铂+依托泊苷"是一线治疗

CUP 患者的有效方案，在 93 例患者中，ORR 为 18%，中位 PFS 和 OS 分别为 3.3 个月和 7.4 个月，2 年生存率为 15%。在另一项长期随访的 II 期试验中[94]，接受"紫杉醇 + 卡铂 + 依托泊苷"治疗的患者的 2 年、3 年生存率分别为 20%、14%。

4）多西他赛 + 卡铂或顺铂

Greco 等[95]报道，在接受"多西他赛 + 顺铂"治疗腺癌和分化较差的 CUP 患者中，有 26% 的患者对治疗产生了明显反应，mOS 为 8 个月，1 年生存率为 42%；在接受"多西他赛和卡铂"治疗的患者中，ORR 为 22%，mOS 为 8 个月，1 年生存率为 29%。在这项研究中，"多西他赛和卡铂"的耐受性优于"多西他赛 + 顺铂"。

希腊合作肿瘤学组（Hellenic Cooperative Oncology Group）的一项 II 期研究发现[96]，对 PS 为 0~2 分的腺癌或分化不良的 CUP 患者，"多西他赛和卡铂"每 3 周一次的治疗，mPFS 为 5.5 个月，OS 为 16.2 个月。

"多西他赛 + 顺铂"在一组 29 例 CUP 患者中进行了研究[97]，51.7% 的患者是分化良好至中度的腺癌，未分化癌（27.6%）和鳞癌（13.8%）患者也包括在内；ORR 为 37.9%，mPFS、OS 分别为 6 个月、16 个月。

因此，"多西他赛 + 顺铂/卡铂"亦是不明原发肿瘤腺癌患者的推荐治疗方案。

5）吉西他滨 + 顺铂

"吉西他滨 + 顺铂"常用于治疗非小细胞肺癌和膀胱癌[98-99]。"吉西他滨 + 顺铂"治疗 CUP 的疗效在随机 II 期 GEFCAPI01 研究中进行了评估[54]，组织学上最常见的是未分化腺癌，25% 的患者只有一个转移部位，在接受"吉西他滨 + 顺铂"治疗的患者中，55% 的患者（$n=21$）出现了客观反应，mOS 为 8 个月。

GEFCAPI02 试验以 1:1 的比例随机分配 52 例患者接受"吉西他滨 + 顺铂"或单用顺铂治疗[53]。"吉西他滨 + 顺铂"治疗组的 mOS 和 1 年生存率分别为 11 个月、46%，而单用顺铂治疗组的 mOS、1 年生存率分别为 8 个月和 35%。"吉西他滨 + 顺铂"治疗组的 mPFS 为 5 个月，顺铂治疗组为 3 个月；1 年 PFS 率分别为 29%、15%。

值得注意的是，在高度怀疑原发肿瘤为胃腺癌、结直肠腺癌中，不推荐使用"吉西他滨 + 顺铂"方案。

第七章 CUP治疗与预后

6）吉西他滨+多西他赛

研究发现[100]，"吉西他滨+多西他赛"作为CUP患者的一线疗法具有良好疗效和耐受性。在35例CUP患者中，1例达到CR、13例为PR，ORR为40%，mPFS为2个月，mOS为10个月。

值得注意的是，在高度怀疑原发肿瘤为胃腺癌、结直肠腺癌中，不推荐使用"吉西他滨+多西他赛"方案。

7）卡培他滨+奥沙利铂

"卡培他滨+奥沙利铂"方案在用于CUP患者一线和二线治疗的Ⅱ期研究中进行了评估。

在一项有51例原发肿瘤不明腺癌患者参与的Ⅱ期试验中[101]，"卡培他滨+奥沙利铂"一线治疗的ORR为11.7%，mPFS为2.5个月，OS为7.5个月，耐受性良好。在一项对48例CUP患者进行的Ⅱ期试验中[102]，"卡培他滨+奥沙利铂"二线治疗，ORR为19%，mPFS为3.7个月，OS为9.7个月，大多数(65%)患者为原发肿瘤不明的腺癌。

值得一提的是，"卡培他滨+奥沙利铂"主要用于胃肠道腺癌的术后辅助、晚期一线治疗；在高度怀疑原发肿瘤为肺腺癌患者一般不做推荐。

8）伊立替康+卡铂/吉西他滨

在一项针对45例CUP患者的Ⅱ期研究中[103]，对"伊立替康+卡铂"进行了评估，结果显示，ORR为41.9%，mPFS为4.8个月，OS为12.2个月，1年、2年生存率分别为44%和27%。但方案存在严重毒性反应，包括Ⅲ级或以上白细胞减少(21%)、中性粒细胞减少(33%)、贫血(25%)和血小板减少症(20%)。

一项Ⅲ期随机试验发现[60]，"伊立替康+吉西他滨"是一线治疗CUP患者的有效方案，ORR为18%，mPFS和OS分别为5.3个月、8.5个月。

值得注意的是，在高度怀疑原发肿瘤为胃腺癌、结直肠腺癌中，不推荐使用"伊立替康+吉西他滨"方案。

9）氟尿嘧啶和亚叶酸钙和伊立替康(FOLFIRI)

"氟尿嘧啶+亚叶酸钙+伊立替康"联合疗法常用于晚期胃肠道腺癌的一线和二线治疗[104-105]。但FOLFIRI治疗CUP患者的数据很有限。一项回顾性研究确定了32例通过分子图谱推测为结肠直肠起源部位的CUP患者[41]，这些患者接受了包括FOLFIRI在内的结肠直肠癌治疗方案。结果显示，与用于治疗CUP的经验性方案相比，接受FOLFIRI等部位特异性方案治疗的患者 ORR 明显提高(50% 对 17%；$P = 0.0257$)。

由于结直肠原发部位是 CUP 最常见的原发部位之一[107]，建议将 FOLFIRI 作为 CUP 患者一线或二线治疗的首选方案。

10) 其他方案

单药卡培他滨、单药氟尿嘧啶可作为不明原发肿瘤腺癌患者的治疗推荐，虽然氟尿嘧啶/亚叶酸钙和奥沙利铂(FOLFOX)尚未在 CUP 患者中进行前瞻性评估，但在治疗结直肠癌方面，FOLFOX 已被证明与 CapeOx(卡培他滨 + 奥沙利铂)相当，FOLFOX(mFOLFOX6)方案可作为不明原发肿瘤腺癌患者的首选治疗方案。如果有临床指征，mFOLFOX6 可与 RT 同时使用。

关于 FOLFIRINOX 治疗 CUP 亦缺乏数据。因此，FOLFIRINOX 应仅限于 PS 评分为 0~1 分且推测为消化道原发部位的 CUP 患者。

2. 鳞癌

不明原发肿瘤鳞癌的化学治疗方案选择主要有"顺铂 + 氟尿嘧啶"、"紫杉醇 + 顺铂 + 5 - 氟尿嘧啶""多西他赛 + 顺铂 + 5 - 氟尿嘧啶"。

虽然"顺铂 + 氟尿嘧啶"是原发肿瘤不明鳞癌患者最常用的治疗方案[108-109]，但"紫杉醇 + 顺铂 + 5 - 氟尿嘧啶"与"顺铂 + 氟尿嘧啶"方案Ⅲ期临床试验比较，结果显示，疗效更好，CR 分别为 33%、14%，"多西他赛 + 顺铂 + 5 - 氟尿嘧啶"与"顺铂 + 氟尿嘧啶"方案Ⅲ期临床试验比较，ORR 分别为 82.8%、60.8%，有显著性差异。

总体而言，目前仅有少数几项小型研究评估了不同化学治疗方案对不明原发肿瘤鳞癌患者的疗效。因此，根据对已知原发性肿瘤鳞癌患者的研究证据以及对不明原发肿瘤鳞癌患者的小型研究，本书列出了可选择的治疗方案，除列出的治疗方案外，还可考虑其他治疗方案。

1) 紫杉醇 + 卡铂

在希腊肿瘤合作组对"紫杉醇 + 卡铂"治疗 CUP 患者的Ⅱ期研究中[93]，有 3 例患者的肿瘤组织学类型为鳞癌，这些患者的 ORR 为 30%，中位反应持续时间为 3 个月。

2) 紫杉醇 + 顺铂

"紫杉醇 + 顺铂"常用于治疗食管癌、头颈癌和非小细胞肺癌(包括腺癌、鳞癌)，一项"紫杉醇 + 顺铂"治疗 37 例不良预后型 CUP 患者Ⅱ期研究的结果显示[110]，ORR 为 42%，mPFS 为 4 个月，mOS 为 11 个月，37 例患者中有 3 例为鳞癌患者。

3）多西他赛+卡铂/顺铂

Pentheroudakis 等[96]开展了一项"多西他赛+卡铂"治疗 CUP 患者的 Ⅱ 期临床试验，有 24 例患者疾病风险较高（定义为主要为结节性疾病或非黏液性腹膜癌），23 例患者疾病风险较低（内脏转移），平均 ORR 为 32%，mPFS 为 5.5 个月，mOS 为 16.2 个月。风险较高的患者 ORR 为 46%（风险较低的患者为 17%），mOS 为 22.6 个月（风险较低的患者仅为 5.3 个月）。结果提示，对于疾病风险较高的 CUP 患者，疗效更好。

一项针对 45 例 CUP 患者的试验评估了"多西他赛+顺铂"的疗效[111]，ORR 为 65.1%，mPFS 为 5 个月，mOS 为 11.8 个月，这项研究中有 2 例患者肿瘤组织学类型为鳞癌，对该方案产生了部分反应。在 Demirci 等[97]对 29 例 CUP 患者进行"多西他赛+顺铂"治疗的研究中，有 4 例患者肿瘤组织学类型为鳞癌，总体 ORR 为 37.9%，mPFS、OS 分别为 6 个月、16 个月。

4）顺铂+氟尿嘧啶

有学者对不明原发肿瘤的鳞癌患者进行了"顺铂+氟尿嘧啶"的回顾性评估[108-109]，Kusaba 等[112]对 11 例接受过该方案治疗的 CUP 患者进行了回顾性分析，结果显示，ORR 为 54.5%，mPFS 为 3 个月，mOS 为 10 个月。

5）多西他赛+顺铂+氟尿嘧啶（DCF）

"多西他赛+顺铂+氟尿嘧啶"常用于治疗胃癌、食管癌和头颈部肿瘤，目前还缺乏在 CUP 中的临床研究，一般可类推于原发肿瘤为高度可疑的食管、头颈部鳞癌患者。

在一项针对 213 例头颈部晚期鳞癌患者的随机试验中[113]，患者接受"顺铂和氟尿嘧啶±多西他赛"治疗后再接受放射治疗，三药治疗组和二药治疗组的 ORR 分别为 80% 和 59.2%（$P=0.002$）。

一项涉及 501 例晚期头颈部鳞癌患者的试验报道显示[114]，单用 DCF 或"顺铂+氟尿嘧啶"治疗患者的 ORR 分别为 72% 和 64%，但 DCF 与包括 Ⅳ 级发热性中性粒细胞减少症在内的严重毒性相关，因此应仅限于 PS 评分为 0~1 的患者。

6）其他方案

根据 CUP 腺癌的证据，可将单药卡培他滨、单药氟尿嘧啶、mFOLFOX6 用于原发肿瘤不明的鳞癌治疗。若有临床指征，单药卡培他滨或氟尿嘧啶可与 RT 同时使用。

3. 神经内分泌癌

不明原发肿瘤的转移性神经内分泌癌临床少见，是预后良好型 CUP，恶性程度高，对化学治疗反应良好，部分患者可长期生存[115]。

Hainsworth 等[116]评估了"紫杉醇 + 卡铂 + 依托泊苷"对未接受过治疗的转移性神经内分泌癌患者的疗效，在这些患者中，有 62% 的患者为原发肿瘤不明的神经内分泌癌，ORR 为 53%，mOS 为 14.5 个月，2 年和 3 年 OS 率分别为 33%、24%。

通常情况下，小细胞肺癌系统治疗方案也可用于原发肿瘤不明的转移性神经内分泌癌。在一项随机Ⅲ期试验（JCOG9702）中[117]，对于老年小细胞肺癌患者或既往未接受过治疗的低危患者，"卡铂 + 依托泊苷"与"顺铂 + 依托泊苷"同样有效，在 ORR 率（两种方案均为 73%）和 mOS（卡铂 + 依托泊苷为 10.6 个月，顺铂 + 依托泊苷为 9.9 个月）方面没有发现明显差异。

因此，对于分化差的（高级别或未分化）或除肺神经内分泌肿瘤以外的小细胞亚型 CUP，可参照小细胞肺癌治疗指南；对于中高分化神经内分泌肿瘤 CUP，可参照神经内分泌肿瘤治疗指南。

（二）靶向治疗

为确定 CUP 分子基因治疗的靶点，许多大 panel NGS 研究对预后不良型 CUP 的突变情况进行了评估[118-122]。有研究报道[119,120,123-124]，CUP 中有 37% ~ 55% 的患者存在 TP53 突变，有 18% ~ 22% 的患者存在 KRAS 突变；亦有经常发生酪氨酸激酶家族成员突变，如 ALK、EGFR、RET、FGFR1 和 NTRK1 等[125]。

Kato 等[126]通过对 442 例 CUP 进行循环肿瘤 DNA 检测，发现 65.6% 的病例基因发生改变，最常见的突变是 TP53、KRAS 和 PIK3CA，其中 5.9% 的病例发现 EGFR 突变、3.6% 的病例 HER - 2 改变、1.6% 的病例 BRAFV600E 突变、1.6% 病例检测到错配修复基因变化。

一项对 200 例 CUP 患者标本进行基因检测的大型前瞻性研究发现[120]，95% 的标本中至少存在 1 个基因改变，85% 的病例发现了潜在治疗靶点。

因此，CUP 肿瘤组织中基因异常改变的发现为部分 CUP 患者提供了靶向治疗的可能性，对靶向治疗潜在获益的 CUP 人群的选择具有重要意义。

一项前瞻性Ⅱ期临床研究纳入了 194 例 CUP 患者[83]，旨在评估 GEP 检测指导 CUP 患者进行特异性治疗的临床疗效，结果显示，mOS 为 12.5

个月(95% CI：9.1～15.4个月)，其中对治疗敏感的肿瘤患者中位 OS 显著优于治疗耐药的患者(13.4个月 vs 7.6个月，P=0.04)。

另一项多中心、非随机对照Ⅱ期临床研究纳入 97 例预后不良的 CUP 患者[127]，接受特异性治疗的 CUP 患者获得了良好预后，1 年生存率为 53.1%，mOS、mPFS 分别为 13.7 个月、5.2 个月，ORR 为 39%。一项小样本研究发现[128]，11 例接受靶向治疗的 CUP 患者中，有 4 例获得≥4 个月的 PFS。

对于携带基因改变提示原发肿瘤的患者，分子靶向治疗已成为其标准治疗。EGFR 突变、ALK 与 ROS1 融合阳性的 CUP 患者强烈暗示 NSCLC 为原发肿瘤，TKIs 是其治疗的首选[17]。多项研究显示[129-130]，对于高度疑似肺腺癌的 EGFR 敏感突变的 CUP 患者，临床给予 EGFR-TKI 或联合治疗，显示出了较好疗效。

相关指南建议，对于 NTRK 融合阳性的 CUP 患者，可选择 larotrectinib、entrectinib[131-132]；对于 BRAF V600E 基因突变的 CUP 患者，可以选择从二线开始使用 BRAF 抑制剂，如果肺部是推定的原发肿瘤部位，可以考虑将 BRAF 抑制剂用于一线治疗[133-135]。

Ross 等[120]报道了伴有 ALK 融合基因突变的 CUP 病例，患者在 ALK 抑制剂克唑替尼靶向治疗后达到 PR。

塞尔帕替尼(Selpercatinib)是一种 RET 激酶抑制剂，于 2022 年获得美国 FDA 批准，用于治疗在既往系统治疗中或治疗后出现进展或无其他满意治疗方案的晚期或转移性 RET 基因融合阳性实体瘤；据此，亦可用于转移性 RET 基因融合阳性 CUP 患者。

值得一提的是，2009 年，Hainsworth 等[136]报道，将 47 例 CUP 患者使用"贝伐单抗+厄洛替尼"作为二线治疗，ORR 仅为 10%，mOS 亦只有 7 个月；其后 Hainsworth 等[137]又报道，对 60 例 CUP 患者给予"紫杉醇+卡铂"一线化学治疗联合或不联合贝伐单抗和厄洛替尼作为维持治疗，其 ORR 率是 53%，mOS 为 13 个月。

目前，仅少数靶向药物适用于 CUP 一线单药治疗，在许多 CUP 治疗中，联合化学治疗仍然发挥着重要作用[138]，CUP 单一靶向治疗有效性仍需进一步临床验证。

(三) 免疫治疗

随着对免疫检查点抑制剂(immune checkpoint inhibitors, ICIs)预测生

物标记物的识别,免疫检查点抑制剂治疗已成为 CUP 患者另一种选择。

对免疫治疗反应的预测指标目前仍无定论,在已知的肿瘤类型中包括肿瘤突变负荷(tumor mutation burden,TMB)、微卫星不稳定(microsatellite instability,MSI)、错配修复缺陷(deficient mismatch repair,dMMR)和程序性死亡受体配体 1(programmed death ligand 1,PD-L1)表达等。高度微卫星不稳定性(microsatellite instability-high,MSI-H)、PD-L1 高表达和高肿瘤突变负荷(tumor mutation burden-high,TMB-H)已被确定为可用于评估免疫肿瘤疗效的泛癌生物标志物[139]。

Gatalic 等[124]报道,在 389 例 CUP 患者中,约 28% 的病例具有 TMB-H、MSI/dMMR 或 PD-L1 高表达等与免疫治疗疗效相关的分子特征。一项研究比较了头颈部原发肿瘤不明的鳞状细胞癌与口咽部鳞状细胞癌中 PD-L1 的表达[140],发现原发肿瘤不明鳞状细胞癌中 PD-L1 的表达显著高于口咽部鳞状细胞癌,且在 p16 阴性的原发肿瘤不明鳞状细胞癌患者中,PD-L1 高表达是一个独立的预后因素。

CUP 中 PD-L1 的表达与肿瘤浸润淋巴细胞密度相关。一项研究检测了 70 例 CUP 患者[119],结果显示,TILs 中 PD-1 表达和肿瘤细胞 PD-L1 表达率为 63% 和 21%,共表达率为 16%(11/70)。

免疫检查点抑制剂的问世显著提高了多种类型晚期恶性肿瘤患者的生存率,如非小细胞肺癌、胃癌、食管癌、泌尿生殖系统肿瘤和头颈部癌[141],且有可能在 CUP 治疗中发挥作用[142]。一项对 CUP 患者免疫特征及其对 ICIs 治疗的潜在适用性探索性研究显示[143],CUP 患者的免疫特征与 ICIs 反应性已明确的原发肿瘤相似,表明 CUP 患者可能从 ICIs 治疗中获益。已有研究报道显示[126,144],在具有上述分子特征的 CUP 中使用 ICIs 可获得良好的治疗反应。

Raghav 等[145]研究了帕博利珠单抗对于 CUP 患者的疗效和安全性,该研究表明,帕博利珠单抗的应用有着一定的疗效,且安全性可以接受。

有研究探讨了 CUP 患者对 ICIs 的反应性和耐药性与其基因组突变的相关性[146],对 ICIs 反应的基因组,如细胞周期蛋白依赖性激酶 4(cyclin-dependent kinase 4,CDK4)、斑点型锌指结构蛋白(speckle type POZ protein,SPOP)等和 ICIs 抵抗的基因组,如磷酸酶张力蛋白同源物基因(phosphatase and tension homolog,PTEN)、β2 微球蛋白(β-2 microglobulin,β2-MG)等,除 TMB>10 个突变/兆碱基的患者在接受 ICIs

第七章 CUP治疗与预后

治疗时显示出较好疗效外,其他标志物在 CUP 患者中不具有预测疗效的价值。

MSI-H 或错配修复缺陷(dMMR)肿瘤对 ICIs 的反应性已在不同的肿瘤中得到证实[147-149]。

目前,FDA 已批准 pembrolizumab 用于 MSI-H 或 dMMR 肿瘤的二线治疗[150],其中也包括 CUP。

在 MSI-H 或 dMMR 晚期结直肠癌中,pembrolizumab 的无进展生存期(PFS)优于标准治疗化学治疗[151]。KEYNOTE-016 是一项Ⅱ期试验[147],评估了 pembrolizumab 在 41 例转移性难治性 dMMR 结直肠癌、pMMR 结直肠癌或 dMMR 非结直肠癌患者中的疗效,dMMR 结直肠癌患者的免疫相关 ORR 为 40%、PFS 为 78%。在这项研究的扩展中,来自代表 12 种不同肿瘤类型的 86 例 dMMR 肿瘤患者的数据显示,Pembrolizumab 的 ORR 为 53%,21%的患者获得完全应答。欧洲药品管理局(EMA)和美国 FDA 已批准将 pembrolizumab 作为此类患者的一线治疗药物[41]。因此,建议结肠型 CUP 的治疗遵循 mCRC 治疗指南,pembrolizumab 可用作 MSI-H 或 dMMR 结肠样 CUP 的一线治疗。

在 KEYNOTE-158 Ⅱ期试验中,233 例患有 27 种不同 MSI-H/dMMR 肿瘤类型(最常见的是子宫内膜癌、胃癌、胆管肉瘤和胰腺癌)的晚期患者在既往使用了至少一种药物失败后接受了 pembrolizumab 治疗[152],中位随访 13 个月后,ORR 为 34.3%。mPFS 为 4 个月,中位 OS 为 24 个月,64.8%的患者发生了治疗相关不良事件(14.6%为 3~5 级)。

TMB-H 是不同肿瘤对 ICIs 治疗反应的预测指标,FDA 批准 pembrolizumab 用于 TMB-H(≥10 个 mut/Mb)的肿瘤;Marabelle 等[152]对参加 KEYNOTE-158 试验的 102 例被鉴定为 TMB-H 的肿瘤患者使用 pembrolizumab 的疗效进行了回顾性分析,结果显示,ORR 为 29%,其中 CR 为 4%,PR 为 25%,中位应答持续时间未达到,50%的患者应答持续时间为 24 个月或更长。同样,nivolumab 对 TMB 高(≥7.75 mut/Mb)的 CUP 更有效[153]。ICIs 治疗最迟可被视为 TMB-H 的 CUP 二线治疗。

PD-L1 高表达与 ICIs 治疗后某些肿瘤(而非所有癌症)的预后改善有关[154-155],与其他肿瘤一样,PD-L1 阳性 CUP 患者的 PFS 和总生存期往往较好。一项多中心Ⅱ期临床研究[156],评估了纳武利尤单抗治疗 CUP 患者的疗效,结果显示,对于 45 例既往曾接受治疗的患者,ORR 为 22.2%,

mPFS、OS 分别为 4.0 个月、15.9 个月；对于 PD-L1 表达水平较高、TMB 较高和 MSI-H 的肿瘤患者，纳武利尤单抗有更好的疗效。

因此，对于 PD-L1 高表达且无其他治疗选择的复发或难治性 CUP，可考虑选择 ICIs 治疗。

多塔利单抗（Dostarlimab-gxly）是一种抗 PD-1 抗体，于 2021 年获得美国 FDA 批准用于治疗 dMMR 复发性或晚期实体瘤患者。

一项非随机Ⅰ期多队列 GARNET 临床试验评估了 dostarlimab-gxly 在 209 例 dMMR 实体瘤患者中的安全性和抗肿瘤活性[157-158]，多数患者患有子宫内膜癌或胃肠道癌，ORR 为 42%，其中 CR 为 9%，PR 为 33%，中位应答持续时间为 35 个月。最常见的治疗相关不良反应是疲劳、贫血、腹泻和恶心，免疫相关不良事件也时有发生，包括肺炎、结肠炎、肝炎、内分泌病、肾炎和皮肤毒性。

根据以上数据，dostarlimab-gxly 可用于治疗腺癌伴 MSI-H/dMMR 的不明原发肿瘤患者。

表 7-4 CUP 系统治疗方案——腺癌

分类	方案组成、剂量、用法
首选方案	卡培他滨 + 奥沙利铂 奥沙利铂：130mg/m²，ivd，d1；卡培他滨：850~1000mg/m²，po，2 次/d，d1~14。q3w
	吉西他滨 + 顺铂 吉西他滨：1000~1250mg/m²，ivd，d1、8；顺铂：75mg/m²，ivd，d1。q3w
	FOLFIRI 伊立替康：180mg/m²，ivd，d1；亚叶酸钙：400mg/m²，ivd，d1；氟尿嘧啶：400mg/m²，静脉推注，d1，然后氟尿嘧啶 2400 mg/m²，静脉持续输注 46~48h。q2w
	mFOLFOX6 奥沙利铂：85mg/m²，ivd，d1；亚叶酸钙：400mg/m²，ivd，d1；氟尿嘧啶：400mg/m²，静脉推注，d1，然后氟尿嘧啶 2400mg/m²，静脉持续输注 46~48h。q2w
	紫杉醇 + 卡铂 紫杉醇：175~200mg/m²，ivd，d1；卡铂：AUC 5~6，ivd，d1。q3w 或紫杉醇：80mg/m²，ivd，d1、8、15；卡铂：AUC 2，ivd，d1、8、15。q4w

续表

分类	方案组成、剂量、用法
其他推荐方案	卡培他滨 卡培他滨：850~1250mg/m², po, 2次/d, d1~14。q3w
	多西他赛 + 卡铂 多西他赛：65mg/m², ivd, d1；卡铂 AUC 5~6, ivd, d1。q3w
	多西他赛 + 顺铂 多西他赛：60~75mg/m², ivd, d1；顺铂：75mg/m², ivd, d1。q3w
	Roswell Park 方案 亚叶酸钙：500mg/m², ivd, d1、8、15、22、29、36；氟尿嘧啶：500mg/m², 亚叶酸钙开始后1小时 ivd, d1、8、15、22、29、36。q8w
	sLV5FU2 方案 亚叶酸钙：400mg/m², ivd, d1；然后 5-氟尿嘧啶：400mg/m², 静脉推注, d1，然后 5-氟尿嘧啶 2400mg/m², 静脉持续输注 46~48h。q2w
	氟尿嘧啶每周方案 亚叶酸钙：20mg/m², ivd, d1；氟尿嘧啶：500mg/m², ivd, 在亚叶酸钙开始后1小时。q1w； 或亚叶酸钙：500mg/m², ivd, d1；氟尿嘧啶 2600mg/m², 24小时持续输注。q1w
	吉西他滨 + 卡铂 吉西他滨 1000mg/m², ivd, d1、8；卡铂：AUC 5, ivd, d8。q3w
	吉西他滨 + 多西他赛 吉西他滨：1000mg/m², ivd, d1、8；多西他赛：75mg/m², ivd, d18。q3w
	伊立替康 + 卡铂 伊立替康：60mg/m², ivd, d1、8、15；卡铂：AUC 5~6, ivd, d1。q4w
	卡培他滨 + 放射治疗 卡培他滨：625~825 mg/m², po, 2次/d, d1~5, q1w, 持续5周，同时放射治疗
	氟尿嘧啶 + 放射治疗 氟尿嘧啶：200~250mg/m², 静脉持续输注 24h, d1~5, q1w, 持续5周，同时放射治疗

续表

分类	方案组成、剂量、用法
在特定条件下的推荐方案	BRAFV600E 突变阳性：达拉非尼 + 曲美替尼 达拉非尼：150mg，po，2 次/d；曲美替尼：2mg，po，1 次/d。q4w
	NTRK 基因融合阳性 恩曲替尼 600mg，po，1 次/d，q4w。或拉罗替尼 100mg，po，2 次/d，q4w
	RET 基因融合阳性：塞尔帕替尼 体重 <50kg：120mg，2 次/d；体重≥50kg：160mg，ivd，2 次/d。
	dMMR/MSI-H 或 TMB-H≥10 突变/Mb 帕博利珠单抗：200mg，ivd，d1，q3w；或 400mg，ivd，d1，q6w
	FOLFIRINOX 奥沙利铂：85mg/m²，ivd，d1；伊立替康：180mg/m²，ivd，d1；亚叶酸钙：400mg/m²，ivd，d1；氟尿嘧啶：400mg/m²，静脉推注，d1；2400mg/m²，静脉持续输注 46~48h。q2w
	伊立替康 + 吉西他滨 伊立替康 100mg/m²，ivd，d1、8；吉西他滨 1000mg/m²，ivd，d1、8。q3w
	mFOLFIRINOX 奥沙利铂：85mg/m²，ivd，d1；伊立替康：150mg/m²，ivd，d1；亚叶酸钙：400mg/m²，ivd，d1；氟尿嘧啶：2400mg/m²，静脉持续输注 46~48h。q2w
	紫杉醇、卡铂 + 依托泊苷 紫杉醇：175~200mg/m²，ivd，d1；卡铂：AUC 5~6，ivd，d1；依托泊苷：50mg/d 与 100mg/d 交替，po，d1~10。q3w

表 7-6 CUP 系统治疗方案——鳞癌、神经内分泌肿瘤

鳞癌	方案组成、剂量、用法
首选方案	mFOLFOX6 奥沙利铂：85mg/m²，ivd，d1；亚叶酸钙：400mg/m²，ivd，d1；氟尿嘧啶：400mg/m²，静脉推注，d1，然后氟尿嘧啶 2400mg/m²，静脉持续输注 46~48h。q2w
	紫杉醇 + 卡铂 紫杉醇：175~200mg/m²，ivd，d1；卡铂：AUC 5~6，ivd，d1。q3w；或紫杉醇：80mg/m²，ivd，d1、8、15；卡铂：AUC 2，ivd，d1、8、15。q4w

第七章 CUP治疗与预后

续表

鳞癌	方案组成、剂量、用法
其他推荐方案	卡培他滨 卡培他滨：850~1250 mg/m^2，po，2 次/d，d1~14。q3w
	顺铂 + 氟尿嘧啶 顺铂：20mg/m^2，ivd，d1~5；氟尿嘧啶：700mg/m^2，ivd，d1~5。q4w
	多西他赛 + 卡铂 多西他赛：75 mg/m^2，ivd，d1；卡铂 AUC 5~6，ivd，d1。q3w
	多西他赛 + 顺铂 多西他赛：60~75mg/m^2，ivd，d1；顺铂：75mg/m^2，ivd，d1。q3w
	吉西他滨 + 卡铂 吉西他滨 1000mg/m^2，ivd，d1、d8；卡铂：AUC 5，ivd，d8。q3w
	吉西他滨 + 顺铂 顺铂 75mg/m^2，ivd，d1；吉西他滨 1000~1250mg/m^2，ivd，d1、d8。q3w
	Roswell Park 方案 亚叶酸钙：500mg/m^2，ivd，d1、d8、d15、d22、d29、d36；氟尿嘧啶 500mg/m^2，亚叶酸钙开始后 1 小时 ivd，d1、d8、d15、d22、d29、d36。q8w
	sLV5FU2 方案 亚叶酸钙：400mg/m^2，ivd，d1；然后：氟尿嘧啶：400mg/m^2 静脉注射，然后氟尿嘧啶：400mg/m^2，静脉推注，d1，然后氟尿嘧啶 2400mg/m^2，静脉持续输注 46~48h。q2w
	氟尿嘧啶每周方案 亚叶酸钙：20mg/m^2，ivd，d1；氟尿嘧啶：500mg/m^2，ivd，在亚叶酸钙开始后 1h。q1w
	紫杉醇 + 顺铂 紫杉醇 175mg/m^2，ivd，d1；顺铂 60mg/m^2，ivd，d1。q3w
	卡培他滨 + 放射治疗 卡培他滨：625~825 mg/m^2，po，2 次/d，d1~5，q1w，持续 5 周，同时放射治疗
	氟尿嘧啶 + 放射治疗 氟尿嘧啶：200~250mg/m^2，静脉持续输注 24h，d1~5，q1w，持续 5 周，同时放射治疗
	氟尿嘧啶、顺铂 + 放射治疗 顺铂：75~100mg/m^2，ivd，d1、d29，d1~4，d29~32；氟尿嘧啶：750~1000mg/m^2，24 小时静脉持续输注，与顺铂同步。q7w，同步放射治疗；或顺铂：15mg/m^2，ivd，d1~5；氟尿嘧啶：800mg/m^2，24 小时持续静脉注射，d1~5。q3w×2，同时放射治疗

续表

鳞癌	方案组成、剂量、用法
在特定条件下的推荐方案	BRAFV600E 突变阳性：达拉非尼 + 曲美替尼 达拉非尼：150mg，po，2 次/d；曲美替尼：2mg，po，1 次/d。q4w
	NTRK 基因融合阳性 恩曲替尼 600mg，po，1 次/d，q4w。或拉罗替尼 100mg，po，2 次/d，q4w
	RET 基因融合阳性：塞尔帕替尼 体重 <50kg：120mg，2 次/d；体重 ≥50kg：160mg，ivd，2 次/d
	dMMR/MSI-H 或 TMB-H≥10 突变/Mb 帕博利珠单抗：200mg，ivd，d1，q3w；或 400mg，ivd，d1，q6w
	多西他赛 + 顺铂 + 氟尿嘧啶 多西他赛：75mg/m², ivd, d1；顺铂：75mg/m², ivd, d1；氟尿嘧啶：750mg/m², ivd, d1~5。q3w
神经内分泌肿瘤	分化不良（高级别）或小细胞亚型 —— 参考小细胞肺癌 CACA 治疗指南
	分化良好 —— 参考神经内分泌肿瘤 CACA 治疗指南

第二节 预 后

一、总体预后

CUP 为一类异质性很强的恶性肿瘤，具有侵袭性强、在"早期"即发生转移、转移方式难以预测等特征[159-160]。虽然 CUP 占所有肿瘤的比例 <5%，但其死亡率在所有肿瘤中排名第 4[161]。一般而言，CUP 患者的根治性治疗机会较少，多数患者预后不良[1]。约 50% 的死亡患者发生在确诊后的 3 个月内，与鳞癌相比，腺癌和未分化癌的生存率更低（1 年生存率分别低于 20% 和 36%）[162]。

相关研究报道[4,14,16,81,163-168]，CUP 患者平均生存期 2~10 个月，OS 为 8~11 个月，仅 20% 左右预后良好的亚型患者生存期超过 1 年，中位 OS 可达 12~36 个月。

接受系统化学治疗后的 CUP 患者中位生存时间为 4~12 个月，1 年、2 年、3 年、5 年生存率分别为 50%、17.8%、11%、6%[169-170]。

二、预后相关因素

(一)一般预后因素

根据目前的研究报道[171-176],影响 CUP 患者预后的因素众多,如性别、年龄、ECOG-PS 评分、组织学类型(如腺癌、鳞癌)、预后分型(预后良好型、预后不良型)、转移部位(淋巴结转移、内脏转移等)、转移灶数量、生化指标、免疫治疗疗效预测指标等。

独立不良预后因素[19,177],一般包括男性、ECOG-PS 评分差(≥2分)、CUP 预后不良亚型、转移累及器官数量较多、存在肝转移或其他内脏转移、腺癌,以及碱性磷酸酶(ALP)升高、乳酸脱氢酶(LDL)升高、低血清白蛋白和淋巴细胞减少,或反映炎症状态的中性粒细胞与淋巴细胞比值(NLR)升高等。

Algin 等[178]对 68 例原发肿瘤部位不明的肝转移性腺癌进行多因素分析,结果显示,ECOG-PS 评分、接受化学治疗、血清白蛋白、血清 CA-199 为独立预后因子,且 39 例接受化学治疗患者的 mOS 明显长于未化学治疗患者(12.5 个月 vs. 4 个月,$P = 0.026$)。Raghav 等[179]通过对 47 例年轻 CUP 患者进行多因素分析,其结果显示,乳酸脱氢酶升高、转移灶≥3 个、未检测出组织起源为不良预后因子。Burgers 等[180]及 Bendardaf 等[181]报道,白细胞数增高以及肿瘤标志物异常在多种实体瘤中与患者的预后相关,但其在原发肿瘤不明的转移癌患者预后方面的作用尚有待进一步研究。Seve 等[171]认为,低血清白蛋白和淋巴细胞减少是独立的不良预后影响因素。

一项研究纳入了原发肿瘤不明的转移性头颈部鳞癌患者[182],多因素分析显示,年龄、人乳头瘤病毒状态、N 分期、淋巴结外转移为其预后相关因素。

Raghav 等[183]开发了一个强大的预后模型和列线图来预测 CUP 患者的 OS,并通过一个包含 926 例患者的大型多中心队列进行了外部验证,确定了 5 个独立的预后因素,包括性别、ECOG-PS 评分、组织学类型、转移部位数量和中性粒细胞-淋巴细胞比率。在 Cox 回归模型中,男性、ECOG-PS 评分差、腺癌、转移部位多和中性粒细胞-淋巴细胞比率高与生存率降低有关,其中 ECOG-PS 评分和中性粒细胞-淋巴细胞比值是预测 OS 的最强指标（$P < 0.001$）。

有研究报道[184-185]，大多数恶性肿瘤 SUVmax 值越高预后越差。刘红红等[186]认为，SUVmax、受转移灶影响的器官及其数目是影响 CUP 预后的重要因素，原发肿瘤 $SUV_{max} \leq 6.5$ 的患者预后好于 $SUV_{max} > 6.5$ 的患者（$AUC = 0.627$）。

另外，Davis 等[187]的回顾性研究表明，与未发现原发肿瘤的患者相比，明确原发肿瘤部位的患者总体生存率更高。

分子预测标志物多变量分析显示[173]，Kirsten 大鼠肉瘤病毒（KRAS）或神经母细胞瘤 RAS 病毒癌基因同源物（NRAS）激活、细胞周期蛋白依赖性激酶抑制剂 2A（CDKN2A）缺失为独立的不良预后因素；肿瘤抑制蛋白 p53（TP53）突变或染色体 17p 缺失亦与 CUP 不良预后相关[188]。

另外，神经营养酪氨酸受体激酶（NTRK）重排可预测 CUP 对 NTRK 抑制剂的治疗反应[132]；TMB-H、MSI-H 是对 ICIs 治疗反应良好的预测标志物[151-152,189-190]；在 CUP 中，较高水平的 PD-L1 表达和较高的 TMB 亦与先前接受 nivolumab 单药治疗患者更好的应答率和更长的生存期有关[156]。

（二）预后分型

有学者根据 CUP 预后的不同，将其分为预后良好型与预后不良型[19,191]，预后不良型是最常见的临床亚型，占所有 CUP 的 75%～85%，其特征一般包括男性、年龄较大（≥65 岁）、体能状态不佳（PS 评分 > 2 分）、伴有多种合并症（如心肺功能不全、严重糖尿病等）、转移累及多个器官（如肝、肺、骨）、多发性脑转移、非乳头状腹膜转移性腺癌（包括恶性腹水形成）与腹腔广泛种植转移（可形成不完全性或完全性肠梗阻），以及腺癌伴多发性肺/胸膜病变（如恶性胸腔积液等）或骨病变（如病理性骨折、脊髓压迫等）、骨髓转移[192-193]。

预后良好型仅占所有 CUP 的 15%～25%，主要包括孤立的、体积较小且可能切除的肿瘤，中线分布的低分化癌、颈淋巴结转移性鳞癌、腋窝淋巴结转移性腺癌、腹股沟淋巴结转移性腺癌或鳞癌、男性伴 PSA 升高的成骨转移性腺癌、具有结直肠癌免疫表型（CK20 阳性，CK7 阴性，CDX2 阳性）的腺癌，以及分化差的神经内分泌癌等。

PetrakisD 等[191]对 311 例 CUP 患者的疗效分析发现，预后不良组（217 例）与预后良好组（94 例）中位 PFS 分别为 4 个月、8 个月，中位 OS 为 7 个月、21个月,均有显著性差异。

(三)骨转移患者预后

叶矗飞[194]报道了已明确原发肿瘤骨转移患者408例,中位OS为18.45个月,6个月、12个月和24个月生存率分别为61.27%、27.70%和10.29%。一般而言,不同原发肿瘤骨转移患者的生存期有一定差异。有学者报道,肺癌骨转移患者中位OS为10.6个月[195]、乳腺癌骨转移患者中位OS为34.0个月[196]、胃癌骨转移患者中位OS为38.3个月[197]、肾癌骨转移患者中位OS为27.7个月[198],肺癌骨转移患者生存期最短。

然而,不明原发肿瘤骨转移患者生存期更短,平均生存期仅3~12个月[16,199-201];且怀疑的原发肿瘤不同,生存期亦显著差异,怀疑肺起源的骨转移癌患者预后较差,生存期只有3个月;而考虑乳腺和前列腺起源的预后较好,生存期有15~23个月[202-206]。

(四)骨髓转移癌患者预后

骨髓转移癌患者治疗极为困难,其预后极差,mOS仅1.5~3个月。不同肿瘤类型的骨髓转移患者生存期有所差异,据报道[207-209],乳腺癌、前列腺癌、胃癌、小细胞肺癌、结肠癌骨髓转移患者mOS分别为6~19个月、4.6个月、1~4个月、3.6个月、14天,原发于乳腺或前列腺的骨髓转移癌患者的预后要优于其他部位的肿瘤患者。

多数学者认为,造成骨髓转移患者死亡的原因往往不是抗肿瘤治疗所致,而是疾病进展所导致的骨髓衰竭、出血、感染、血栓等并发症。

有研究表明[210],积极的抗肿瘤治疗可持久控制疾病进展、明显改善患者预后。Demir等[211]的研究发现,乳腺癌骨髓转移后接受全身治疗的患者较未接受治疗的患者存活时间明显延长(分别为17.3个月、0.93个月)。Hung等[9]报道,83例骨髓转移患者中抗肿瘤治疗组患者的mOS为87天,支持治疗组为21天。Kucukzeybek等[10]报道了39例已知原发肿瘤的患者,最佳支持治疗组mOS为28天,化学治疗组mOS为418天。Zhou等[212]的研究表明,全身系统治疗组中位OS为9个月,最佳支持治疗组mOS仅为1个月。

对于乳腺癌,有报道接受化学治疗的患者中位OS为1.78年,明显长于未化学治疗患者的0.08年[213];对于小细胞肺癌骨髓转移预后的研究提示[209],化学治疗是独立预后因素,化学治疗可延长疾病进展时间。

Nakashima 等[214]回顾了分析既往文献中 12 例结肠癌骨髓转移患者,3 例(25%)接受化学治疗中位生存期为 83 天,而 9 例(75%)未接受化学治疗的患者的中位生存期为 12 天,化学治疗显著延长了患者的预后。

靶向药物 TKI 治疗可延长合并骨髓转移的 EGFR 突变肺腺癌患者生存期[215],抗雄激素治疗在前列腺癌骨髓转移患者也证实了可以改善生存[216]。

无论原发肿瘤是否明确,肿瘤骨髓转移系统治疗主要有化学治疗、靶向治疗、内分泌治疗等,但目前没有标准治疗方案;对于 CUP 骨髓转移患者,可根据患者性别、临床表现特点、影像学检查、骨髓活检病理、肿瘤标志物等推测其原发肿瘤,从而采取相应的系统治疗方案,这些系统治疗方法可以延长患者生存。

(五)转移性卵巢肿瘤患者预后

转移性卵巢肿瘤的预后与年龄,月经、腹腔积液、包块大小、包块囊实性、原发灶位置、组织学分类,组织学分级、术中癌灶残留多少、术后辅助治疗均有相关性,最重要的影响因素是原发灶的位置、病理类型和细胞减灭术。

不同原发肿瘤的转移性卵巢肿瘤预后有明显差异,肿瘤细胞的不同分类和分级决定肿瘤细胞倍增速度,高分化管状腺癌恶性度相对印戒细胞癌和黏液细胞癌低,故预后最好。

三、随访

目前对于 CUP 患者综合治疗后的随访没有统一标准,一般可根据预后分型确定基本随访间隔时间。预后良好型患者,建议 3~6 个月随访 1 次,预后不良型患者,建议每 3 个月随访 1 次。

对于正在接受治疗且预后不佳的 CUP 患者,停止治疗后,如果认为患者适合继续治疗,应每隔 3 个月通过 CT 或 MRI 进行重新分期和随访。

接受消融手术/放射治疗的单发或少转移 CUP 患者,以及其他亚型 CUP 患者,如孤立腋窝结节转移的女性,亦有长期生存者[19]。

由于早期诊断出局部复发可使患者获得更多的局部消融治疗机会[177],故在最初的 2 年中,应每隔 3~6 个月进行一次 CT 或 MRI 随访,然后在第 3~5 年中每隔 6~12 个月进行一次随访。

下篇 不明原发肿瘤

第七章 CUP治疗与预后

鉴于 CUP 继发其他恶性肿瘤的风险较高,故 CUP 长期存活者可遵守为普通人群推荐的癌症筛查指南,其中包括结肠癌、乳腺癌、前列腺癌和皮肤癌等。若有家族病史和(或)分子检查怀疑存在种系癌症易感基因突变,则应提供遗传咨询和检测。如果得到证实,种系癌症诱发突变应进行额外筛查。

一般而言,预后不良型 CUP 患者生存期较短,其康复的重点在于综合治疗结束后加强支持治疗与对症处理,以期有较高的生活质量。

预后良好型 CUP 患者一般生存期较长,社会心理支持、症状管理、身体功能康复等尤为重要,其康复方法与已知原发肿瘤患者综合治疗后的康复基本一致。

参考文献

[1] Rassy E, Assi T, Pavlidis N. Exploring the biological hall marks of cancer of unknown primary: where do we stand today? [J]. Br J Cancer, 2020, 122(8): 1124-1132.

[2] Hainsworth JD, Fizazi K. Treatment for patients with unknown primary cancer and favorable prognostic factors[J]. Semin Oncol, 2009, 36(1): 44-51.

[3] Golfinopoulos V, Pentheroudakis G, Salanti G, et al. Comparative survival with diverse chemotherapy regimens for cancer of unknown primary site: multiple-treatments meta analysis [J]. Cancer Treat Rev, 2009, 35(7): 570-573.

[4] Greco FA, Pavlidis N. Treatment for patients with unknown primary carcinoma and unfavorable prognostic factors[J]. Semin Oncol, 2009, 36(1): 65-74.

[5] Fung KY, Law SW. Management of malignant atlanto-axial tumours[J]. J Orthop Surg (Hong Kong), 2005, 13(3): 232-239.

[6] Piccioli A, Maccauro G, Spinelli MS, et al. Bone metastases of unknown origin: epidemiology and principles of management[J]. J Orthop Traumatol, 2015, 16(2): 81-86.

[7] Oken MM, Creech RH, Tormey DC, et al. Toxicity and response criteria of the Eastern Cooperative Oncology Group[J]. Am J Clin Oncol, 1982, 5(6): 649-655.

[8] Simon MA, Bartucci EJ. The search for the primary tumor in patients with skeletal metastases of unknown origin[J]. Cancer, 1986, 58(5): 1088-1095.

[9] Hung YS, Chou WC, Chen TD, et al. Prognostic factors in adult patients with solid cancers and bone marrow metastases[J]. Asian Pac J Cancer Prev, 2014, 15(1): 61-67.

[10] Kucukzeybek BB, Calli AO, Kucukzeybek Y, et al. The prognostic significance of bone

marrow metastases: evaluation of 58 cases[J]. Indian J Pathol Microbiol, 2014, 57(3): 396-399.

[11] McGill F, Ritter DB, Rickard C, et al. Management of Krukenberg tumors: an 11-year experience and review of the literature[J]. Prim Care Update Ob Gyns, 1998, 5(4): 157-158.

[12] Taylor AE, Nicolson VM, Cunningham D. Ovarian metastases from primary gastrointestinal malignancies: the Royal Marsden Hospital experience and implications for adjuvant treatment [J]. Br J Cancer, 1995, 71(1): 92-96.

[13] Etrakis D, Pentheroudakis G, Voulgaris E, et al. Prognostication in cancer of unknown primary(CUP): development of a prognostic algorithm in 311 cases and review of the literature[J]. Cancer Treat Rev, 2013, 39(7): 701-708.

[14] Pavlidis N, Khaled H, Gaafar R. A mini review on cancer of unknown primary site: A clinical puzzle for the oncologists[J]. J Adv Res, 2015, 6(3): 375-382.

[15] Massard C, Loriot Y, Fizazi K. Carcinomas of an unknown primary origin-diagnosis and treatment[J]. Nat Rev Clin Oncol, 2011, 8(12): 701-710.

[16] Fizazi K, Greco FA, Pavlidis N, et al. Cancers of unknown primary site: ESMO Clinical Practice Guidelines for diagnosis, treatment and follow up[J]. Ann Oncol, 2015, 26(suppl 5): 133-138.

[17] Planchard D, Popat S, Kerr K, et al. Metastatic non-small cell lungcancer: ESMO Clinical Practice Guidelines for diagnosis, reatmentand follow-up[J]. Ann Oncol, 2018, 29(suppl 4): iv192-iv237.

[18] Lievens Y, Guckenberger M, Gomez D, et al. Defining oligometastatic disease from a radiation oncology perspective: an ESTRO-ASTRO consensus document[J]. Radiother Oncol, 2020, 148: 157-166.

[19] Pavlidis N, Petrakis D, Golfinopoulos V, et al. Long-term survivors among patients with cancer of unknown primary[J]. Crit Rev Oncol Hematol, 2012, 84(1): 85-92.

[20] Pouyiourou M, Wohlfromm T, Kraft B, et al. Local ablative treatment with surgery and/or radiotherapy in single-site and oligometastatic carcinoma of unknown primary[J]. Eur J Cancer, 2021, 157: 179-189.

[21] Rudà R, Borgognone M, Benech F, et al. Brain metastases from unknown primary tumour: a prospective study[J]. J Neurol, 2001, 248(5): 394-398.

[22] Bartelt S, Lutterbach J. Brain metastases in patients with cancer of unknown primary[J]. J Neurooncol, 2003, 64(3): 249-253.

[23] Galloway TJ, Ridge JA. Management of squamous cancer metastatic to cervical nodes with an unknown primary site[J]. J Clin Oncol, 2015, 33(29): 3328-3337.

[24] Matsuyama S, Nakafusa Y, Tanaka M, et al. Iliac lymph node metastasis of an unknown

primary tumor: report of a case[J]. Surg Today, 2006, 36(7): 655-658.

[25] Machiels JP, René Leemans C, Golusinski W, et al. Squamous cell carcinoma of the oral cavity, larynx, oropharynx and hypopharynx: EHNS-ESMO-ESTRO Clinical Practice Guidelines for diagnosis, treatment and follow-up[J]. Ann Oncol, 2020, 31(11): 1462-1475.

[26] de Bresser J, de Vos B, vander Ent F, et al. Breast MRI in clinically and mammographically occult breast cancer presenting with an axillary metastasis: a systematic review[J]. Eur J Surg Oncol, 2010, 36(2): 114-119.

[27] Pentheroudakis G, Lazaridis G, Pavlidis N. Axillary nodal metastases from carcinoma of unknown primary (CUPAx): a systematic review of published evidence[J]. Breast Cancer Res Treat, 2010, 119(1): 1-11.

[28] Gennari A, André F, Barrios CH, et al. ESMO Clinical Practice Guideline for the diagnosis, staging and treatment of patients with metastatic breast cancer[J]. Ann Oncol, 2021, 32(12): 1475-1495.

[29] Walker GV, Smith GL, Perkins GH, et al. Population-based analysis of occult primary breast cancer with axillary lymph node metastasis[J]. Cancer, 2010, 116(17): 4000-4006.

[30] Rueth NM, Black DM, Limmer AR, et al. Breast conservation in the setting of contemporary multimodality treatment provides excellent outcomes for patients with occult primary breast cancer[J]. Ann Surg Oncol, 2015, 22(1): 90-95.

[31] Macedo FI, Eid JJ, Flynn J, et al. Optimal surgical management for occult breast carcinoma: a meta-analysis[J]. Ann Surg Oncol, 2016, 23(6): 1838-1844.

[32] Kim H, Park W, Kim SS, et al. Prognosis of patients with axillary lymphnode metastases from occult breast cancer: analysis of multicenter data[J]. Radiat Oncol J, 2021, 39(2): 107-112.

[33] Motz K, Qualliotine JR, Rettig E, et al. Changes in Unknown Primary Squamous Cell Carcinoma of the Head and Neck at Initial Presentation in the Era of Human Papilloma virus[J]. JAMA Otolaryngol Head Neck Surg, 2016, 142(3): 223-228.

[34] Pentheroudakis G, Pavlidis N. Serous papillary peritoneal carcinoma: unknown primary tumour, ovarian cancer counterpart or a distinctentity? A systematic review[J]. Crit Rev Oncol Hematol, 2010, 75(1): 27-42.

[35] Kim J, Park EY, Kim O, et al. Cell origins of high-grade serous ovarian cancer[J]. Cancers (Basel), 2018, 10(11): 433.

[36] Finch A, Beiner M, Lubinski J, et al. Salpingo-oophorectomy and the risk of ovarian, fallopian tube, and peritoneal cancers in women witha BRCA1 or BRCA2 Mutation[J]. JAMA, 2006, 296(2): 185-192.

[37] Ben-Baruch G, Sivan E, Moran O, et al. Primary peritoneal serous papillary carcinoma: a study of 25 cases and comparison with stage Ⅲ-Ⅳ ovarian papillary serous carcinoma[J]. Gynecol Oncol, 1996, 60(3): 393-396.

[38] Ray-Coquard I, Pautier P, Pignata S, et al. Olaparib plus bevacizumabas first-line maintenance in ovarian cancer[J]. N Engl J Med, 2019, 381(25): 2416-2428.

[39] Tomuleasa C, Zaharie F, Muresan MS, et al. How to Diagnose and Treat a Cancer of Unknown Primary Site[J]. J Gastrointestin Liver Dis, 2017, 26(1): 69-79.

[40] Varadhachary GR, Raber MN, Matamoros A, et al. Carcinoma of unknown primary with a colon-cancer profile-changing paradigm and emerging definitions[J]. Lancet Oncol, 2008, 9(6): 596-599.

[41] Hainsworth JD, Schnabel CA, Erlander MG, et al. A retrospective study of treatment outcomes in patients with carcinoma of unknown primary site and a colorectal cancer molecular profile[J]. Clin Colorectal Cancer, 2012, 11(2): 112-118.

[42] Hodroj K, Barthelemy D, Lega JC, et al. Issues and limitations of available biomarkers for fluoropyrimidine-based chemotherapy toxicity, a narrative review of the literature[J]. ESMO Open, 2021, 6(3): 100125.

[43] Trullas A, Delgado J, Genazzani A, et al. The EMA assessment of pembrolizumab as monotherapy for the first-line treatment of adult patients with metastatic microsatellite instability-high or mismatch repair deficient colorectal cancer[J]. ESMO Open, 2021, 6(3): 100145.

[44] McGregor DK, Wu TT, Rashid A, et al. Reduced expression of cytokeratin 20 in colorectal carcinomas with high levels of microsatellite instability[J]. Am J Surg Pathol, 2004, 28(6): 712-718.

[45] Parker C, Castro E, Fizazi K, et al. Prostate cancer: ESMO Clinical Practice Guidelines for diagnosis, treatment and follow-up[J]. Ann Oncol, 2020, 31(9): 1119-1134.

[46] Greco FA, Hainsworth JD. Renal cell carcinoma presenting as carcinoma of unknown primary site: recognition of a treatable patient subset[J]. Clin Genitourin Cancer, 2018, 16(4): E893-E898.

[47] Overby A, Duval L, Ladekarl M, et al. Carcinoma of unknown primarysite (CUP) With metastatic renal-cell carcinoma (mRCC) histologic and immunohistochemical characteristics (CUP-mRCC): results from consecutive patients treated with targeted therapy and review of literature[J]. Clin Genitourin Cancer, 2019, 17(1): E32-E37.

[48] Stoyianni A, Pentheroudakis G, Pavlidis N. Neuroendocrine carcinoma of unknown primary: a systematic review of the literature and a comparative study with other neuroendocrine tumors[J]. Cancer Treat Rev, 2011, 37(5): 358-365.

[49] Losa F, Soler G, Casado A, et al. ESMO clinical guideline on unknown primary cancer

(2017)[J]. Clin Transl Oncol, 2018, 20(1): 89-96.

[50] Pentheroudakis G, Stoyianni A, Pavlidis N. Cancer of unknown primary patients with midline nodal distribution: midway between poor and favourable prognosis?[J]. Cancer Treat Rev, 2011, 37(2): 120-126.

[51] Bugat R, Bataillard A, Lesimple T, et al. Summary of the Standards, Options and Recommendations for the management of patients with carcinoma of unknown primary site (2002)[J]. Br J Cancer, 2003, 89(suppl 1): S59-S66.

[52] Levy A, Massard C, Gross-Goupil M, et al. Carcinomas of an unknown primary site: a curable disease?[J]. Ann Oncol, 2008, 19(9): 1657-1658.

[53] Gross-Goupil M, Fourcade A, Blot E, et al. Cisplatin alone or combined with gemcitabine in carcinomas of unknown primary: results of the randomised GEFCAPI 02 trial[J]. Eur J Cancer, 2012, 48(5): 721-727.

[54] Culine S, Lortholary A, Voigt JJ, et al. Cisplatin in combination with either gemcitabine or irinotecan in carcinomas of unknown primary site: results of a randomized phase II study-trial for the French Study Group on Carcinomas of Unknown Primary (GEFCAPI 01)[J]. J Clin Oncol, 2003, 21(18): 3479-3482.

[55] Huebner G, Link H, Kohne CH, et al. Paclitaxel and carboplatin vs gemcitabine and vinorelbine in patients with adeno- or undifferentiated carcinoma of unknown primary: a randomised prospective phase II trial[J]. Br J Cancer, 2009, 100(1): 44-49.

[56] Lee J, Hahn S, Kim DW, et al. Evaluation of survival benefits by platinums and taxanes for an unfavourable subset of carcinoma of unknown primary: a systematic review and meta-analysis[J]. Br J Cancer, 2013, 108(1): 39-48.

[57] Pavlidis N. Forty years experience of treating cancer of unknown primary[J]. Acta Oncologica, 2007, 46(5): 592-601.

[58] Piga A, Nortilli R, Cetto GL, et al. Carboplatin, doxorubicin and etoposide in the treatment of tumours of unknown primary site[J]. Br J Cancer, 2004, 90(10): 1898-1904.

[59] Greco FA, Burris HA, Litchy S, et al. Gemcitabine, carboplatin, and paclitaxel for patients with carcinoma of unknown primary site: a Minnie Pearl Cancer Research Network study[J]. J Clin Oncol, 2002, 20(6): 1651-1656.

[60] Hainsworth JD, Spigel DR, Clark BL, et al. Paclitaxel/carboplatin/etoposide versus gemcitabine/irinotecan in the first-line treatment of patients with carcinoma of unknown primary site: a randomized, phase III Sarah Cannon Oncology Research Consortium Trial [J]. Cancer J, 2010, 16(1): 70-75.

[61] Pauli C, Bochtler T, Mileshkin L, et al. A Challenging Task: Identifying Patients with Cancer of Unknown Primary (CUP) According to ESMO Guidelines: The CUPISCO Trial Experience[J]. Oncologist, 2021, 26(5): E769-E779.

[62] Lee CS, Jung CH. Metastatic spinal tumor[J]. Asian Spine J, 2012, 6(1): 71-78.

[63] 王丰, 伦登兴, 张浩, 等. 脊柱转移瘤481例的流行病学分析[J]. 中国脊柱脊髓杂志, 2017, 27(9): 787-794.

[64] 吴银松, 王臻. 联合化疗治疗原发灶不明转移癌的Meta分析[J]. 中国骨肿瘤骨病, 2003, 2(4): 225-228.

[65] Wu YY, Chang JY, Chao TY. Paclitaxel and carboplatin-induced complete remission in peritoneal carcinomatosis of unknown origin: a report of two cases and review of the literature[J]. Tumori, 2010, 96(2): 336-339.

[66] Cerezo L, Raboso E, Ballesteros AI. Unknown primary cancer of the head and neck: a multidisciplinary approach[J]. Clin Transl Oncol, 2011, 13(2): 88-97.

[67] Kakhki VR, Anvari K, Sadeghi R, et al. Pattern and distribution of bone metastases in common malignant tumors[J]. Nucl Med Rev Cent East Eur, 2013, 16(2): 66-69.

[68] Granieri S, Bonomi A, Frassini S, et al. Prognostic impact of cytoreductive surgery (CRS) with hyperthermic intraperitoneal chemotherapy (HIPEC) in gastric cancer patients: a meta-analysis of randomized controlled trials[J]. Eur J Surg Oncol, 2021, 47(11): 2757-2767.

[69] Quénet F, Elias D, Roca L, et al. Cytoreductive surgery plus hyperthermic intraperitoneal chemotherapy versus cytoreductive surgery alone for colorectal peritoneal metastases (PRODIGE 7): a multicentre, randomised, open-label, phase 3 trial[J]. Lancet Oncol, 2021, 22(2): 256-266.

[70] Delhorme JB, Ohayon J, Gouy S, et al. Ovarian and peritoneal psammocarcinoma: results of a multicenter study on 25 patients[J]. EurJ Surg Oncol, 2020, 46(5): 862-867.

[71] Sebbag G, Shmookler BM, Chang D, et al. Peritoneal carcinomatosis from an unknown primary site, Management of 15 patients[J]. Tumori, 2001, 87(2): 67-73.

[72] Mugerwa S, Lekharaju V, Kiire CF. Management of peritoneal carcinomatosis secondary to metastatic cancer of unknown primary in men[J]. Eur J Cancer Care (Engl), 2009, 18(1): 22-27.

[73] Huo YR, Richards A, Liauw W, et al. Hyperthermic intraperitoneal chemotherapy (HIPEC) and cytoreductive surgery (CRS) in ovarian cancer: a systematic review and meta-analysis[J]. Eur J Surg Oncol, 2015, 41(12): 1578-1589.

[74] Kamal M, Mohamed ASR, Fuller CD, et al. Outcomes of patients diagnosed with carcinoma metastatic to the neck from an unknown primary source and treated with intensity-modulated radiation therapy[J]. Cancer, 2018, 124(7): 1415-1427.

[75] Mourad WF, Hu KS, Shasha D, et al. Initial experience with oropharynx-targeted radiation therapy for metastatic squamous cell carcinoma of unknown primary of the head and neck[J]. Anticancer Res, 2014, 34(1): 243-248.

[76] Janssen S, Glanzmann C, Huber G, et al. Individualized IMRT treatment approach for cervical lymph node metastases of unknown primary[J]. Strahlenther Onkol, 2014, 190(4): 386-393.

[77] 黎立喜, 张娣, 马飞. 原发灶不明肿瘤治疗的新策略[J]. 中华肿瘤杂志, 2023, 45(1): 44-49.

[78] Amela EY, Lauridant-Philippin G, Cousin S, et al. Management of "unfavourable" carcinoma of unknown primary site: synthesis of recent literature[J]. Crit Rev Oncol Hematol, 2012, 84(2): 213-223.

[79] Matsubara N, Mukai H, Nagai S, et al. Review of primary unknown cancer: cases referred to the National Cancer Center Hospital East[J]. Int J Clin Oncol, 2010, 15(6): 578-582.

[80] Hainsworth JD, Greco FA. Cancer of Unknown Primary Site: New Treatment Paradigms in the Era of Precision Medicine[J]. Am Soc Clin Oncol Educ Book, 2018, 38: 20-25.

[81] Hainsworth JD, Daugaard G, Lesimple T, et al. Paclitaxel/carboplatin with or without belinostat as empiric first-line treatment for patients with carcinoma of unknown primary site: a randomized, phase 2 trial[J]. Cancer, 2015, 121(10): 1654-1661.

[82] Hasegawa H, Ando M, Yatabe Y, et al. Site-specific chemotherapy based on predicted primary site by pathological profile for carcinoma of unknown primary site[J]. Clin Oncol (R Coll Radiol), 2018, 30(10): 667-673.

[83] Hainsworth JD, Rubin MS, Spigel DR, et al. Molecular gene expression profiling to predict the tissue of origin and direct site-specific therapy in patients with carcinoma of unknown primary site: a prospective trial of the Sarah Cannon research institute[J]. J Clin Oncol, 2013, 31(2): 217-223.

[84] Hayashi H, Kurata T, Takiguchi Y, et al. Randomized phase Ⅱ trial comparing site-specific treatment based on gene expression profiling with carboplatin and paclitaxel for patients with cancer of unknown primary site[J]. J Clin Oncol, 2019, 37(7): 570-579.

[85] Nishikawa K, Hironaka S, Inagaki T, et al. A multicentre retrospective study comparing site-specific treatment with empiric treatment for unfavourable subset of cancer of unknown primary site[J]. Jpn J Clin Oncol, 2022, 52(12): 1416-1422.

[86] Rassy E, Bakouny Z, Choueiri TK, et al. The role of site-specific therapy for cancers of unknown of primary: A meta-analysis[J]. Eur J Cancer, 2020, 127: 118-122.

[87] van der Gaast A, Verweij J, Henzen-Logmans SC, et al. Carcinoma of unknown primary: identification of a treatable subset?[J]. Ann Oncol, 1990, 1(2): 119-122.

[88] Hainsworth JD, Johnson DH, Greco FA. Cisplatin-based combination chemotherapy in the treatment of poorly differentiated carcinoma and poorly differentiated adenocarcinoma of unknown primary site: results of a 12-year experience[J]. J Clin Oncol, 1992, 10(6):

912-922.

[89] Greco FA, Gray J, Burris HA, et al. Taxane-based chemotherapy for patients with carcinoma of unknown primary site[J]. Cancer J, 2001, 7(3): 203-212.

[90] Mikhail S, Lustberg MB, Ruppert AS, et al. Biomodulation of capecitabine by paclitaxel and carboplatin in advanced solid tumors and adenocarcinoma of unknown primary[J]. Cancer Chemother Pharmacol, 2015, 76(5): 1005-1012.

[91] van Hagen P, Hulshof MC, van Lanschot JJ, et al. Preoperative chemoradiotherapy for esophageal or junctional cancer[J]. N Engl J Med, 2012, 366(22): 2074-2084.

[92] Greco FA, Rodriguez GI, Shaffer DW, et al. Carcinoma of unknown primary site: sequential treatment with paclitaxel/carboplatin/etoposide and gemcitabine/irinotecan: a Minnie Pearl Cancer Research Network phase II trial[J]. Oncologist, 2004, 9(6): 644-652.

[93] Briasoulis E, Kalofonos H, Bafaloukos D, et al. Carboplatin plus paclitaxel in unknown primary carcinoma: a phase II Hellenic Cooperative Oncology Group Study[J]. J Clin Oncol, 2000, 18(17): 3101-3107.

[94] Greco FA, Burris HA, Erland JB, et al. Carcinoma of unknown primary site[J]. Cancer, 2000, 89(12): 2655-2660.

[95] Greco FA, Erland JB, Morrissey LH, et al. Carcinoma of unknown primary site: phase II trials with docetaxel plus cisplatin or carboplatin[J]. Ann Oncol, 2000, 11(2): 211-215.

[96] Pentheroudakis G, Briasoulis E, Kalofonos HP, et al. Docetaxel and carboplatin combination chemotherapy as outpatient palliative therapy in carcinoma of unknown primary: a multicentre Hellenic Cooperative Oncology Group phase II study[J]. Acta Oncol, 2008, 47(6): 1148-1155.

[97] Demirci U, Coskun U, Karaca H, et al. Docetaxel and cisplatin in first line treatment of patients with unknown primary cancer: a multicenter study of the Anatolian Society of Medical Oncology[J]. Asian Pac J Cancer Prev, 2014, 15(4): 1581-1584.

[98] Schiller JH, Harrington D, Belani CP, et al. Comparison of four chemotherapy regimens for advanced non-small-cell lung cancer[J]. N Engl J Med, 2002, 346(2): 92-98.

[99] von der Maase H, Hansen SW, Roberts JT, et al. Gemcitabine and cisplatin versus methotrexate, vinblastine, doxorubicin, and cisplatin in advanced or metastatic bladder cancer: results of a large, randomized, multinational, multicenter, phase III study[J]. J Clin Oncol, 2000, 18(17): 3068-3077.

[100] Pouessel D, Culine S, Becht C, et al. Gemcitabine and docetaxel as front-line chemotherapy in patients with carcinoma of an unknown primary site[J]. Cancer, 2004, 100(6): 1257-1261.

[101] Schuette K, Folprecht G, Kretzschmar A, et al. Phase II trial of capecitabine and

oxaliplatin in patients with adeno - and undifferentiated carcinoma of unknown primary[J]. Oncologie, 2009, 32(4): 162-166.

[102] Hainsworth JD, Spigel DR, Burris HA, et al. Oxaliplatin and capecitabine in the treatment of patients with recurrent or refractory carcinoma of unknown primary site: a phase 2 trial of the Sarah Cannon Oncology Research Consortium[J]. Cancer, 2010, 116(10): 2448-2454.

[103] Yonemori K, Ando M, Yunokawa M, et al. Irinotecan plus carboplatin for patients with carcinoma of unknown primary site[J]. Br J Cancer, 2009, 100(1): 50-55.

[104] Guimbaud R, Louvet C, Ries P, et al. Prospective, randomized, multicenter, phase Ⅲ study of fluorouracil, leucovorin, and irinotecan versus epirubicin, cisplatin, and capecitabine in advanced gastric adenocarcinoma: a French intergroup (Federation Francophone de Cancerologie Digestive, Federation Nationale des Centres de Lutte Contre le Cancer, and Groupe Cooperateur Multidisciplinaire en Oncologie) study[J]. J Clin Oncol, 2014, 32(31): 3520-3526.

[105] Sebbagh S, Roux J, Dreyer C, et al. Efficacy of a sequential treatment strategy with GEMOX - based followed by FOLFIRI - based chemotherapy in advanced biliary tract cancers[J]. Acta Oncol, 2016, 55(9-10): 1168-1174.

[106] Hainsworth JD, Schnabel CA, Erlander MG, et al. A retrospective study of treatment outcomes in patients with carcinoma of unknown primary site and a colorectal cancer molecular profile[J]. Clin Colorectal Cancer, 2012, 11(2): 112-118.

[107] Varadhachary GR, Talantov D, Raber MN, et al. Molecular profiling of carcinoma of unknown primary and correlation with clinical evaluation[J]. J Clin Oncol, 2008, 26(27): 4442-4448.

[108] Jeremic B, Zivic DJ, Matovic M, et al. Cisplatin and 5 - fluorouracil as induction chemotherapy followed by radiation therapy in metastatic squamous cell carcinoma of an unknown primary tumor localized to the neck. A phase II study[J]. J Chemother, 1993, 5(4): 262-265.

[109] Khansur T, Allred C, Little D, et al. Cisplatin and 5 - fluorouracil for metastatic squamous cell carcinoma from unknown primary[J]. Cancer Invest, 1995, 13(3): 263-266.

[110] Park YH, Ryoo BY, Choi SJ, et al. A phase II study of paclitaxel pluscisplatin chemotherapy in an unfavourable group of patients with cancer of unknown primary site[J]. Jpn J Clin Oncol, 2004, 34(11): 681-685.

[111] Mukai H, Katsumata N, Ando M, et al. Safety and efficacy of a combination of docetaxel and cisplatin in patients with unknown primary cancer[J]. Am J Clin Oncol, 2010, 33(1): 32-35.

[112] Kusaba H, Shibata Y, Arita S, et al. Infusional 5 - fluorouracil and cisplatin as first - line

chemotherapy in patients with carcinoma of unknown primary site[J]. Med Oncol, 2007, 24(2): 259 – 264.

[113] Pointreau Y, Garaud P, Chapet S, et al. Randomized trial of induction chemotherapy with cisplatin and 5 – fluorouracil with or without docetaxel for larynx preservation[J]. J Natl Cancer Inst, 2009, 101(7): 498 – 506.

[114] Posner MR, Hershock DM, Blajman CR, et al. Cisplatin and fluorouracil alone or with docetaxel in head and neck cancer[J]. N Engl J Med, 2007, 357(17): 1705 – 1715.

[115] Spigel DR, Hainsworth JD, Greco FA. Neuroendocrine carcinoma of unknown primary site [J]. Semin Oncol, 2009, 36(1): 52 – 59.

[116] Hainsworth JD, Spigel DR, Litchy S, et al. Phase II trial of paclitaxel, carboplatin, and etoposide in advanced poorly differentiated neuroendocrine carcinoma: a Minnie Pearl Cancer Research Network Study[J]. J Clin Oncol, 2006, 24(22): 3548 – 3554.

[117] Okamoto H, Watanabe K, Kunikane H, et al. Randomised phase III trial of carboplatin plus etoposide vs split doses of cisplatin plus etoposide in elderly or poor – risk patients with extensive disease small – cell lung cancer: JCOG 9702[J]. Br J Cancer, 2007, 97(2): 162 – 169.

[118] Tothill RW, Li J, Mileshkin L, et al. Massively – parallel sequencing assists the diagnosis and guided treatment of cancers of unknown primary[J]. J Pathol, 2013, 231(4): 413 – 423.

[119] Gatalica Z, Millis SZ, Vranic S, et al. Comprehensive tumor profiling identifies numerous biomarkers of drug response in cancers of unknown primary site: analysis of 1806 cases[J]. Oncotarget, 2014, 5(23): 12440 – 12447.

[120] Ross JS, Wang K, Gay L, et al. Comprehensive genomic profiling of carcinoma of unknown primary site: new routes to targeted therapies[J]. JAMA Oncol, 2015, 1(1): 40 – 49.

[121] Löffler H, Pfarr N, Kriegsmann M, et al. Molecular driver alterations and their clinical relevance in cancer of unknown primary site[J]. Oncotarget, 2016, 7(28): 44322 – 44329.

[122] Clynick B, Dessauvagie B, Sterrett G, et al. Genetic characterisation of molecular targets in carcinoma of unknown primary[J]. J Transl Med, 2018, 16(1): 185.

[123] Varghese AM, Arora A, Capanu M, et al. Clinical and molecular characterization of patients with cancer of unknown primary in the modern era[J]. Ann Oncol, 2017, 28 (12): 3015 – 3021.

[124] Gatalica Z, Xiu J, Swensen J, et al. Comprehensive analysis of cancers of unknown primary for the biomarkers of response to immune checkpoint blockade therapy[J]. Eur J Cancer, 2018, 94: 179 – 186.

[125] Drilon A, Siena S, Ou SI, et al. Safety and Antitumor Activity of the Multitargeted Pan-

[125] TRK, ROS1, and ALK Inhibitor Entrectinib: Combined Results from Two Phase I Trials (ALKA-372-001 and STARTRK-1)[J]. Cancer Discov, 2017, 7(4): 400-409.

[126] Kato S, Krishnamurthy N, Banks KC, et al. Utility of Genomic Analy–sis In Circulating Tumor DNA from Patients with Carcinoma of Un–known Primary[J]. Cancer Res, 2017, 77(16): 4238-4246.

[127] Hayashi H, Takiguchi Y, Minami H, et al. Site-Specific and Targeted Therapy Based on Molecular Profiling by Next-Generation Sequencing for Cancer of Unknown Primary Site: A Nonrandomized Phase 2 Clinical Trial[J]. JAMA Oncol, 2020, 6(12): 1931-1938.

[128] Subbiah IM, Tsimberidou A, Subbiah V, et al. Next generation sequencing of carcinoma of unknown primary reveals novel combinatorial strategies in a heterogeneous mutational landscape[J]. Oncoscience, 2017, 4(5/6): 47-56.

[129] Yamasaki M, Funaishi K, Saito N, et al. Putative lung adeno-carcinoma with epidermal growth factor receptor mutation presenting as carcinoma of unknown primary site: A case report[J]. Medicine (Baltimore), 2018, 97(7): E9942.

[130] Tan DS, Montoya J, Ng QS, et al. Molecular profiling for drug gable genetic abnormalities in carcinoma of unknown primary[J]. J Clin Oncol, 2013, 31(14): E237-E239.

[131] Ardini E, Siena S. Entrectinib approval by EMA reinforces options for ROS1 and tumour agnostic NTRK targeted cancer therapies[J]. ESMO Open, 2020, 5(5): E000867.

[132] Farago AF, Demetri GD. Larotrectinib, a selective tropomyosin receptor kinase inhibitor for adult and pediatric tropomyosin receptor kinase fusion cancers[J]. Future Oncol, 2020, 16(9): 417-425.

[133] Adashek JJ, Menta AK, Reddy NK, et al. Tissue–agnostic activity of BRAF plus MEK inhibitor in BRAF V600–mutant tumors[J]. Mol Cancer Ther, 2022, 21(6): 871-878.

[134] Subbiah V, Wolf J, Konda B, et al. Tumour–agnostic efficacy and safety of selpercatinib in patients with RET fusion–positive solid tumours other than lung or thyroid tumours (LIBRETTO–001): a phase 1/2, open–label, basket trial[J]. Lancet Oncol, 2022, 23(10): 1261-1273.

[135] Subbiah V, Cassier PA, Siena S, et al. Pan–cancer efficacy of pralsetinib in patients with RET fusion–positive solid tumors from the phase 1/2 ARROW trial[J]. Nat Med, 2022, 28(8): 1640-1645.

[136] Hainsworth JD, Spigel DR, Farley C, et al. Phase II trial of bevacizumab and erlotinib in carcinomas of unknown primary site: the Minnie Pearl Cancer Research Network[J]. J Clin Oncol, 2007, 25(13): 1747-1752.

[137] Hainsworth JD, Spigel DR, Thompson DS, et al. Paclitaxel/carboplatin plus bevacizumab/erlotinib in the first–line treatment of patients with carcinoma of unknown primary site[J]. Oncologist, 2009, 14(12): 1189-1197.

[138] Lombardo R, Tosi F, Nocerino A, et al. The quest for improving treatment of cancer of unknown primary (CUP) through molecularly-driven treatments: asystematic review[J]. Front Oncol, 2020, 10: 533.

[139] Chowell D, Yoo Sk, Valero C, et al. Improved prediction of immune checkpoint blockade efficacy across multiple cancer types[J]. Nat Biotechnol, 2022, 40(4): 499-506.

[140] Schmidl B, Vossenkämpe KA, Stark L, et al. Comparison of PD-L1 expression in squamous cell cancer of unknown primary and oropharyngeal squamous cell carcinoma[J]. Eur Arch Otorhino laryngol, 2023, 280(4): 1991-1997.

[141] Ribas A, Wolchok JD. Cancer immunotherapy using checkpoint blockade[J]. Science, 2018, 359(6382): 1350-1355.

[142] Goodman AM, Kato S, Bazhenova L, et al. Tumor Mutational Burden as an Independent Predictor of Response to Immunotherapy in Diverse Cancers[J]. Mol Cancer Ther, 2017, 16(11): 2598-2608.

[143] Haratani K, Hayashi H, Takahama T, et al. Clinical and immune profiling for cancer of unknown primary site[J]. J Immunother Cancer, 2019, 7(1): 251.

[144] Groschel S, Bommer M, Hutter B, et al. Integration of genomics and histology revises diagnosis and enables effective therapy of refractory cancer of unknown primary with PD-L1 amplification[J]. Cold Spring Harb Mol Case Stud, 2016, 2(6): A001180.

[145] Raghav KP, Stephen B, Karp DD, et al. Efficacy of pembrolizumab in patients with advanced cancer of unknown primary (CUP): a phase 2 non-randomized clinical trial [J]. J Immunother Cancer, 2022, 10(5): E004822.

[146] Rassy E, Boussios S, Pavlidis N. Genomic correlates of response and resistance to immune checkpoint inhibitors in carcinomas of unknown primary[J]. Eur J Clin Invest, 2021, 51(9): E13583.

[147] Le DT, Uram JN, Wang H, et al. PD-1 Blockade in tumors with mismatch-repair deficiency[J]. N Engl J Med, 2015, 372(26): 2509-2520.

[148] Overman MJ, Mc Dermott R, Leach JL, et al. Nivolumab in patients with metastatic DNA mismatch repair-deficient or microsatellite instability-high colorectal cancer (CheckMate 142): an open-label, multicentre, phase 2 study[J]. Lancet Oncol, 2017, 18(9): 1182-1191.

[149] Luchini C, Bibeau F, Ligtenberg MJL, et al. ESMO recommendations on microsatellite instability testing for immunotherapy in cancer, and itsrelationship with PD-1/PD-L1 expression and tumour mutational burden: a systematic review-based approach[J]. Ann Oncol, 2019, 30(8): 1232-1243.

[150] Marcus L, Lemery SJ, Keegan P, et al. FDA approval summary: pembrolizumab for the treatment of microsatellite instability-high solid tumors[J]. Clin Cancer Res, 2019, 25

(13): 3753-3758.

[151] Diaz LA Jr, Shiu KK, Kim TW, et al. Pembrolizumab versus chemotherapy for microsatellite instability-high or mismatch repair-deficient metastatic colorectal cancer (KEYNOTE-177): final analysis of a randomised, openlabel, phase 3 study[J]. Lancet Oncol, 2022, 23(5): 659-670.

[152] Marabelle A, Fakih M, Lopez J, et al. Association of tumour mutational burden with outcomes in patients with advanced solid tumours treated with pembrolizumab: prospective biomarker analysis of the multicohort, open-label, phase 2 KEYNOTE-158 study[J]. Lancet Oncol, 2020, 21(10): 1353-1365.

[153] Hellmann MD, Ciuleanu TE, Pluzanski A, et al. Nivolumab plus ipilimumab in lung cancer with a high tumor mutational burden[J]. N Engl J Med, 2018, 378(22): 2093-2104.

[154] Reck M, Rodríguez-Abreu D, Robinson AG, et al. Pembrolizumab versus chemotherapy for PD-L1 positive non-small-cell lung cancer[J]. N Engl J Med, 2016, 375(19): 1823-1833.

[155] Sati N, Boyne DJ, Cheung WY, et al. Factors modifying the associations of single or combination programmed cell death 1 and programmed cell death ligand 1 inhibitor therapies with survival outcomes in patients with metastatic clear cell renal cell carcinoma: a systematic review and meta-analysis[J]. JAMA Netw Open, 2021, 4(1): E2034201.

[156] Tanizaki J, Yonemori K, Akiyoshi K, et al. Open-label phase Ⅱ study of the efficacy of nivolumab for cancer of unknown primary[J]. Ann Oncol, 2022, 33(2): 216-226.

[157] Oaknin A, Tinker AV, Gilbert L, et al. Clinical activity and safety of the anti-programmed death 1 monoclonal antibody dostarlimab for patients with recurrent or advanced mismatch repair-deficient endometrial cancer: a nonrandomized phase 1 clinical trial[J]. JAMA Oncology, 2020, 6(11): 1766-1772.

[158] Berton D, Banerjee SN, Curigliano G, et al. Antitumor activity of dostarlimab in patients with mismatch repair-deficient/microsatellite instability-high tumors: A combined analysis of two cohorts in the GARNET study[J]. J Clin Oncol, 2021, 39(15 suppl): 2564-2564.

[159] Van't-Veer LJ, Weigelt B. Road map to metastasis[J]. Nat Med, 2003, 9(8): 999-1000.

[160] Rassy E, Pavlidis N. Progress in refining the clinical management of cancer of unknown primary in the molecular era[J]. Nat Rev Clin Oncol, 2020, 17(9): 541-554.

[161] Avlidis N, Pentheroudakis G. Cancer of unknown primary site[J]. The Lancet, 2012, 379(9824): 1428-1435.

[162] Hemminki K, Bevier M, Hemminki A, et al. Survival in cancer of unknown primary site:

population – based analysis by site and histology[J]. Ann Oncol, 2012, 23(7): 1854 – 1863.

[163] Deron PB, Bonte KM, Vermeersch HF, et al. Lymph node metastasis of squamous cell carcinoma from an unknown primary in the upper and middle neck: impact of ^{18}F – fluorodeoxyglucose positron emission tomography/computed tomography[J]. Cancer Biother Radiopharm, 2011, 26(3): 331 – 334.

[164] Yoo J, Henderson S, Walker – Dilks C. Evidence – based guideline recommendations on the use of positron emission tomography imaging in head and neck cancer[J]. Clin Oncol (R Coll Radiol), 2013, 25(4): E33 – E66.

[165] Bochtler T, Loffler H, Kramer A. Diagnosis and management of metastatic neoplasms with unknown primary[J]. Semin Diagn Pathol, 2018, 35(3): 199 – 206.

[166] Pavlidis N. Forty years experience of treating cancer of unknown primary[J]. Acta Oncologica, 2007, 46(5): 592 – 601.

[167] 王金艳, 仲悦娇, 陈凌翔, 等. 原发灶不明肿瘤的诊断与治疗[J]. 中华全科医学, 2018, 16(12): 2067 – 2071.

[168] Pelosi E, Pennone M, Deandreis D, et al. Role of whole body positron emission tomography/computed tomography scan with ^{18}F – fluorodeoxyglucose in patients with biopsy proven tumor metastases from unknown primary site[J]. Q J Nucl Med Mol Imaging, 2006, 50(1): 15 – 22.

[169] Seve P, Sawyer M, Hanson J, et al. The influence of comorbidities, age, and performance status on the prognosis and treatment of patients with metastatic carcinomas of unknown primary site: a population – based study[J]. Cancer, 2006, 106(9): 2058 – 2066.

[170] Culine S, Fabbro M, Ychou M, et al. Alternative bimonthly cycles of doxorubicin, cyclophosphamide, and eptoposide, cisplatin with hematopoietic growth factor support in patients with carcinoma of unknown primary site[J]. Cancer, 2002, 94(3): 840 – 846.

[171] Seve P, Ray – Coquard I, Trillet – Lenoir V, et al. Low serum albumin levels and liver metastasis are powerful prognostic markers for survival inpatients with carcinomas of unknown primary site[J]. Cancer, 2006, 107(11): 2698 – 2705.

[172] Huang CY, Lu CH, Yang CK, et al. A simple risk model to predict survival in patients with carcinoma of unknown primary origin[J]. Medicine (Baltimore), 2015, 94(47): e2135.

[173] Bochtler T, Reiling A, Endris V, et al. Integrated clinicomolecular characterization identifies RAS activation and CDKN2A deletion as independent adverse prognostic factors in cancer of unknown primary[J]. Int J Cancer, 2020, 146(11): 3053 – 3064.

[174] Raghav K, Hwang H, Jácome AA, et al. Development and validation ofa novel nomogram

for individualized prediction of survival in cancer of unknown primary[J]. Clin Cancer Res, 2021, 27(12): 3414-3421.

[175] Schneider BJ, El-Rayes B, Muler JH, et al. Phase Ⅱ trial of carboplatin, gemcitabine, and capecitabine in patients with carcinoma of unknowm primary site[J]. Cancer, 2007, 110(4): 770-775.

[176] Vande Wouw AJ, Jansen RL, Griffioen AW, et al. Clinical and immunohistochemical analysis of patients with unknown primary rumour. A search for prognostic factors in UPT[J]. Anticancer Res, 2004, 24(1): 297-301.

[177] Culine S, Kramar A, Saghatchian M, et al. Development and validation of a prognostic model to predict the length of survival in patients with carcinomas of an unknown primary site[J]. J Clin Oncol, 2002, 20(24): 4679-4683.

[178] Algin E, Ozet A, Gumusay O, et al. Liver metastases from adenocarcinomas of unknown primary site: management and prognosis in 68 consecutive patients[J]. Wien Klin Wochenschr, 2016, 128(1-2): 42-47.

[179] Raghav K, Mhadgut H, McQuade JL, et al. Cancer of unknown primary in adolescents and young adults: clinicopathological features, prognostic factors and survival outcomes[J]. PLoS One, 2016, 11(5): E0154985.

[180] Burgers JA, Damhuis RA. Prognostic factors in malignant mesothelioma[J]. Lung Cancer, 2004, 45(1): S49-54.

[181] Bendardaf R, Lamlum H, Pyrhönen S. Prognostic and predictive molecular markers in colorectal carcinoma[J]. Anticancer Res, 2004, 24(4): 2519-2530.

[182] Schroeder L, Boscolo-Rizzo P, Dal Cin E, et al. Human papilloma virusas prognostic marker with rising prevalence in neck squamous cell carcinoma of unknown primary: a retrospective multicentre study[J]. Eur J Cancer, 2017, 74: 73-81.

[183] Raghav K, Hwang H, Jacome AA, et al. Development and validation of a novel nomogram for individualized prediction of survival in cancer of unknown primary[J]. Clin Cancer Res, 2021, 7(12): 3414-3421.

[184] 梁颖, 吴宁, 方艳, 等. ^{18}F-FDG PET/CT 显像 SUVmax、MTV 和 TLG 判断弥漫性大B 细胞淋巴瘤的预后价值[J]. 中华核医学与分子影像杂志, 2015, 35(2): 97-101.

[185] Kim YS, Kim SJ, Kim YK, et al. Prediction of survival and cancer recurrence using ^{18}F-FDG PET/CT in patients with surgically resected early stage (Stage I and II) non-small cell lung cancer[J]. Neoplasma, 2011, 58(3): 245-250.

[186] 刘红红, 兰晓莉, Anand Gungadin, 等. ^{18}F-FDG PET/CT 对原发灶不明颈部淋巴结转移癌的诊断及预后价值[J]. 中华核医学与分子影像杂志, 2016, 36(1): 48-53.

[187] Davis KS, Byrd JK, Mehta V, et al. Occult primary head and neck squamous cell carcinoma: utility of discovering primary lesions[J]. Otolaryngol Head Neck Surg, 2014,

151(2): 272-278.

[188] Bochtler T, Wohlfromm T, Hielscher T, et al. Prognostic impact of copy number alterations and tumor mutational burden in carcinoma of unknown primary[J]. Genes Chromosomes Cancer, 2022, 61(9): 551-560.

[189] Samstein RM, Lee CH, Shoushtari AN, et al. Tumor mutational load predicts survival after immunotherapy across multiple cancer types[J]. Nat Genet, 2019, 51(2): 202-206.

[190] Le DT, Durham JN, Smith KN, et al. Mismatch repair deficiency predicts response of solid tumors to PD-1 blockade[J]. Science, 2017, 357(6349): 409-413.

[191] Petrakis D, Pentheroudakis G, Voulgaris E, et al. Prognosication in cancer of unknown primary (CUP): development of prognostic algorithm in 311 cases and review of the literature[J]. Cancer Treat Rev, 2013, 39(7): 701-708.

[192] Bochtler T, Lffler H, Krmer A. Diagnosis and management of meta-static neoplasms with unknown primary[J]. Semin Diagn Pathol, 2018, 35(3): 199-206.

[193] Losa F, Iglesias L, Pané M, et al. 2018 consensus statement by the Spanish Society of Pathology and the Spanish Society of Medical Oncology on the diagnosis and treatment of cancer of unknown primary[J]. Clin Transl Oncol, 2018, 20(11): 1361-1372.

[194] 叶勰飞, 王斌, 代丽, 等. 408例恶性肿瘤骨转移临床特征分析[J]. 中国肿瘤临床, 2013, 40(4): 217-220.

[195] 唐顺, 郭卫, 杨荣利. 127例肺癌骨转移患者随访的预后因素分析[J]. 中国肿瘤临床, 2008, 35(23): 1335-1338.

[196] 吴凯南, 孔令泉. 乳腺癌骨转移若干影响因素的分析[J]. 中国肿瘤临床, 2005, 32(24): 1396-1399.

[197] 王龙, 刘巍, 吕雅蕾, 等. 食管胃结合部腺癌及胃癌Cox模型预后影响因素分析[J]. 中国肿瘤临床, 2012, 39(19): 1420-1425.

[198] Yuasa T, Urakami S, Yamamoto S, et al. Treatment outcome and prognostic factors in renal cell cancer patients with bone metastasis[J]. Clin Exp Metastasis, 2011, 28(4): 405-411.

[199] Biermann JS, Holt GE, Lewis VO, et al. Metastatic bonedisease: diagnosis, evaluation, and treatment[J]. J Bone Joint Surg Am, 2009, 91(6): 1518-1530.

[200] Ettinger DS, Handorf CR, Agulnik M, et al. Occult primary, version 3.2014[J]. J Natl Compr Canc Netw, 2014, 12(7): 969-974.

[201] Jacobsen S, Stephensen SL, Paaske BP, et al. Skeletal metastases of unknown origin: a retrospective analysis of 29 cases[J]. Acta Orthop Belg, 1997, 63(1): 15-22.

[202] Piccioli A, Rossi B, Scaramuzzo L, et al. Intramedullary nailing for treatment of pathologic femoral fractures due to metastases[J]. Injury, 2014, 45(2): 412-417.

[203] Piccioli A. Breast cancer bone metastases: an orthopedic emergency[J]. J Orthop

Traumatol, 2014, 15(2): 143-144.

[204] Hemminki K, Riihimaki M, Sundquist K, et al. Site-specific survival rates for cancer of unknown primary according tolocation of metastases[J]. Int J Cancer, 2013, 133(1): 182-189.

[205] Forsberg JA, Eberhardt J, Boland PJ, et al. Estimating survival in patients with operable skeletal metastases: an application of a bayesian belief network[J]. PLoS One, 2011, 6(5): 1995-1996.

[206] Snee MP, Vyramuthu N. Metastatic carcinoma from unknown primary site: the experience of a large oncology centre[J]. BrJ Radiol, 1985, 58(695): 1091-1095.

[207] Shinden Y, Sugimachi K, Tanaka F, et al. Clinicopathological characteristics of disseminated carcinomatosis of the bone marrow in breast cancer patients[J]. Mol Clin Oncol, 2018, 8(1): 93-98.

[208] Kwon JY, Yun J, Kim HJ, et al. Clinical outcome of gastric cancer patients with bone marrow metastases[J]. Cancer Res Treat, 2011, 43(4): 244-249.

[209] Che Y, Luo Y, Wang D, et al. Clinical Analysis of Small Cell Lung Cancer with Bone Marrow Metastases[J]. Zhongguo Fei Ai Za Zhi, 2018, 21(5): 403-407.

[210] Kopp HG, Krauss K, Fehm T, et al. Symptomatic bone marrow involvement in breast cancer - clinical presentation, treatment, and prognosis: a single institution review of 22 cases[J]. Anticancer Res, 2011, 31(11): 4025-4030.

[211] Demir L, Akyol M, Bener S, et al. Prognostic evaluation of breast cancer patients with evident bone marrow metastasis[J]. Breast J, 2014, 20(3): 279-287.

[212] Zhou MH, Wang ZH, Zhou HW, et al. Clinical outcome of 30 patients with bone marrow metastases[J]. J Cancer Res Ther, 2018, 14(Supplement): S512-S515.

[213] 车轶群, 王迪, 沈迪, 等. 乳腺癌骨髓转移的临床特征和预后分析[J]. 癌症进展, 2018, 16(7): 870-873, 877.

[214] Nakashima Y, Takeishi K, Guntani A, et al. Rectal cancer with disseminated carcinomatosis of the bone marrow: report of a case[J]. Int Surg, 2014, 99(5): 518-522.

[215] Wang D, Luo Y, Shen D, et al. Clinical features and treatment of patients with lung adenocarcinoma with bone marrow metastasis[J]. Tumori, 2019, 105(5): 388-393.

[216] Hiroshige T, Eguchi Y. Prostate cancer with disseminated carcinomatosis of the bone marrow: Two case reports[J]. Mol Clin Oncol, 2017, 7(2): 233-236.

附　录

附录1　主要名词术语英文缩写、全称、中文名

英文缩写	英文全称	中文名
ACS	American Cancer Society	美国癌症协会
AE1/AE3	cytokeratin AE1/AE3	角蛋白 AE1/AE3
AFP	alpha-fetoprotein	甲胎蛋白
AJCC	American joint committee on cancer	美国癌症联合委员会
ALK	anaplastic lymphoma kinase	间变性淋巴瘤激酶
AML	acute myeloid leukemia	急性髓系白血病
BM-CUP	bone metastases from cancer of unknown primary	不明原发肿瘤骨转移
BM-CUP	brain metastasis of unknown primary cancer	不明原发肿瘤脑转移
BRCA	breast cancer susceptibility genes	乳腺癌易感基因
CD10	cluster of differentiation-10	白细胞分化抗原-10
CDK4	cyclin-dependent kinase 4	细胞周期蛋白依赖性激酶4
CDX2	caudal-related homeobox-2	尾型同源框转录因子-2
CgA	chromogranin	嗜铬蛋白
CK	cytokeratin	细胞角蛋白
CK20	cytokeratin 20	细胞角蛋白20
CK7	cytokeratin 7	细胞角蛋白7
CUP	carcinomas of unknown primary	不明原发肿瘤
dMMR	deficient mismatch repair	错配修复基因缺失
EC	endometrial cancer	子宫内膜癌
EMT	epithelial-mesenchymal transition	上皮-间质转化
ER	estrogen receptor	雌激素受体
ESMO	european society for medical oncology	欧洲肿瘤内科学会

续表

英文缩写	英文全称	中文名
GATA3	GATA Binding Protein 3	GATA结合蛋白3
GCDFP-15	gross cystic disease fluid protein-15	巨大囊肿病液体蛋白-15
GEP	gene expression profiling	基因表达谱
HBOC	hereditary breast-ovarian cancer syndrome	遗传性乳腺癌-卵巢癌综合征
HCG	human chorionic gonadotropin	人绒毛膜促性腺激素
HepPar-1	hepatocyte Par-1	肝细胞抗原1
HL	Hodgkin's lymphoma	霍奇金淋巴瘤
HMB-45	human melanoma black-45	黑色素瘤相关抗原
HNPCC	hereditary nonpolyposis colorectal cancer	遗传性非息肉性结直肠肿瘤综合征
HNSCC	head and neck squamous cell carcinoma	头颈部鳞癌
HPV	human papilloma virus	人乳头状瘤病毒
HSCT	hematopoietic stem cell transplant	造血干细胞移植
ICIs	immune checkpoint inhibitors	免疫检查点抑制剂
IDM	intracranial dural matastasis	硬脑膜转移瘤
IHC	immunohistochemistry	免疫组化
KRAS	kirsten rat sarcoma viral proto-oncogene	鼠类肉瘤病毒癌基因
LCA	leukocyte common antigen	淋巴细胞共同抗原
LDH	lactate dehydrogenase	乳酸脱氢酶
LFS	Li-Fraumeni syndrome	李-佛美尼综合征
LS	Lynch syndrome	林奇综合征
M-BPBC	metachronous bilateral primary breast cancer	异时性双侧原发性乳腺癌
MCs	multiplicity carcinomas	多重癌
MG	mammaglobin	乳腺球蛋白
M-MPLCs	metachronous MPLCs	异时性多原发肺内癌
M-MPNs	metachronous multiple primary neoplasms	异时性多原发肿瘤
MMR	mismatch repair	DNA错配修复基因
MPCs	multiple primary cancers	多原发癌
MPEC	multiple primary esophageal carcinoma	多原发食管癌
MPLCs	multiple primary lung cancers	肺内多原发肺癌

续表

英文缩写	英文全称	中文名
MPNs	multiple primary neoplasms	多原发肿瘤
MSI	micro satellite instability	微卫星不稳定性
MSI-H	microsatellite in stability-high	高度微卫星不稳定性
NAACCR	the North American Association of Central Cancer Registries	北美癌症登记中心协会
NCCN	national comprehensive cancer network	（美国）国家综合癌症网络
NCI	National Cancer Institute	美国国家癌症研究所
NGS	next generation sequencing	二代测序
NHL	non Hodgkin's lymphoma	非霍奇金淋巴瘤
NICE	national institute for health and clinical excellence	国家卫生与临床优化研究所
NSE	neuron-specific enolase	神经特异性烯醇化酶
NS-MPNs	multiple primary neoplasms of nervous	神经系统多原发肿瘤
OCT4	octamer-binding transcription factor-4	八聚体结合转录因子-4
OPT	occult primary tumor	隐匿性原发肿瘤
ORR	objective response rate	客观缓解率
OS	overall survival	总生存期
PAP	prostate acid phosphatase	前列腺酸性磷酸酶
PAR-1	proteinase activated receptor-1	蛋白酶激活受体-1
PCI	peritoneal cancer index	腹膜癌指数
PD-L1	programmed death ligand 1	程序性死亡受体配体1
PFS	progression free survival	无进展生存期
PM	peritoneal metastases	腹膜转移
PR	progesterone receptor	孕激素受体
PSA	prostate specific antigen	前列腺特异性抗原
PTEN	phosphatase and tension homolog	磷酸酶张力蛋白同源物基因
RCC	renal cell carcinoma	肾细胞癌
RT-PCR	real-time polymerase chain reaction	实时聚合酶链式反应
S-BPBC	synchronous bilateral primary breast cancer	同时性双侧原发性乳腺癌
SEER	surveillance, epidemiology, and end results	监测、流行病学和结果数据库

续表

英文缩写	英文全称	中文名
S-MPLCs	synchronous MPLCs	同时性多原发肺内癌
S-MPNs	synchronous multiple primary neoplasms	同时性多原发肿瘤
SPOP	speckle type POZ protein	斑点型锌指结构蛋白
Syn	synaptophsin	突触素
TBI	total body irradiation	全身照射
TG	thyroglobulin	甲状腺球蛋白
TILs	tumor infiltrating lymphocytes	肿瘤浸润性淋巴细胞
TMB	tumor mutation burden	肿瘤突变负荷
TMB-H	tumor mutation burden – high	高肿瘤突变负荷
TSH	thyroid stimulating hormone	促甲状腺激素
TTF-1	thyroid transcription factor – 1	甲状腺转录因子-1
UICC	union for international cancer control	国际抗癌联盟
Vim	vimentin	波形蛋白
WT-1	Wilm's tumor gene – 1	Wilm瘤基因-1
β2-MG	β-2 microglobulin	β2微球蛋白
β-hCG	β-human chorionic gonadotrophin	人绒毛膜促性腺激素β亚基

附录2 体能状态(ECOG-PS)评分

评分	标准
0	身体状态良好,能够不受限制地进行患病前的所有活动
1	在体力活动方面受到限制,但可以活动,能够从事轻体力劳动或久坐不动的工作,如轻体力家务劳动、办公室工作等
2	可以活动,能够自理,但无法从事任何工作活动。醒着的时候有50%以上的时间在外面活动
3	只能进行有限的自我护理,50%以上的清醒时间只能躺在床上或椅子上
4	完全残疾;无法进行任何自我护理;完全只能躺在床上或椅子上